S0-BWW-848

ADVANCED
IMMUNOCHEMISTRY

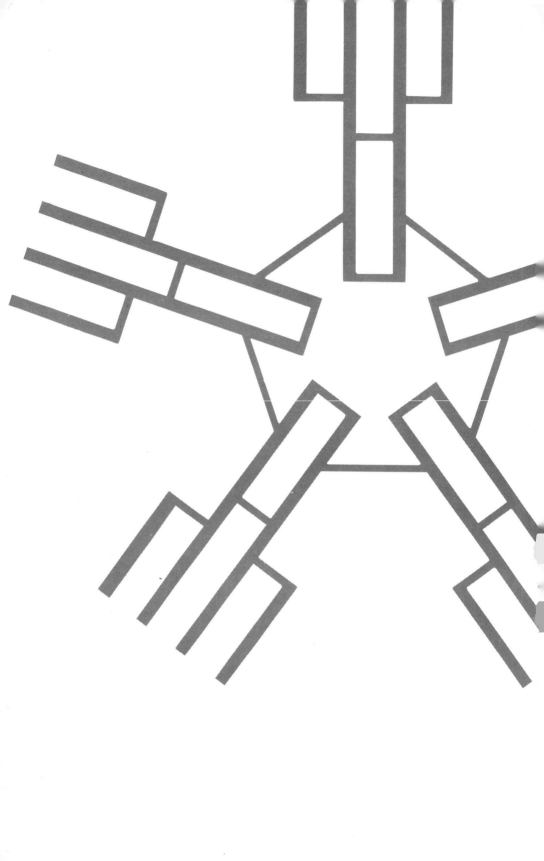

ADVANCED IMMUNOCHEMISTRY

Eugene D. Day, Ph.D.

Professor of Immunology and
Director of Graduate Studies
Department of Microbiology and Immunology
School of Medicine, Duke University
Durham, North Carolina

THE WILLIAMS & WILKINS COMPANY/*Baltimore*

QR
182
.D29
c.2

CHEMISTRY
LIBRARY

Copyright ©, 1972
The Williams & Wilkins Company
428 E. Preston Street
Baltimore, Md. 21202, U.S.A.

All rights reserved. This book is protected by copyright. No part of this book may be reproduced in any form or by any means, including photocopying, or utilized by any information storage and retrieval system without written permission from the copyright owner.

Made in the United States of America

Library of Congress Catalog Card Number 70-187539
SBN 683-02416-7

Composed and printed at the
Waverly Press, Inc.
Mt. Royal and Guilford Aves.
Baltimore, Md. 21202, U.S.A.

REPL.-
BOOKS

With love to my Wife and Son

PREFACE

"Having held our previous symposium on the Genetic
Code, it seemed natural to turn directly from that to the
subject of antibodies. The code epitomizes living systems
at their most inflexible ... By way of contrast, the formation of specific antibodies denotes extreme versatility. This
versatility appears, at first sight, to be in direct conflict with
the central dogma of molecular biology which maintains that
the primary structure of proteins is encoded in nucleic
acids, not improvised."

Thus did Dr. John Cairns write in the foreword to the 1967 Cold
Spring Harbor Symposium on *Antibodies*. Dr. Niels Jerne likewise
invoked the analogy of military combat, pointing out that this was the
"moment in history when we are experiencing the massive impact of
molecular biology on immunology and the smaller recoil impact of
immunology on molecular biology"; however, Jerne anticipated a
cease-fire and predicted peace and its benefits: "The definitive
solution of the antibody problem is approaching, and there is no
doubt of the deep effect this will have on medicine, on the understanding of allergic and degenerative disorders and cancer, and on
immunization, transplantation and other disorders." Dr. Jerne might
have added that not only will this resolution of a problem in molecular
diversity serve mankind in his immediate physical needs, but also
in his starving world of ideas. Evolution, biochemical genetics, the
genetic code itself, have already felt the recoil which, though restricted in scope, has certainly been penetrating in thrust. Beyond
are philosophy, religion, and politics which through this revolution in
thought must be brought to understand how individuality can accrue
in the face of law and order.

The introductory chapter to *Foundations of Immunochemistry*
(Day, 1966) was written when the revolution was in full swing but yet
unresolved: "Modern protein chemistry, with its foundations secure
in concepts of molecular biology, is beginning to adapt itself to a fact
of nature that it had previously attempted to avoid—the fact of

individuality among molecules created by *biological variescence*. Giving rise to heterogeneity within a particular functional protein species, variescence (a term invented by C. S. Peirce, 1911, to mean a change that produces an uncompensated increment in the number of independent elements of a situation) merely expresses in a particular molecular way the diversity created by adaptive, genetic, and evolutionary processes in biology." The introductory chapter was concluded with the summary statement: "Thus, it is only now, as protein chemistry begins to divest itself from the confining bonds of Liebig's stoichiometry, that Mulder's word, protein, takes on the true significance of a primary functional element of living matter. Heterogeneity, biological variescence, molecular individuality—these are the essence of the primary stuff of life."

Although Hoffman (1967) took exception to this thesis "which a reader with some background in physical biochemistry might regard as rank heresy, viz. that the notorious heterogeneity of immunoglobulins is the rule, rather than the exception, in protein chemistry," it is now, five years later, abundantly clear that molecular uniformity, as reflected by the general current product of the genetic code, is merely the backbone upon which the codes for molecular diversities are built and transmitted. Although many fewer diversities are permitted within the restricted framework of natural law and order than are undoubtedly attempted, point mutations that do become accepted within the genetic code result in time in an enormous kaleidoscope of amino acid sequence patterns in many different proteins, not just in immunoglobulins alone. For example, in her 1969 *Atlas of Protein Sequence and Structure*, Dayhoff has tabulated the best estimates of the rates of mutation of 18 different proteins (Table P-1) and has shown thereby that the immunoglobulins, *in all their diversity*, have changed not much more rapidly than ribonucleases in the 10^8 years of evolution from cretaceous times; meanwhile, growth hormones have doubled their variety, fibrinopeptides tripled, and only histones resisted much change.

The unexpected event which nature allowed to take place (and nurtured), an event which placed the immunoglobulins in a category different from that of the fibrinopeptides, ribonucleases, and histones, was the phylogenetic development of phenotypic diversity within a single individual. We don't know *how* it happened, but we do know that it *did* happen. Thus, although each single productive lymphocyte within us is committed to producing its own brand of homogeneous antibody combining site in a very faithful manner, and although all the lymphocytes that are produced as a clone by cell

TABLE P-1

Mutation Rate Among Proteins

Protein	PAMs*/ 10^8 years	Protein	PAMs*/ 10^8 years
Fibrinopeptides	90	Myoglobins	9
Growth hormones	60	Gastrins	9
Immunoglobulins	34	Adenohypophyseal hor-	
Constant region, κ-chain	40	mones	9
Variable region, κ-chain	34	Encephalitogenic proteins	7
Constant region, γ-chain	28	Insulins	4
Ribonucleases	30	Cytochromes c	3
Hemoglobins	12	Glyceraldehyde 3-PO$_4$ de-	
β-hemoglobins	13	hydrogenases	2
α-hemoglobins	11	Histones	0.06

* One PAM is one accepted point mutation/100 residues in an amino acid sequence.
(From Dayhoff, 1969.)

division after this commitment is made are also restricted to the production of this same brand of homogeneous antibody combining site, there are a diverse number of senior cells existing side by side each one of which contains a different commitment and the *potential* to generate its own clone when stimulated to proliferate. The extent of the diversity is so vast that Jerne (*op. cit.*) believes that his original estimate of the number of different antibody molecules which one animal can synthesize—1,000,000—may be orders of magnitude too low. But whatever the magnitude, it is yet eminently clear that the primary structure of an individual immunoglobulin molecule is encoded in the nucleic acids of the cell that produce it.

Are there other genetically encoded systems within the body that, like immunoglobulins, have their diversity expressed within the individual? Or are the immunoglobulins unique in not restricting their evolutionary species to orders above the individual? One need only review the history of "molecular disease" [and, incidentally, of the molecular resistance to disease (Knudson and Owen, 1968)] since its beginning in the work of Pauling, Itano, Singer, and Wells (1949) to realize that the hemoglobins, the isozymes, and the immunoglobulins do indeed belong to the same category, and that they represent only a sailor's view of the total iceberg that apparently exists. One of many bathyspheric views is the original one of Thomas (1959) that was reiterated and expanded by Burnet (1967) in his introduction to the Cold Spring Harbor Antibody Symposium. If indeed Thomas is correct in his belief that there is a rational basis for immunological prevention, control, and/or cure of malignant disease, and if, further-more, Burnet is correct in his belief that our heterogeneous immune processes are involved in the surveillance of our heterogeneous population of cell-surface histocompatibility antigens—to "seek and destroy" those unwanted cells that present with unwelcome idiotypes—then it follows that the malignant cells themselves are also encoded in the nucleic acids and represent yet another complex system of diversity, complete with encoded protein, that is generated within the individual and reflected in evolution.

Even though we have at present no more than a dim bathyspheric glimpse of an even more deeply submerged system—brain structure and function—it is certain that here molecular diversity will exhibit its most subtle form. In preparation for the future study of the central nervous system a more than casual glimpse of a more accessible system—the immunoglobulins—may prove to be of invaluable service.

E.D.D.

REFERENCES

Burnet, F. M. (1967). The impact of ideas on immunology. Sym. Quant. Biol. *32:* 1–8.

Cairns, J. (1967). Foreward. Sym. Quant. Biol. *32:* v.

Day, E. D. (1966). *Foundations of Immunochemistry*, The Williams & Wilkins Co. (Baltimore, 209 pp.), pp. 3–7.

Dayhoff, M. O. (1969). *Atlas of Protein Sequence and Structure*, Vol. 4, National Biomedical Research Foundation (Silver Spring, Md., xxvi + 109 text pp. + 252 data pp.), p. 42.

Hoffman, L. G. (1967). Review of *Foundations of Immunochemistry*, Science *155:* 1527–1528.

Jerne, N. K. (1967). Summary: Waiting for the end. Sym. Quant. Biol. *32:* 591–603.

Knudson, A. G., Jr., and Owen, R. D. (1968). Molecular genetics and disease resistance. In *Structural Chemistry and Molecular Biology*, Rich, A., and Davidson, N., eds. Freeman (San Francisco, 907 pp.), pp. 281–284.

Pauling, L., Itano, H. A., Singer, S. J., and Wells, I. C. (1949). Sickle cell anemia, a molecular disease. Science *110:* 543–548.

Peirce, C. S. (1911). Letter to Lady Welby, May 22, 1911. In *Values in a Universe of Chance, Selected Writings of Charles S. Pierce*, Wiener, P. P., ed., Doubleday Anchor Books (Garden City, N. Y., 446 pp., 1958), pp. 428–430.

Thomas, L. (1959). Discussion. In *Cellular and Humoral Aspects of Hypersensitive States*, Lawrence, H. S., ed. Hoeber (New York, 667 pp.), pp. 529–532.

ACKNOWLEDGMENTS

The writing of this book would not have been so easily accomplished had it not been for the professional bibliographic assistance from my wife, Shirley; the faithful and diligent typing of the manuscript by my secretary, Mrs. Geraldine Oalmann; and the very excellent aid and cooperation on the part of my Editor, Miss Sara Finnegan of The Williams & Wilkins Company. The many publishers and authors, cited separately in text and references, are due our sincere thanks for their generous permission to include copyrighted material in these pages. Dr. Don Mickey, Mr. Paul McMillan, and Mr. Lewis Rigsbee are due a special acknowledgment for keeping the laboratory in full swing during this writing.

Special thanks are due Dr. Frank W. Putnam for providing sequence information on immunoglobulin *Ou* in advance of publication.

E.D.D.

CONTENTS

PART ONE
Structure of Antibodies

1. THE LIGHT CHAINS OF IMMUNOGLOBULINS

2. THE HEAVY CHAINS OF IMMUNOGLOBULINS

PART TWO
Reactions of Antibodies

PART ONE

Structure of
Antibodies

1

THE LIGHT CHAINS OF
IMMUNOGLOBULINS

1. Bence-Jones proteins

Protein chemistry as a science had its real beginnings at a time when the influence of the Swedish chemist, Berzelius (1779–1848), was uppermost. His remarkable contributions to chemical formulations through considerations of stoichiometry were so thoroughly felt during his lifetime that the English medical journal, *The Lancet*, in Volume II, 1847, expressed great concern over his ill health. It was in this same volume that the lectures of Professor H. Bence Jones on chemical pathology appeared expressing, as one might expect, great confidence in the Berzelian method.

Professor Jones, although he was sure that a single formulation could be obtained for an elemental protein radical, could not decide whether the Dutch chemist, Mulder, or the German chemist, Liebig, was right (Jones, 1847). Mulder had been responsible for conferring the Greek word προγ $\hat{\eta}$ ιοσ (*proteios*), meaning primary or foremost, upon a group of animal substances including fibrin, albumin, and leucine, but he felt that the primary or protein radical common to all of them was confined to a stoichiometric compound containing carbon, nitrogen, oxygen, and hydrogen, but no sulfur. In cases where extra oxygen or sulfur appeared, these were considered to be derivative of Mulder's protein radical.

Thus Mulder (1838) had written:

"Um die analysirten Körper zu unterscheiden, habe ich die in dem Fibrin u.s.w. enthaltene thierische Materie *Protéin* genannt; Pr + SP ist also Fibrin; Pr + S$_2$P Albumin von Serum u.s.w.—Die Verbindung mit Schwefelsäure könnte *Proteinschwefelsäure* (acide sulpho-protéïque), die gelbe Säure *Xanthoproteinsäure* genannt werden. Zur Unterscheidung der extractartigen Materien habe ich das farblose Extract *Protid*, das rothe Extract *Erythroprotid* genannt."

By 1846 (Moulton, 1942) a bitter controversy had developed be-

3

tween Mulder and Liebig over the question of whether the primary
protein radical should or should not contain sulfur, and finally one of
Liebig's students, after a lengthy analytical presentation (Laskowski,
1846), concluded:

> "...dass, da die Annahme des von Hrn. Mulder unter dem
> namen Proteïn beschriebenen Körpers sich bloss darauf
> gründete, das man denselben schwefelfrei isolirt zu haben
> glaubte,—der von Hrn. Mulder isolirte Körper aber schwefel-
> haltig unter der von ihm beschriebene nicht isolibar ist—,
> selbst kein Grund vorhanden ist. das Proteïn als hypotheti-
> schen Grundstoff anzunehmen."

Mulder's theories were dashed, but the name he chose, protein,
survived.

The reason why H. Bence Jones had become so highly interested in
the spirited chemical discussion across the Channel was at least
partly professional. In 1845 he had received a letter from Dr. Watson,
a general practitioner, which described an accompanying urine
specimen that was obtained from a patient suffering from *mollities
ossium*.* The letter was short and to the point:

> Saturday, Nov. 1st, 1845
>
> Dear Dr. Jones,—The tube contains urine of very high
> specific gravity. When boiled it becomes slightly opaque. On
> the addition of nitric acid, it effervesces, assumes a reddish
> hue, and becomes quite clear; but as it cools, assumes the
> consistence and appearance which you see. Heat reliquefies
> it. What is it?
>
> (Signed) Dr. Watson

Jones (1847) analyzed the specimen and found it to contain a protein
substance (an "oxide of albumen") that was distinguishable from albumin by its solubility in nitric acid and lack of heat coagulability.
After separation by precipitation with alcohol the protein retained its
characteristics of solubility in cold water, increased solubility in
boiling water, coagulation with continued boiling, and return to solution by even further boiling. The substance could then be precipitated
with acid, solubilized by heating, and reprecipitated by cooling.
Jones noted at the end of his analysis: "Each oz. of this urine contained as much nutritive matter as an oz. of the blood. No supply of
food could compensate for such a loss."

---

* Professor Jones was not the only one brought in as a consultant on the case. According to Geshickter and Copeland (1928), McIntyre (1850) and Dalrymple (1848) were
both requested to give opinions, in particular to determine if there was correlation between the fracture of two ribs and other aspects of the case.

Through the years other clinicians found urinary proteins from time to time that exhibited the same solubility characteristics as this one and the name *Bence-Jones proteins* was appended to them. For the diagnosis of multiple myeloma, analysis of urine for Bence-Jones protein became routine because of the high association between the plasma-cell disease and the urinary pattern. Another characteristic of multiple myeloma was the unusually high degree of increased plasma protein levels (hyperproteinemia), unequivocally shown in 1928 by Perlzweig, Delrue, and Geshickter. Later this increase in protein was shown to be due to globulins with β- and γ-mobility (e.g., in the study by Moore, Kabat, and Gutman, 1943) as well as in components similar to urinary Bence-Jones protein (cf. review by Gutman, 1948).

Physicochemical characterization of Bence-Jones proteins developed at the same time as characterization of plasma components, but the large degree of variation exhibited by individual results from different laboratories and/or from individual patients led Putnam and Stelos (1953) to explore the reasons for such divergence. Mobilities, sedimentation coefficients, and diffusion coefficients were determined with extreme precision for 18 different cases of multiple myeloma, but, in spite of the care taken, extreme heterogeneity was observed. Mobilities ranged from 1.0 to 6.9; sedimentation coefficients, 2.05 to 6.30; isoelectric points, 4.6 to 6.7. There was no pattern except diversity itself—and the common peculiar property first noted by Professor Jones, that of precipitating when slowly heated, redissolving on boiling, and reprecipitating when cooled (Putnam, Easley, Lynn, Ritchie, and Phelps, 1959).

Then, in 1955, came the beginning of a solution. Through application of Ouchterlony's (1953) new agar-gel diffusion technique for measuring antigen-antibody reactions, Korngold and Lipari (1955) and Deutsch, Kratochvil, and Reif (1955) established the immunochemical relationship between the relatively small molecules of Bence-Jones proteins (molecular weight of about 40,000), the myeloma immunoglobulins, and normal γ-globulin (γG).

Hektoen as early as 1921 had investigated the immunological properties of specific precipitates formed between antibody and Bence-Jones proteins, and Baynes-Jones and Wilson in that same year had established two different groups on the basis on antigenic specificity. Hektoen and Welker (1940) showed that these two groups could appear at times in the urine of the same patient. Yet 34 years passed before the antigenic relationship between urinary and serum globulin, first seen by Hektoen, was established! Korngold and Lipari in 1956 treated the immunological relationship between the urinary microglobulins and normal and myeloma γG in depth and demonstrated three types. In 1958 Webb, Rose, and Sehon succeeded in immunochemically identifying the microglobulins in normal urine, thus removing Bence-Jones proteins from the category of myeloma specificity, and in 1961 Berggard identified them in normal plasma.

2. Light chains and Bence-Jones proteins

After the separation of subunits of γG into light and heavy chains by Edelman (1959), subsequent events showed that Bence-Jones microglobulins and the light chains from γG were very similar. Poulik and Edelman (1961), by alkylating reduced light chains to prevent them from recombining, and by reducing and alkylating Bence-Jones microglobulins in a similar way, showed that as long as the source of the reduced proteins was from the same patient a common electrophoretic mobility was obtained. Edelman and Gally (1962) then proceeded to demonstrate exquisitely that the light chains from normal γG exhibited the same peculiar thermal properties that H. Bence-Jones had originally observed in 1845 with Dr. Watson's urine specimen!

Reinforcing their views by observing similarities in amino acid analysis of light chains and urinary microglobulins from the same patient, and obtaining homogeneity in ion-exchange chromatography of the two on carboxymethyl (CM)-cellulose, Edelman and Gally concluded that Bence-Jones proteins were, in fact, oligomeric forms of light chains with dimers of 40,000 molecular weight predominating. In terms of the WHO nomenclature the two antigenically distinct types of microglobulins, as dimers of light chains, would be written as κ_2 and λ_2. That dimers did not always form in urine was shown by Deutsch (1963) who obtained a 1.85S Bence-Jones protein from one particular myeloma case. The protein had a molecular weight of 17,000, was able to be crystallized (Fig. 1-1), and had the characteristics of a single light chain.

Previously, Putnam (1962) had very effectively shown by two-dimensional chromatographic and electrophoretic separation of peptides from tryptic digests of Bence-Jones microglobulins that the "fingerprints" were closely similar to the fingerprints of a subunit portion of myeloma or normal globulins obtained from the same individual. Unlike fingerprint heterogeneity that had persistently been displayed from one individual to the next, structural homogeneity by chemical means was now observed for the first time. Significantly this homogeneity was established between the naturally occurring light chain fragment and its counterpart in whole globulin in a given in-

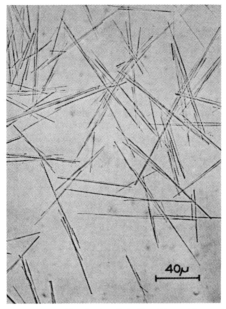

Fɪɢ 1-1. Twice crystalized γ-L-globulin. (From Deutsch, 1963.)

dividual. Schwartz and Edelman (1963) then showed that peptide maps of separated light chains from 6.5S myeloma globulin and those of naturally occurring Bence-Jones light chains from the same individual were similar.

After Porter (1959) had achieved the limited papain-cysteine cleavage of rabbit immunoglobulin into three separable fragments (I, II, and III), there was a period of uncertainty concerning the antigenicity of I and II (each now known collectively as Fab) since many believed that the crystallizable fragment III (now known as Fc) carried the antigenic determinants that made possible the immunization of one species with γG from another. However, when Putnam, Tan, Lynn, Easley, and Migita (1962) showed that each Fab and Fc fragment carried partial determinants of the whole and when Mannick and Kunkel (1962) showed that the macroglobulins could be classified into the same two groups that Korngold and Lipari (1956) had established for γG and Bence-Jones proteins, there was no longer any real question concerning either the antigenicity of Fab nor the unbiquitous appearance of its Bence-Jones antigens among the various isotypes of immunoglobulins. Fleischman, Porter, and Press (1963) finally discovered the actual relationship between the Fab fragments and the light chains of γG originally found by Edelman. This required obtaining light chains that would be soluble in aqueous solution rather than those obtained in urea by the Edelman method which were insoluble when the urea was dialyzed away. By reducing rabbit γG in urea-free solutions and separating the resultant chains in Sephadex-75 in the presence of weak acids (1 N acetic or propionic), Fleischman and colleagues obtained in nearly 100% yield two fractions representing light and heavy chains. This same system, when applied to fragments I and II, gave rise to intact light chains and only a fragment of heavy chain material (now called Fd). The linkage of the light chain to the heavy chain was shown to be that of a single disulfide bond.

Papain cleavage of human γG had been shown to give rise to only two fractions (Edelman, Heremans, Hermans, and Kunkel, 1960), with S (slow) and F (fast) relative mobilities and with distinct antigenic differences as shown by agar-gel immunoelectrophoresis. Franklin and Stanworth (1961) established the antigenic relationship between the S fragment and Bence-Jones protein thereby establishing S as the source of the light chain moiety. Thus, the way was now clear to obtain light chains from fragments as well as from intact normal human immunoglobulins and myeloma proteins, and to begin comparing their structures with each other and with the urinary Bence-Jones proteins. Perhaps of even greater significance was the final realization that the Bence-Jones proteins were not just a mere scientific curiosity but in themselves held the key to immunoglobulin structure and diversity. When Putnam and Udin boldly suggested in 1953 that the massive production of one globulin with a high degree of molecular and electrical homogeneity in the usual case of multiple myeloma was actually a random selection from the family of normal globulins, there was little feedback in the scientific literature. Likewise, when Putnam and Hardy (1955) suggested that Bence-Jones proteins were not degradative products but rapidly synthesized precursors of immunoglobulins, there was still relatively little response. However, when it was established that there were many points of identity between the light chains of normal immunoglobulins and their urinary counterpart, many an attitude among the scientific community was changed. Suddenly there was a surge of sequencing and almost a plethora of data.

3. Amino acid sequences of κ- and λ-light chains

Putnam, Titani, and Whitley published the first complete sequence analysis of a Bence-Jones protein (Ag) in 1966. That sequence (Table 1-1), except for very minor revisions in the positioning of certain amino acids, became the standard by which all subsequent light chain sequence analyses would be compared. According to the two

TABLE 1-1

Amino Acid Sequence and Composition of Human Bence-Jones Protein, Ag (κ)

Sequence*						Residue Position
DIQMT	QSPSS	LSASV	GDRVT	ITCQA	SQDIN	1–30
HYLNW	YQQGP	KKAPK	ILIYD	ASNLE	TGVPS	31–60
RFSGS	GFGTD	FTFTI	SGLQP	EDIAT	YYCQQ	61–90
YDTLP	RTFGQ	GTKLE	IKRTV	AAPSV	FIFPP	91–120
SNEQL	KSGTA	SVVCL	LNNFY	PREAK	VQWKV	121–150
DNALQ	SGNSQ	ESVTE	QDSKD	STYSL	SSTLT	151–180
LSKAD	YEKHK	VYACE	VTHQG	LSSPV	TKSFN	181–210
RGEC						211–214

Composition							
12	A	ala	alanine	1	M	met	methionine
5	C	cys	cysteine	9	N	asn	asparagine
11	D	asp	aspartic	11	P	pro	proline
10	E	glu	glutamic acid	16	Q	gln	glutamine
9	F	phe	phenylalanine	6	R	arg	arginine
13	G	gly	glycine	27	S	ser	serine
3	H	his	histidine	19	T	thr	threonine
9	I	ile	isoleucine	13	V	val	valine
13	K	lys	lysine	2	W	trp	tryptophan
15	L	leu	leucine	10	Y	tyr	tyrosine

* The revised sequence of *Ag* as it appears in up-to-date form in the *Atlas of Protein Sequence and Structure* (Dayhoff, 1969, p. D-98).

The N-terminal group is aspartic acid and the C-terminal is cysteine. The remaining 4 cysteines are at positions 23, 88, 134, and 194.

(From Putnam, Titani, and Whitley, 1966.)

main types of Bence-Jones proteins that had been classified immunologically and had been found to hold for light chains in general (types I and II in the old literature, κ and λ in the new), Bence-Jones protein *Ag* was typed *kappa;* thus, its structure became the prototype sequence of a typical κ-chain. In like manner, the next year, Wikler, Titani, Shinoda, and Putnam (1967) published the first complete sequence analysis of the λ-type light chain, as based upon Bence-Jones protein *Sh* (Table 1-2), and Gray, Dreyer, and Hood (1967) published the first sequence of a non-human κ-type urinary Bence-Jones protein derived from mouse myeloma #41 (Table 1-3). Any remaining doubt concerning the relevance of Bence-Jones protein sequences to the immunoglobulin problem was completely dispelled when Gottlieb, Cunningham, Rutishauser, and Edelman (1970) published the complete and unambiguous sequence of κ-light chains, obtained from human γG (Table 1-4), that confirmed the preliminary sequence given by Cunningham, Gottlieb, Konigsberg, and Edelman (1968).

4. Symmetry in light chain and importance of sulfur

The main point upon which Mulder and Liebig disagreed, as we have seen, was concerned with the central importance of sulfur in the protein radical, but how important it was with respect to the particular urinary protein which Bence Jones pondered took 120 years to realize. The Berzelian formula for a λ-chain, $C_{986}H_{1537}$ $N_{274}O_{326}S_5$, as given Putnam, Titani, Wikler, and Shinoda (1967), provides little clue and merely confirms Liebig's graduate student that it is an integral part of a protein. The amino acid analysis likewise offers only little additional information, i.e., that the sulfur appears in its usual place in five cysteine residues.

Milstein (1964, 1966a–c; Milstein, Frangione, and Pink, 1967) perhaps more than anyone else addressed himself to this question. One cysteine had already been accounted for in the link between the heavy and light chains, as established by Fleischman, Porter, and Press (1963). But which of the five cysteines was it and what function

TABLE 1-2

Amino Acid Sequence and Composition of Human Bence-Jones Protein, Sh (λ)

Sequence*						Residue Position
SELTQ	DPAVS	VALGQ	TVRIT	CQGDS	LRGYD	1–30
AAWYQ	QKPGQ	APLLV	IYGRN	NRPSG	IPDRF	31–60
SGSSS	GHTAS	LTITG	AQAED	EADYY	CNSRD	61–90
SSGKH	VLFGG	GTKLT	VLGQP	KAAPS	VTLFP	91–120
PSSEE	LQANK	ATLVC	LISDF	YPGAV	TVAWK	121–150
ADSSP	VKAGV	ETTTP	SKQSN	NKYAA	SSYLS	151–180
LTPEQ	WKSHR	SYSCQ	VTHEG	STVEK	TVAPT	181–210
ECS						211–213

Composition†							
20	A	17	G	0	M	28	S
5	C	4	H	6	N	19	T
9	D	5	I	14	P	15	V
10	E	11	K	12	Q	3	W
4	F	15	L	7	R	9	Y

* The revised up-to-date sequence of *Sh* as it appears in the *Atlas* (Dayhoff, 1969, p. D-86). The one-letter notation of amino acids is defined in Table 1-1.

† The empirical formula is $C_{986}H_{1537}N_{274}O_{326}S_5$, a total of 3,128 atoms and a formula weight of 22,607 (Putnam *et al.*, 1967). Both the N-terminal and the C-terminal groups are serine. The 5 cysteine residues are at positions 21, 86, 135, 195, and 212.

(From Wikler, Titani, Shinoda, and Putnam, 1967.)

TABLE 1-3

Amino Acid Sequence and Composition of Mouse Bence-Jones Protein, #41 (κ)

Sequence*						Residue Position
DIQMT	QSPSS	LSASL	GERVS	LTCRA	SQBIG	1–30
SLSBW	LZZBP	GZTIK	RLIYA	TSSLB	SGVPK	31–60
RFSGS	RSGSD	YSLTI	SSLES	EDFVD	YXCLQ	61–90
YASSP	WTFGG	GTKLE	IKRAB	AAPTV	SIFPP	91–120
SSEQL	TGGSA	SVVCF	LNNFY	PKDIN	VKWKI	121–150
DGSER	QBGVL	ZSBTB	WDSKD	STYSM	SSTLT	151–180
LTKBZ	YZRHB	SYTCZ	ATHKT	STSPI	VKSFN	181–210
RNEC						211–214

Composition							
9	A	13	G	5	N	9	V
10	B	2	H	9	P	4	W
5	C	10	I	6	Q	1	X
8	D	11	K	9	R	8	Y
7	E	16	L	38	S	7	Z
7	F	2	M	18	T		

* From the *Atlas* presentation (Dayhoff, 1969, p. D-107).

    B = undesignated form of asparaginyl residue, D or N

    Z = undesignated form of glutamyl residues, E or Q or pyrrolidonyl

    X = uncertain identity.

The remainder of the one-letter notations are described in Table 1-1.

The N-terminal and C-terminal ends are the same as human *Ag.* κ-chain, i.e., aspartic acid and cysteine. Likewise, the remaining 4 cysteines are at residues 23, 88, 134, and 194 in the same positions as in *Ag.*

(From Gray, Dreyer, and Hood, 1967.)

did the other four have? Through isolation and evaluation of many overlapping peptides, Milstein was able to establish that the first two cysteines (e.g., 23 and 88 in human *Ag* and *Eu* and in mouse #41 and #70; 21 and 86 in human *Sh*) were joined covalently to form an intrachain disulfide bridge; that the next two cysteines were likewise linked (e.g., 134 and 194 in human *Ag* and *Eu* and in mouse #41 and #70; 135 and 195 in human *Sh*); and that the last cysteine (C-terminal in κ-chains, penultimate in λ) was reserved for the interchain bridging of light-heavy and light-light dimers.

The resultant overall structure is a relatively symmetrical double-looped chain in which each loop remains independent of the other. The contrast with the dependent covalent loops of ribonuclease (Fig. 1-2) was pointed out by Welscher (1969) who noted that the double-loop formation provides a mechanism of globular folding that is both space-filling and nonoverlapping. Thus the light chain is free from the demands for excessive residues in high energy conformation.

TABLE 1-4

Amino Acid Sequence and Composition of Kappa Chain from Human γG, Eu

Sequence*						Residue Position
DIQMT	QSPST	LSASV	GDRVT	ITCRA	SQSIN	1–30
TWLAW	YQQKP	GKAPK	LLMYK	ASSLE	SGVPS	31–60
RFIGS	GSGTE	FTLTI	SSLQP	DDFAT	YYCQQ	61–90
YNSDS	LMFGQ	GTKVE	VKGTV	AAPSV	FIFPP	91–120
SDEQL	KSGTA	SVVCL	LNNFY	PREAK	VQWKV	121–150
DNALQ	SGNSQ	ESVTE	QDSKD	STYSL	SSTLT	151–180
LSKAD	YEKHK	VYACE	VTHQG	LSSPV	TKSFN	181–210
RGEC						211–214

Composition

A	13	G	13	M	3	S	32
C	5	H	2	N	7	T	18
D	10	I	6	P	10	V	15
E	10	K	15	Q	15	W	3
F	8	L	15	R	5	Y	9

* The sequence for *Eu* given by Gottlieb, Cunningham, Rutishauser, and Edelman (1970) up-dates the presentation in any previous source, and eliminates all ambiguity such as given in the preliminary data of the *Atlas* (Dayhoff, 1969, p. D-96) or of Cunningham *et al.* (1968).

The one-letter amino acid notation is described in Table 1-1.

The N-terminal and C-terminal ends are the same in *Eu* as they are in human *Ag* κ-chain, i.e., aspartic acid and cysteine. Likewise, the remaining 4 cysteines are at residues 23, 88, 134, and 194 in the same position as *Ag*.

Thermodynamic stability must be provided, however, and the only way to do so, while still maintaining rotational freedom, is to place heavy restrictions upon the sequence pattern of amino acids. A random coil will not do. Thus the globular conformation of the light chain is almost wholly dependent upon its primary structure, and most importantly upon the placement of the intrachain disulfide bridges. It is to be expected, therefore, that the most conservative of all residues in the evolving immunoglobulins are these loop-forming cysteines.

5. Asymmetry in light chains—variable and constant halves

As a result of clear-cut investigations on the extent of sequence homology among the light chains of man, and between those of man and mouse, it was proved what had long been felt: that there was a distinct difference between the N-terminal and the C-terminal halves (Hilschmann and Craig, 1965; Titani and Putnam, 1965; Milstein, 1966d; Perham, Appella, and Potter, 1966; and Gray, Dreyer, and

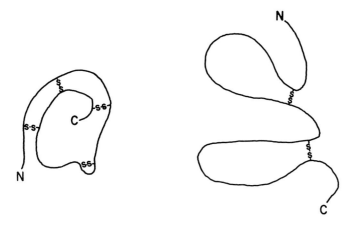

RNAase   **Ig Light Chain**

Fig. 1-2. Drawings suggestive of the structure of ribonuclease (*left*) and immuno-globulin light chain (*right*). Ribonuclease: 124 residues and 4 S—S bridges forming spiralling dependent covalent loops. Ig light chain: 213–221 residues and 2 S—S bridges forming two independent covalent loops.

Hood, 1967). Since no two Bence-Jones proteins out of hundreds had ever been found that had the same peptide patterns, there was no surprise that the sequences of the first one hundred seven or eight residues, reading from the amino-terminal end, confirmed what had long been known—the fact of heterogeneity. What created excite-ment was the dramatic departure from the heterogeneous pattern midway through the chain and the obvious onset of protein homology. To be sure there were minor variations in pattern in the latter half, but these existed to such a much lesser degree that the term *constant* region or C_L was coined to contrast its limited heterogeneity with the *variable* region or V_L. So unequivocal was the concept of re-gional mutual exclusiveness that WHO deemed it most proper to designate the formulas of κ- and λ-chains as $V_\kappa C_\kappa$ and $V_\lambda C_\lambda$ (WHO, 1969).

The contrasts are immediately seen in the maximum-homology alignments of 6 human κ-chains (Table 1-5), 6 human λ-chains (Table 1-6), and 2 mouse κ-chains (Table 1-7) according to the alignment scheme of Dayhoff (1969). By arranging the aligned sequences in 5 consecutive parts,

   (a) a variable N-terminal region (e.g., the first 23 residues of κ)
   (b) a variable loop region (e.g., 72 residues of κ closed by 2 cysteines)

TABLE 1-5

Alignment of κ-Chain Sequences According to Maximum Homology

Region*	Protein	Sequence†									Residue Position (Eu Numbering)
(a)	Ag	-DIQM	TQSPS	SLSAS	VGDRV	TIT					0–22
	Roy	-DIQM	TQSPS	SLSAS	VGDRV	TIT					
	Eu	-DIQM	TQSPS	TLSAS	VGDRV	TIT					
	Ti	-EIVL	TQSPG	TLSLS	PGERA	TLS					
	Cum	EDIVM	TQTPL	SLPVT	PGEPA	SIS					
	Mil	-DIVL	TQSPL	SLPVT	PGEPA	SIS					
(b1)	Ag	CQASQ	-----	-DINH	YLNWY	QQGPK	KAPKI	LIYDA	S		23–52 (a–f insertion between 27 and 28)
	Roy	CQASQ	-----	-DISI	FLNWY	QQKPG	KAPKL	LIYDA	S		
	Eu	CRASQ	-----	-SINT	WLAWY	QQKPG	KAPKL	LMYKA	S		
	Ti	CRASQ	S----	-VSNS	FLAWY	QQKPG	QAPRL	LIYVA	S		
	Cum	CRSSQ	SLLDS	GDGNT	YLNWY	LQKAG	QQPSL	LIYTL	S		
	Mil	CRSSQ	NLLZ-	-SBGB	YLDWY	LZKPG	ZSPZL	LIYLG	S		
(b2)	Ag	NLETG	VPSRF	SGSGF	GTDFT	FTISG	LQPED	IATYY	C		53–88
	Roy	KLEAG	VPSRF	SGTGS	GTDFT	FTISS	LQPED	IATYY	C		
	Eu	SLESG	VPSRF	IGSGS	GTEFT	LTISS	LQPDD	FATYY	C		
	Ti	SRATG	IPDRF	SGSGS	GTDFT	LTISR	LEPED	FAVYY	C		
	Cum	YRASG	VPDRF	SGSGS	GTDFT	LKISR	VQAED	VGVYY	C		
	Mil	NRASG	VPNRF	SGSGS	GTBFT	LKISR	VZAZB	VGVYY	C		
(c)	Ag	QQYDT	LPRTF	GQGTK	LEIKR	TVAAP	SVFIF	PPSNE	QLKSG	TASVV	89–133
	Roy	QQFDN	LPLTF	GGGTK	VDFKR	TVAAP	SVFIF	PPSDE	QLKSG	TASVV	
	Eu	QQYNS	DSKMF	GQGTK	VEVKG	TVAAP	SVFIF	PPSDE	QLKSG	TASVV	
	Ti	QQYGS	SPSTF	GQGTK	VELKR	TVAAP	SVFIF	PPSDE	QLKSG	TASVV	
	Cum	MQRLE	IPYTF	GQGTK	LEIRR	TVAAP	SVFIF	PPSDE	QLKSG	TASVV	
	Mil	MQALQ	TPLTF	GGGTN	VEIKR	TVAAP	SVFIF	PPSBZ	ZLKSG	TASVV	

14

(d1)								134–164
Ag	CLLNN	FYPRE	AKVQW	KVDNA	LQSGN	SQESV	T	
Roy	CLLNN	FYPRE	AKVQW	KVDNA	LQSGN	SQESV	T	
Eu	CLLNN	FYPRE	AKVQW	KVDNA	LQSGN	SQESV	T	
Ti	CLLNN	FYPRE	AKVQW	KVDNA	LQSGN	SQESV	T	
Cum	CLLNN	FYPRE	AKVQW	KVDNA	LQSGN	SQESV	T	
Mil	CLLNN	FYPRE	AKVQW	KVBBA	LZSGB	SZZSV	T	

(d2)							165–194
Ag	EQDSK	DSTYS	LSSTL	TLSKA	DYEKH	KVYAC	
Roy	QQDSK	DSTYS	LSSTL	TLSKA	DYEKH	KLYAC	
Eu	EQDSK	DSTYS	LSSTL	TLSKA	DYEKH	KVYAC	
Ti	ZZBSK	DSTYS	LSSTL	TLSKA	DYEKH	KVYAC	
Cum	QQDSK	DSTYS	LSSTL	TLSKA	DYEKH	KVYAC	
Mil	ZZBSK	DSTYS	LSSTL	TLSKA	BYZKH	KVYAC	

(e)					195–214
Ag	EVTHQ	GLSSP	VTKSF	NRGEC	
Roy	EVTHQ	GLSSP	VTKSF	NRGEC	
Eu	EVTHQ	GLSSP	VTKSF	NRGEC	
Ti	EVTHQ	GLSSP	VTKSF	NRGEC	
Cum	EVTHQ	GLSSP	VTKSF	NRGEC	
Mil	ZVTHZ	GLSSP	VTKSF	NRGEC	

* (a) N-terminal region of 23 residues; (b) variable loop region with insertion a–f; (c) switch region; (d) constant loop region; and (e) C-terminal region.

† Alignment according to Dayhoff (1969, p. D-220). B, undesignated asparaginyl, D or N; Z, undesignated glutamyl, E or Q or pyrrolidonyl; see Table 1-1 for other notation.

TABLE 1-6

Alignment of λ-Chain Sequences According to Maximum Homology

Region*	Protein	Sequence†											Residue Position (Eu Numbering)
(a)	New	-ZSVL	TQPP-	SVSAA	PGQKV	TIS							0-22
	Ha	-ZSVL	TQPP-	SVSGT	PGQRV	TIS							
	Bau	--YGL	TQPP-	SLSVS	PGQTA	SIT							
	Kern	--YAL	TQPP-	SVSVS	PGQTA	VIT							
	Bo	-ZSAL	TQPP-	SASGS	PGQSV	TIS							
	Sh	--SEL	TQDP-	AVSVA	LGQTV	RIT							
(b1)	New	CSGGS	TN---	-IGNN	YVSWH	QHLPG	TAPKL	LIYED	N				23-52 (a–f insertion between 27 and 28)
	Ha	CSGGS	SNG--	-TGNN	YVYWY	QQLPG	TAPKL	LIYRD	D				
	Bau	CSGDK	-----	-LGEQ	YVCWY	QQKPG	QSPVL	VIYHD	S				
	Kern	CSGDN	-----	-LEKT	FVSWF	QQRPG	QSPLL	VIYHT	S				
	Bo	CTGTS	SDV--	-GNDK	YVSWY	QQHPG	RAPKL	VIFEV	S				
	Sh	CQGDS	-----	-LRGY	DAAWY	QQKPG	QAPLL	VIYGR	N				
(b2)	New	KRPSG	IPDRI	SASKS	GTSAT	LGITG	LRTGD	EADYY	C				53-88
	Ha	KRPSG	VPDRF	SGSKS	GTSAS	LAISG	LRSED	EAHYH	C				
	Bau	KRPSG	IPERF	SGSNS	GTTAT	LTISG	TQAMD	EADYY	C				
	Kern	ERPSE	IPERF	SGSSS	GATAT	LTISG	AQSVD	EADYF	C				
	Bo	QRPSG	VPDRF	SGSKS	NDTAS	LTVSG	LRAED	EADYY	C				
	Sh	NRPSG	IPDRF	SGSSS	GHTAS	LTITG	AQAED	EADYY	C				
(c)	New	ATWDS	SLNAV	VFGGG	TKVTV	LGQPK	AAPSV	TLFPP	SSEEL	QANKA	TLV		89-133 (a–b insertion between 97 and 98; a, between 107 and 106)
	Ha	AAWDY	RLSAV	VFGGG	TQLTV	LRQPK	AAPSV	TLFPP	SSEEL	QANKA	TLV		
	Bau	QAWDS	YTVI-	-FGGG	TKLTV	LGQPK	AAPSV	TLFPP	SSZZL	ZABKA	TLV		
	Kern	QTWDT	ITAI-	-FGGG	TKLTV	LSQPK	AAPSV	TLFPP	SSEEL	QANKA	TLV		
	Bo	SSYVD	NNNFV	VFGGG	TKLTV	LRQPK	AAPSV	TLFPP	SSEEL	QANKA	TLV		
	Sh	NSRDS	SGKHV	LFGGG	TKLTV	LGQPK	AAPSV	TLFPP	SSEEL	QANKA	TLV		

(d1)								134–164
New	CLISD	FYPGA	VTVAW	KADSS	PVKAG	V-ETT	T	
Ha	CLISD	FYPGA	VTVAW	KADSS	PVKAG	V-ETT	T	
Bau	CLISD	FYPGA	VTVAW	KADSS	PVKAG	V-ETT	T	
Kern	CLISD	FYPGA	VTVAW	KADGS	PVKAG	V-ETT	T	
Bo	CLISD	FYPGA	VTVAW	KADSS	PVKAG	V-ETT	T	
Sh	CLISD	FYPGA	VTVAW	KADSS	PVKAG	V-ETT	T	

(d2)							165–190
New	PSKQS	NNKYA	ASSYL	SLTPE	QWKSH	RSYSC	
Ha	PSKQS	NNKYA	ASSYL	SLTPE	QWKSH	RSYSC	
Bau	PSKZS	BBKYA	ASSYL	SLTPZ	ZWKSH	RSYSC	
Kern	PSKQS	NNKYA	ASSYL	SLTPE	QWKSH	RSYSC	
Bo	PSKQS	NNKYA	ASSYL	SLTPE	QWKSH	RSYSC	
Sh	PSKQS	NNKYA	ASSYL	SLTPE	QWKSH	RSYSC	

(e)						195–215
New	QVTHE	GST—	VEKTV	APTEC	S	
Ha	QVTHE	GST—	VEKTV	APTEC	S	
Bau	QVTHZ	GST—	VZKTV	APTEC	S	
Kern	QVTHE	GST—	VEKTV	APTEC	S	
Bo	QVTHE	GST—	VEKTV	APTEC	S	
Sh	QVTHE	GST—	VEKTV	APTEC	S	

* See Table 1-5 for designation of region.

† Bau sequence taken from Baczko, Braun, Hess, and Hilschmann (1970). Part of Kern sequence reported by Hilschmann to Smith, Hood, and Fitch (1971). The remaining sequences are taken from the *Atlas*, Dayhoff (1969, p. D-220). Z stands for Glx which can be Glu or Gln. B stands for Asx which can be Asp or Asn. See Table 1-1 for other notations. The numbering system is in keeping with the current practice (e.g., Wu and Kabat, 1970) of assigning letters to insertions or gap regions between 27 and 28, 97 and 98, and 106–107. Homology gaps also appear in λ-chain at 0, 9, 160, 203, and 204 to keep in line with κ-chain homology.

17

TABLE 1-7
Alignment of Mouse κ-Chain Sequences According to Maximum Homology

Region*		Sequence†	Residue Position (Eu Numbering)
(a)	#41	-DIQM TQSPS SLSAS LGERV SLT	0-22
	#70	-DIVL TQSPA SLAVS LGQRA TIS	
(b1)	#41	CRASQ ----- -BIGS LSBWL ZZBPG ZTIKR LIYAT S	23-52 (a-f insertion between 27 and 28)
	#70	CRASE SVBB- -SGIS FMNWF ZZKPG ZPPKL LIYAA S	
(b2)	#41	SLBSG VPKRF SGSRS GSDYS LTISS LESED FVDYX C	53-88
	#70	NQGSG VPARF SGSGS GTDFS LNIHP MZZBB TAMYF C	
(c)	#41	LQYAS SPWT- -FGGG TKLEI -KRAB AAPTV SIFPP SSEQL TGGSA SVV	89-133 (a-b insertion between 97 and 98; a, between 107 and 106)
	#70	ZZSKE VPWT- -FGGG TKLEI -KRAB AAPTV SIFPP SSZZL TGGSA SVV	
(d1)	#41	CFLNN FYPKD INVKW KIDGS ERQBG VLZSB T	134-164
	#70	CFLBB FYPKD INVKW KIDGS ERZBG VLZSB T	
(d2)	#41	BWDSK DSTYS MSSTL TLTKB ZYZRH BSYTC	165-190
	#70	BWDSK DSTYS MSSTL TLTKB ZYZRH BSYTC	
(e)	#41	ZATHK TSTSP IVKSF NRNEC	195-214
	#70	ZATHK TSTSP IVKSF NRNEC	

* See Table 1-5 for designation of region.
† According to Dayhoff alignment (1969, p. D-220). Z is undesignated glutamyl; B is undesignated asparaginyl; one-letter notation for amino acids is described in Table 1-1.

18

    (c) a "switch" peptide region (45 residues in κ)

    (d) a constant loop region (61 residues in κ closed by 2
       cysteines)

    (e) a constant C-terminal region (20 residues in κ)

one can readily observe the asymmetry. For example, perfect homology characterizes all 6 κ-chains in the constant C-terminal region, whereas moderate heterogeneity defines the N-terminal region with only 6 out of 23 residues unchanged. Only by subdividing the 6 N-terminal regions can one find a semblance of subgroup homology. Likewise, perfect homology in the constant loop region is marred by only 2 interchanges at the 32nd and 58th residues of κ, whereas extreme heterogeneity is obtained in the variable loop region with 54 out of 72 residues (75%) experiencing interchanges. Finally, within the switch peptide region, only 4 out of the first 20 remain homologous as opposed to perfect homology in the remaining 25. Overall the first 115 residues of the 6 κ-chains display only 24% homology under maximum alignment conditions, whereas the remaining 106 residues exhibit 98%.

6. Genetic polymorphism in constant loop region

In 1961 Ropartz, Lenoir, and Rivat had discovered a new inheritable property of immunoglobulins that was confined to Fab fragments. The factor was named InV because of the capacity of immunoglobulin from patient V that carried the factor to inhibit a typing serum but the V is no longer capitalized. Fudenberg and Franklin (1963) then established that Inv was restricted to Bence-Jones proteins and light chains. There were three specificities Inv(1), Inv(a), and Inv(b), now known as Inv(1), Inv(2), and Inv(3), respectively, which were responsible for the original immunological classification described by Korngold and Lipari (1956) and were confined to the κ-chains.[*] The specificity of the factor was very importantly noted to be allelic in nature (Inv[1, 2] vs. Inv[3]) and subject to simple Mendelian heredity. An Inv[1, 2] gene controlled Inv(1) and Inv(2), and an Inv[3] gene controlled Inv(3). Thus, a single individual that gave rise to Inv(3) could not form Inv(1) or Inv(2) regardless of the cellular source of his heterogeneous collection of κ-chains. When structural homology studies were made of 27 κ-type Bence-Jones proteins (Baglioni, Zonta, Cioli, and Carbonara, 1966), the Inv loci were found to control the amino acid residue at the 58th position of the constant

---

[*] At one time Inv(3) appeared to be associated with λ- as well as κ-chains (Lawler and Cohen, 1965), but the report was later found to be in error due to an unreliable typing serum (Cohen and Milstein, 1967b).

loop region with leucine characteristic of Inv(1) and Inv(2), valine responsible for Inv(3). In terms of residue numbering from the N-terminus of the complete light chain this would place Inv anywhere from position 189 to 198 in known κ sequences, but always fixed as the third residue before cysteine IV, now designated as position 191 according to Eu numbering.

As a result of analyses by Mannik and Kunkel (1963) and by Fahey (1963) it had been determined that all normal human individuals carried both κ- and λ-chains even though any one myeloma protein would be either κ or λ, but not both. When the genetic polymorphism of the κ-chain Inv factor was found to distinguish individuals, a similar segregation was looked for and found among individuals with respect to λ-chain types. Genetic polymorphism was indeed found, but the case for proved allelism remained open and in doubt. When Ein and Fahey (1967) produced a rabbit antiserum to λ-type Bence-Jones protein, Oz, and found that the antiserum could distinguish two groups Oz(+) and Oz(−), there was hope that an allelism for λ-chains had been found comparable to Inv. Virtual certainty of proving allelism was assured when the structural identity of Oz was found at the 56th residue of the 60-residue-long constant loop region of λ. (From the N-terminus the position would be placed anywhere from position 190 to 194, but now designated as position 190 according to Eu numbering and always fixed as the 4th residue before cysteine IV.) Oz(+) was associated with lysine, Oz(−) with arginine (Appella and Ein, 1967). Unlike Inv, however, Oz could *not* be proved to be allelic, to distinguish individuals, and by itself, unassociated with other residue positions, to follow the laws of simple Mendelian heredity. In fact, when Ein (1968) found 10 consecutive normal sera containing both Oz(+) and Oz(−) light chain types, the likelihood of proving allelism for λ on the basis of Oz was very remote indeed.

At the 19th residue of the constant loop region of λ, 18 residues after cysteine III, Ponstingl, Hess, and Hilschmann (1968) found a substitution of glycine for serine in Bence-Jones protein Kern. Hess and Hilschmann (1970) determined that this structure was genetically polymorphic and labeled the factor *Kern*(+) for glycine, *Kern*(−) for serine. It will be interesting to find out, as further studies with *Kern* unfold, whether the simple pattern of Inv or the more complex one of Oz is repeated.

The importance of having established genetic polymorphism in the constant region of the light chain cannot be overestimated, but is yet not enough for many studies. The subsequent developments in the molecular biology of immunoglobulins have demanded at least one clear-cut example of allelism to settle theoretical matters. Dreyer and Bennett pointed out the paradox in 1965:

"That one end of the light chain behaves as if it were made by the genetic code contained in any one of more than 1000 genes while the other end of the L chains can be shown to be the product of a single gene."

To show that the constant half of a κ- or a λ-chain is indeed under the control of a single locus, three kinds of evidence really ought to be presented: that the chain can undergo mutation, i.e., exhibit allotypes; that the chain will segregate according to simple Mendelian law; and that the phenotypic amino acid sequence, whenever produced, is rigidly constant. As one can see, the κ constant region does display these requirements for single gene encodment. The λ-chain by very strong analogy is presumed to meet the same requirements although evidence for simple Mendelian segregation is still lacking due to the absence of allotypes.

7. Allelism in light chain of rabbit immunoglobulins (IgG)

Alloantigenic determinants in rabbit IgG that resulted in the production of anti-IgG in other rabbits were discovered by Oudin (1956). It was established in subsequent studies by Oudin (1960), by Dray and Young (1958), and by Dubiski, Dudziak, Skalba, and Dubiska (1959) that the determinants were truly allelic and subject to genetic segregation, i.e., that the genome carried only one of each pair of heritable traits; in work by Dubiski, Dubiska, Skalba, and Kelus (1961), Marrack, Richards, and Kelus (1961), and Leskowitz (1963) that the allotypic specificities were localized on Fab fragments; and in a report by Gilman, Nisonoff, and Dray (1964) that the alloantigens were definitely restricted to Fab. Each of two loci, a and b, not closely linked, had three allelic forms a^1, a^2, a^3 and b^4, b^5, b^6 which controlled the six antigenic specificities a1, a2, a3, b4, b5, and b6 (Oudin, 1960; Dubiski, Dudziak, Skalba, and Kelus, 1961; and Dray, Young, and Gerald, 1963). The a locus controlled specificities in the heavy chain fragment Fd, a matter that will be discussed when heavy chain structure is described. The b locus was found to control light chain allotypic specificities (Feinstein, Gell, and Kelus, 1963; Stemke, 1964; and Reisfeld, Dray, and Nisonoff, 1965) and thus is pertinent to the present discussion. As shown in Table 1–8, regardless of the a allotype, the rabbits doubly homozygous for b^4 and any a differed from b^5 and any a with remarkable uniformity. Threonine (-4.0) and valine (-2.4) were evidently interchanged in b4 structures for leucine ($+2.5$), lysine ($+0.8$), proline ($+1.1$), serine ($+1.2$), and alanine

TABLE 1-8

Differences in Amino Acid Composition of Rabbit γG-Immunoglobulin Light Chains of Different Allotypes

Amino Acid*	Homozygous Rabbits Residues/190									Average Difference
	$a^2a^2b^5b^5$ vs. $a^2a^2b^4b^4$			$a^1a^1b^5b^5$ vs. $a^1a^1b^4b^4$			$a^3a^3b^5b^5$ vs. $a^3a^3b^4b^4$			
	b5	b4	Diff.	b5	b4	Diff.	b5	b4	Diff.	
D	17.0	17.4	−0.4	16.4	17.0	−0.6	16.7	16.6	0.1	−0.3
L	12.6	10.5	+2.1	12.5	9.9	2.6	12.7	9.8	2.9	**+2.5**
K	8.8	8.1	+0.7	8.8	8.2	0.6	9.4	8.4	1.0	**+0.8**
P	12.3	10.9	+1.4	12.5	11.4	1.1	12.5	10.7	1.8	**+1.1**
S	20.1	20.7	−0.6	22.6	19.3	3.3	20.3	19.4	0.9	**+1.2**
T	23.3	26.4	−3.1	23.9	28.4	−4.5	23.2	27.4	−4.2	**−4.0**
V	17.2	19.3	−2.1	16.5	19.3	−2.8	17.3	19.6	−2.3	**−2.4**
A	15.2	13.9	+1.3	15.0	14.8	0.2	15.6	14.7	0.9	**+0.9**
R	2.9	3.0	−0.1	3.0	2.9	0.1	2.9	2.9	0.0	+0.0
C	7.4	7.3	+0.1	7.3	6.9	0.4	inc.	inc.		+0.2
E	18.8	18.5	+0.3	18.2	18.0	0.2	17.8	18.5	−0.7	−0.1
G	16.8	16.4	+0.4	16.4	16.6	−0.2	16.9	16.7	0.2	+0.1
H	1.4	1.3	+0.1	1.4	1.2	0.2	1.3	1.3	0.0	+0.1
I	6.7	6.7	0.0	6.4	6.6	−0.2	7.0	7.0	0.0	−0.1
M	0.6	0.6	0.0	0.6	0.7	−0.1	0.8	0.8	0.0	+0.0
F	5.9	5.8	+0.1	5.9	5.9	0.0	6.1	6.0	0.1	+0.0
T	9.3	9.3	0.0	8.6	8.8	−0.2	8.5	9.4	−0.9	−0.4

* One-letter notation for amino acids is given in Table 1-1.

(From Reisfeld, Dray, and Nisonoff, 1965.)

(+0.9) in b5 structures. It is thus apparent, even before sequencing proves it, that a complex allotypic ordering of amino acids is to be expected.

An indication of at least a partial C-region locale for the three allelic varieties has been presented by Frangione (1969). In spite of a previous hint by Appella and Perham (1967) that the C-terminal heptapeptide of rabbit κ-light chains might be as constant as those in the human and not under the influence of allotypic control, Frangione (1969) found that each of the three allelic forms of the *b* locus specified a different C-terminal pentapeptide:

b4: -N-R-G-D-C
b5: -S-R-K-N-C
b6: -S-R-K-S-C

Of the three sequences only b4 had been given previously as representative of rabbit κ-chain (Appella and Perham, 1967; Hood, Gray, Sanders, and Dreyer, 1967; Dayhoff, 1969, p. D-97). No relation to a rabbit λ C-terminal hexapeptide was at all obvious. It is expected, in view of the large amino acid differences already noted between b4 and b5 specificities, that these C-terminal sequences will prove to be only a small part of the total encoded structures and that, like Oz, will fail in themselves to segregate among individuals.

In retrospect it is indeed fortunate to have had such a clear-cut example of simple allelism in Inv. It remains the only unambiguous identified structure among all the light chains that serves as a single-gene marker. Much depends on that point in the pages that follow.

Meanwhile, a second light chain locus, the c locus with c^7 and c^{21} alleles has been identified (Mage, Young, and Reisfeld, 1968; Gilman-Sachs, Mage, Young, Alexander, and Dray, 1969) which offers additional insight into the varieties possible under allotypic control. All rabbits thus far reported have either c^7, c^{21}, or both allotypes, and none lack both. The two specificities may thus be considered as codominant alleles, inheritable on occasion as a phenogroup, and suggestively linked quite closely. Vice, Hunt, and Dray (1970), by utilizing the technique of allotype suppression in the newborn through the use of specific alloantisera (Dray, 1962; Dubiski, 1967; Mage, 1967), partially suppressed b5 specificity in b^5b^5 homozygous rabbits of phenotype c^7c^{21}, precipitated the immunoglobulins with specific anti-b5, anti-c^7, and anti-c^{21} antisera, and tested each fractionated protein for cross-reactivity with the other two antisera. No two allotypic specificities were cross-reactive, i.e., each light chain was controlled by a separate allele. The genetic polymorphism was thus quite analogous to Oz in the human. According to Appella, Mage, Dubiski, and Reisfeld (1968) and to Rejnek, Mage, and Reisfeld (1969), those b(−) rabbit light chains that were lacking in b allotypic specificities through the mechanism of immunosuppression were very closely akin to human λ-chains, whereas rabbit light chains under b(+) control were comparable to κ-chains. The λ-chain population in its N- and C-terminal regions even had considerable homology with the λ-chains of man and mouse. With b(+) control relegated to κ-chains one is reminded that Frangione's (1969) findings concerning the three different C-terminal pentapeptides for b4, b5, and b6 are indeed specifically directed toward rabbit κ-chains.

Probably more than any other drawback in obtaining meaningful structural identity of the allotypes of a rabbit light chain has been the lack of myelomas and thus of homogeneous rabbit immunoglobulins with which to determine extensive sequences. Now that homogeneous rabbit antibodies can be obtained in quantity (cf. Chapter 6) and allelic expression can be controlled through immunosuppression it is to be expected that the identities will soon be forthcoming.

8. Conformational allotypes and the problem of Inv(1) and Inv(2)

Polmar and Steinberg (1967) opened their attack on the problem of the quaternary structure of IgG by showing how some heavy chain allotypes are dependent upon heavy and light chain interaction to achieve their full expression. The light chain, moreover, must be specifically ordered. Thus, various homogeneous Bence-Jones light chains differed in their ability to restore Gm(3) and Gm(4) anti-genicity, but not according to any known light chain type. In like manner Inv(1) depended for its full expression upon the interaction of heavy and light chains. Litwin and Kunkel (1965, 1967) had encountered this phenomenon in the case of Inv in their earlier studies of isolated light chains where typing had become a problem, and then showed in the later work the dependence of Inv(1) and Inv(2) upon the multichain conformation. Inv(1) and Inv(2) appeared together in all myeloma and Bence-Jones molecules in the study as coexisting antigens in the same structures and obviously were not secreted by separate cell populations. Finally Solomon, McLaughlin, and Steinberg (1970) determined that Inv antigenicity depended at the very least upon the intact κ-light chain molecule. One may conclude therefore that the Inv residue in the constant loop region must be only a primary sequence marker and not at all the full antigen that was once thought.

9. Subgroups of variable N-terminal didecapeptide

During the initial excitement over the high degree of contrast between the constant and the variable halves there was a tendency to ascribe all matters of diversity to all parts of the variable region. Since it is the intention in these pages and the ones to follow to identify as clearly as possible those structural components of the immunoglobulin molecule that are built for actual binding, it is equally important to dissociate from our model of the active site those regions of the molecule that are unlikely to be involved even if the sequences form an integral part of the total V-region. One must exercise such precaution in analyzing the function of the light chain variable half, V_L, at this point, and one must continue the practice of foresight in viewing the heavy chain variable quarter, V_H, later on.

The most misleading concept in the current literature is the assumption that the N-terminal didecapeptide is a suitable measure of binding-site diversity. Any attempt to read meaning into specific ligand interaction on the basis of the sequential arrangement of the first 20 amino acids would be in error should the assumption not be true. In fact, if one "ascribes only a role in three-dimensional folding to the first 23 N-terminal amino acid residues of the light chain", as Wu and Kabat (1970) have done, "all recombinational theories of antibody formation [Smithies, 1963; Edelman and Gally, 1967] become uninformative since they are based exclusively on sequence data in this region and thus are probably not dealing with a region involving antibody complementarity." The discovery of subgroups of the variable region, based upon the sequences of the N-terminal didecapeptides of κ-chains (Niall and Edman, 1967; Milstein, 1967; and Hilschmann, 1967) and λ-chains (Hilschmann, Ponstingl, Baczko, Braun, Hess, Suter, Barnikol, and Watanabe, 1969) has thus done much to clarify our thinking concerning the rôle of the N-terminal sequence in molecular affairs.

A hint of subgroup classification of the N-terminal sequences has already been given. In Table 1–5 the first three proteins, Ag, Roy, and Eu belong to one group, Ti to a second, and Cum and Mil to a third. The signatories* of a memorandum drafted for WHO (1969) have devised not only a useful nomenclature for these three κ subgroups and for five λ subgroups, but have also accepted standard prototype sequences for the N-terminal didecapeptides that are representative of the subgroups (Table 1–9).

An evolutionary basis for the origin of variable regions became almost mandatory after the recognition of subgroups. Somatic hyper-

TABLE 1-9

Subgroup Classification of Human Light Chains and Their N-terminal Didecapeptide Sequences

Human Light Chain	Subgroup Designation	Residue Sequence (Positions 1–20)			
κ	$V_{\kappa I}$	DIQMT	QSPSS	LSASV	GDRVT
	$V_{\kappa II}$	EIVLT	QSPGT	LSLSP	GERAT
	$V_{\kappa III}$	DIVMT	QSPLS	LPVTP	GEPAS
λ	$V_{\lambda I}$	ZSVLT	QPP–S	VSGAP	GQRVT
	$V_{\lambda II}$	ZSALT	QPA–S	VSGSP	GQSIT
	$V_{\lambda III}$	–YVLT	QPP–S	VSVSP	GQTAS
	$V_{\lambda IV}$	ZSALT	QPP–S	ASGSP	GQSVT
	$V_{\lambda V}$	–SELT	QPP–A	VSVAL	GQTVR

Z = pyrrolid-2-one-5-carboxylic acid derived from glutamic acid. The subgroups are numbered in order of prevalence in 1969 (WHO, 1969).

*Asofsky, Binaghi, Edelman, Goodman, Heremans, Hood, Kabat, Rejnek, Rowe, Small, and Trnka.

mutation hypotheses, which had previously been offered to describe the *whole* of V-region diversity, were scrapped in favor of step-by-step evolutionary ones, and the "predominant share of antibody variability, as reflected in subgroup specific sequences" was interpreted as having its orgin most conservatively in evolution (Hilschmann *et al.*, 1969). In fact, there was every indication that the subgroups might represent only the main branches of an evolutionary tree growing into diversity (as drawn for λ-chains by Baczko, Braun, Hess, and Hilschmann, 1970); in that event subdivision of the subgroups should also be expected. Although a full discussion of evolution and germ line theory as it pertains to antibody formation must be postponed until the next chapter on heavy chain structures, it is now appropriate to reexamine the paradox posed by Dreyer and Bennett (1965) which was referred to earlier.

The paradox remains intact even though the N-terminal didecapeptide sequence does not represent the bulk of antibody diversity; in fact, the paradox becomes reinforced because somatic differentiation is discounted thereby. Only one gene is required to encode for the constant half of a κ-chain, but at least three genes are required to encode even for the three known subgroups and many more for the expected subdivisions. Since the complete light chain is synthesized on a single template from the N- to the C-terminus and not assembled by subsequent peptide fusion of variable and constant halves (Lennox, Knopf, Munro, and Parkhouse, 1967), one of man's favorite dogmas must be shattered—the concept of one-gene-one-polypeptide. Regardless of what one's favorite scheme might be to account for the assembly of light chains, one must include a step for the fusion of two sources of genetic material, one constant and the other variable, both of which are present in the germ line prior to any specific cell commitment.

10. Question of randomness or nonrandomness of variable and constant gene fusion

The observations that Oz^+ and Oz^- in humans and c^7 and c^{21} in rabbits are nonallelic in individuals; that the alleles Ab^4 and Ab^5 in rabbits involve a number of amino acid exchanges; and that even $Inv^{1, 2}$, which segregates so simply from Inv^3, controls much more than leucine at position 191 all lead to the question of whether the fusion of V and C genetic material is really as random as was once thought. Obviously the homology in the constant region is so near perfect, to say nothing of the amino acid balance, that the constant region gene, if it were to exert complete control over Oz, Kern, and

Inv, would have to extend its influence into the variable region. The only way to do so would be through some nonrandom selection of variable subgroups by constant alleles at the time of genetic fusion. In essence the result would be a single germ line that coded for an entire light chain of a subdivision of a subgroup. In this light, the fact that Kern[(+)] constant regions have so far been fused to λ variable regions of subgroup IV is of extreme interest (Hess and Hilschmann, 1970).

Tischendorf (1969) has found an antigenic marker, *St*, within the variable region of 52 Bence-Jones and myeloma proteins. The St(+) proteins were all from subgroup $V_{\lambda I}$; St(−), from $V_{\lambda II}$ and $V_{\lambda III}$ (and presumably IV and V). No correlation was found between St and Oz and no evidence for unigenic control of λ-chains was obtained: 20% of 15 St(+) proteins were Oz(+) and 80% were Oz(−); 38% of 29St(−) were Oz(+) and 62% were Oz(−). To answer the question of allelism in the case of Oz, Tischendorf offered the possibility that a fused V-C gene for λ might segregate among individuals. Thus one single indivual could be Oz(+)St(+) and Oz(−)St(−), whereas another would be Oz(−)St(+) and Oz(+)St(−), and yet both individuals would contain a mixture of Oz(+) and Oz(−) light chains.

Such a hypothesis is easily approached by experiment and no doubt will soon be tested. Whatever the answer there does appear to be a tendency for less than random pairing of V and C halves. The tendency toward restricted pairing is reinforced by the fact that the variable-chain subgroups of κ-chains are all confined to κ isotypes and not present in λ, and that λ subgroups are restricted to λ isotypes and not present in κ.

11. Stability, flexibility, and complementarity of light chains

It is now generally accepted that of all the forces contributing to the total free conformational energy of a globular protein—electrostatic interactions, hydrophobic interactions, London forces, and hydrogen bonding—hydrophobic interactions contribute the major share. Moreover, those nonpolar side chains and individual residues of a sequence that are not required to maintain internal tertiary configurations are free to make external contacts with other hydrophobic regions. Tanford (1962) has provided a measure of side chain contributions of individual amino acids which has come to be known as *hydrophobicity* (Table 1–10).

Welscher (1969) has calculated the total hydrophobicities of the constant and variable regions of a number of light chains, as well as

TABLE 1-10

Hydrophobicities of Amino Acid Side Chains

Amino Acid	Cal/Mole/Side Chain	Amino Acid	Cal/Mole/Side Chain
W	3000	K	1500
I	2970	M	1300
Y	2870	C	1000*
F	2650	A	730
P	2600	R	730
L	2420	T	440
V	1690	G	0

* Quoted from Bigelow (1967).
(From Tanford, 1962.)

the average hydrophobicity and fractional charge per residue. The result is most enlightening (Table 1–11).

The following conclusions may be drawn:

   (a) Hydrophobicities and fractional charges are essentially independent in V and C regions.

   (b) Spontaneous association is expected because of the relatively high content of nonpolar residues and low number of ionized residues.

   (c) An increase in temperature will enhance association and encourage dimerization even without disulfide bond formation. Further increases in temperature will then favor redissolution. The peculiar heat-induced properties first observed by H. Bence Jones (1848) are thus explained.

   (d) Since the interchanges of amino acids in one sequence site are compensated for by appropriate interchanges at another in order to maintain uniform total hydrophobicity and fractional charge, a random arrangement cannot be tolerated despite high sequence variability.

   (e) Globular folding of a chain is achieved after synthesis of the N-terminal half.

   (f) V and C regions are similar in form even though structurally distinct.

   (g) The total structural appearance is virtually independent of isotypic, allotypic, and idiotypic variations.

The overall conclusion is perhaps best said in the words of Milstein, Frangione, and Pink (1967): "One remarkable feature of the immunoglobulin structure is the constancy of its basic structure in spite of its chemical heterogeneity. Heterogeneity within a common

TABLE 1-11

Total Hydrophobicities and Fractional Charges of Variable and Constant Regions of Immunoglobulin Light Chains

Source of Light Chain	Formula	No. of Residues	Nonpolar Residues	$H\phi_{Av}$ per Residue	Fractional Charge per Residue
			%	cal	units
Human	C_κ	106	44.3	970	0.22
Human	C_λ	105	47.6	1020	0.19
Mouse	C_κ	106	40.6	950	0.22
Human	$V_{\kappa I}$, Roy	108	50.9	1100	0.18
Human	$V_{\kappa II}$, Ti	109	51.4	1050	0.17
Human	$V_{\kappa III}$, Cum	115	53.0	1110	0.18
Mouse	V_κ, 41	108	46.3	1000	0.19
Mouse	V_κ, 70	112	52.7	1020	0.18
Human	$V_{\lambda I}$, New	111	54.1	1000	0.15
Human	$V_{\lambda II}$, Bo	112	49.1	940	0.19
Human	$V_{\lambda III}$, Kern	106	51.9	1040	0.14
Human	$V_\kappa C_\kappa$	216	47.0	960	0.20
Human	$V_\lambda C_\lambda$	214	49.5	1030	0.20
Mouse	$V_\kappa C_\kappa$	216	49.3	970	0.20
Horse, pool	$V_\chi C_\chi$	212	49.7	950	0.18
Dog, pool	$V_\chi C_\chi$	210	51.3	1030	0.21
Sheep, $\gamma 1$	$V_\chi C_\chi$	218	47.9	980	0.18
Pig, λ	$V_\lambda C_\lambda$	220	52.7	1000	0.15
Rabbit, pool	$V_\chi C_\chi$	210	51.8	990	0.18
Guinea Pig, $\gamma 1$	$V_\chi C_\chi$	213	48.0	1020	0.20
Chicken, pool	$V_\chi C_\chi$	215	50.2	970	0.18
Bullfrog, IgG	$V_\chi C_\chi$	210	47.6	1010	0.24
Dogfish, 7S	$V_\chi C_\chi$	206	48.8	1060	0.21

(From Welscher, 1969.)

basic structure ideally fulfills the biological function of antibodies, which must be unique in their specific recognition of an indefinite number of antigens and yet maintain properties characteristic of all antibodies." The words were meant to be descriptive of the disulfide bridges of the immunoglobulin chain, which they are, but they could also now apply to regional hydrophobicity balance as well.

Glycine is a structure that lacks a side chain, has little hydrophobic character, and permits wide steric latitude in configurations. Wu and Kabat (1970) have calculated the frequency of glycine occurrence in each position of all available sequences and have thoroughly examined the consequences of such positioning (Table 1-12). Essentially three frequencies are obtained: common, 94–100%: group specific, 35–62%; variable, 4–24%. Glycines in the common and group specific regions are considered to have fundamental structural significance to account for their preservation through evolution to man and mouse—"to confer flexibility unique to antibodies." Glycines in the remaining positions are assumed to have other individual and varied roles not involved in maintaining molecular flexibility. Wu and Kabat strongly believe that the glycines in positions 99–100 function as a pivot to permit optional fitting around the antigenic determinant, and they support their case most convincingly by pointing to an analogous region in the heavy chain that is also reserved for two glycines (Press and Hogg, 1969; Cunningham, Pflumm, Rutishauser, and Edelman, 1969). The remaining glycines are felt to permit wide latitude in nearby substitutions and to encourage variability. Indeed a plot of variability at different amino acid positions for the variable region of the light chains (Wu and Kabat, 1970, figure 2) reveals particularly high

TABLE 1-12
Frequency of Glycine Occurrence in Each Position of Light Chain Sequences

Position	Glycine Occurrence Common no./total	%	Position	Glycine Occurrence Variable no./total	%
16	60/61	99	9	10/63	16
41 (39)	15/16	94	13	14/61	23
57	15/16	94	24	1/26	4
64	15/16	94	26	2/24	8
68	15/16	94	27f	1/22	5
99	20/20	100	28	2/22	9
101	19/19	100	29	4/21	19
Group Specific			30	5/21	24
25	10/25	40	50	3/14	21
66	10/16	62	51	1/14	7
77	6/17	35	55	1/16	6
100	11/20	55	74	1/16	6
			81	1/17	6
			84	1/18	6
			92	3/21	14
			93	1/21	5
			95	1/21	5
			107	2/18	11

(From Wu and Kabat, 1970.)

densities in the 24–34, 50–56, and 89–97 regions. Wu and Kabat point out that the first and third of these "insertion regions" are signaled by invariant cysteines and switched off by invariant tryptophan and phenylalanine, respectively. One must remember that the first and third regions are connected by the disulfide bond between cysteine I and cysteine II; thus there is a continuous stretch of variability,

-W-34-33-32-31-30-29-28-27-26-25-24-C_I-C_{II}-

89-90-91-92-93-94-95-96-97-F-F-G-

which ends in the pivotal region of 100-101. Wu and Kabat have therefore advanced the theory that this stretch is the "complementarity-determining" region of the light chain, the region that is in direct contact with an antigenic determinant, and the one that forms, along with its analogous heavy chain counterpart, the antibody-combining site. As a corollary to the theory they also advance the hypothesis that short linear sequences of episomal nucleotides are inserted into the deoxyribonucleic acid (DNA) of the structural genes of the variable region, that these insertions account for the very high variability in length and makeup of the complementarity-determining region, and that this insertion model is independent of and apart from any theory that describes the generation of diversity whether germ line or somatic.

The "complete insertion hypothesis" is a most important advance in immunochemistry because it "makes certain predictions which also can be used to test its validity." It would be best to keep in mind, however, that "site theory" concerning the location of the complementarity region does not depend upon the validity of the "insertion corollary." Should the latter prove to be invalid, the theory may still prove to be true. Likewise, should the site theory prove to be true the insertion corollary is not automatically proved thereby. Some of the predictions are as follows:

(a) The N-terminal didecapeptide is not involved in complementarity.

(b) Antibody molecules of a given specificity and with a uniform site can occur in any class or subclass of immunoglobulin by the insertion of short linear sequences.

(c) Structurally different antibody molecules with the same binding affinity for a homogeneous determinant have similar or even identical combining sites.

(d) Antibodies of a given qualitative specificity but showing differences in degree of cross-reactivity with analogs would be expected to show smaller differences in their insertion regions than would antibodies of unrelated specificities.

(e) Cases may exist in which several kinds of sequence patterns may produce the same binding affinity and apparent specificity. Unique insertional sequences would not be expected here even with antibodies of homogeneous binding affinity. Thus, in tests of the hypothesis, negative results are less important than positive ones.

In the chapters that follow the evolution of heavy chain structures, their relationship to light chains and to the binding site, the concepts of homogeneous binding, of specificity and cross-reactivity, and of affinity—all of these—will often feed from and feed back to the light chains, their variable regions, and the inserted segments of complementarity. It is indeed fortunate that we can be guided by such a clear-cut working model as that envisioned by Wu and Kabat.

12. Evolution of the light chain

To reiterate, in view of the very clear evaluation of the binding site region of light chains by Wu and Kabat (1970) there is very little one can say about the origins of extensive antibody diversity on the basis of the limited but very real diversity in the sequences of the N-terminal didecapeptides. Thus, for example, the very definitive exposition by Hood and Talmage (1970) is not really a delineation of a germ line mechanism of *antibody* diversity, as the title would have us believe, but rather an excellent and masterful evolutionary account of how heterogeneity has made its appearance among the N-terminal didecapeptides of 64 light chains. At this juncture in our own systematic development of the structural basis of antibody formation, it is certainly enough to consider the evolution of the first 20 amino acids of the N-terminal portion. It does require explanation. And, perhaps because of it, a concept of the combining site, as developed subsequently in Chapter 4, can then be gained all the more clearly.

Milstein (1966c) stated the problem best: "If an ancestor gene gave rise to all the variants which we are discussing, the question to answer is what is the time interval necessary to introduce the changes. If the answer is millions of years, as in the various haemoglobins, cytochromes, and other proteins, then each variant must derive from a different gene and a germ line follows. If the answer is hours to months, the mutations must occur at a very increased rate and a soma theory follows."

The somatic mutation hypothesis of Brenner and Milstein (1966) was developed to fill the negative void that was created in the minds of those who were firm believers in the traditional one-gene-one-chain dogma of protein formation. Thus, logic required the necessary rejection of any multigene-one-chain germ line theories. Cohen and Milstein (1967a) advanced somatic mutation on this basis. Many lines of evidence now make it necessary to accept a multigene-one-chain hypothesis as an explanation of multigene encoded diversity in the N-terminal didecapeptides coupled to single-gene encoded homogeneity in the C-terminal centapeptide portions. One particularly elegant immunological experiment among these removes somatic mutation, it seems, as an important overall process in N-terminal formation. Ruffilli, Compere, and Baglioni (1970), by using a technique similar to antibody suppression of allotype specificity, were able to suppress light chain formation in newborn mice by injection of specific anti-V_L antibodies lacking reactivity for C_L regions, thus proving that V_L antigens are already formed in newborn animals and not created *de novo* later on.

Although logic would have required the acceptance of a somatic theory had the germ line theory been totally rejected, logic does not require conversely the total rejection of a somatic theory if the germ line theory is accepted. Now that the multigene-one-chain idea has gained wide acceptance the human tendency is to reject the somatic alternate, but logic requires that the alternate be examined on its own merits. Soma-based mechanisms may yet have other attributes such as helping to account for variation in the hypervariable insertion-deletion regions that appear to fluctuate independently either of the one-gene encoded C-terminal centadecapeptide or the multigene encoded N-terminal didecapeptide.

Germ line theory has emerged from such formal statements as those of Lederberg (1959), Smithies (1963, 1967), and Dreyer and Bennett (1965). The issue which still has not been resolved is when, how, and where the variable genes, which evolved through one germ line, and the constant genes, which evolved through another, can fuse into effective nucleic acid templates to form protein chains and yet remain relatively independent of each other in continuing evolution. The proposed copy-splice mechanism for production of light chains (Dreyer, Gray, and Hood, 1967) and for membrane-bound receptor molecules (Dreyer, 1970)—in fact, for any family of recognition molecules that requires extreme diversity cast upon a restricted background—is one envisioned process (Fig. 1–3). by which a new stretch of DNA, coding for an intact variable portion, might be inserted

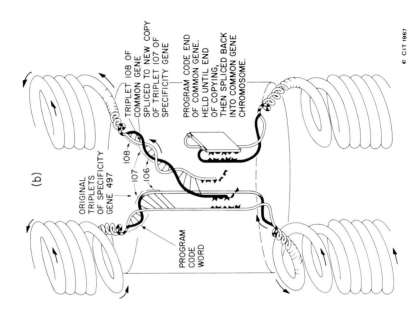

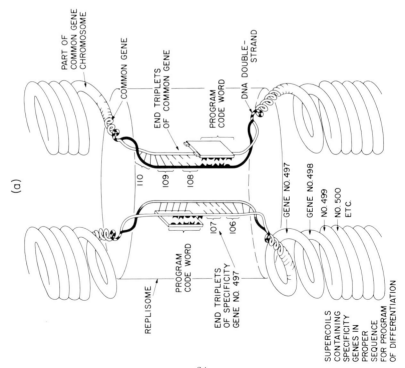

© CIT 1967

34

within an established stretch of DNA. At some step just prior to cell commitment a hypothetical "replisome" organelle with copy-splice capability would function in such a way as to splice a copy of the triplet nucleotides of a particular variable gene, that were responsible for the message of the C-terminal residue of V_L (e.g., triplet 107 in a specific case), to the triplet nucleotides of the common region that were responsible for copying the message of the N-terminal residue of C_L (e.g., triplet 108 in the same specific case). After the reading of a complete copy of a V_L message into the common gene, the program code end of the common gene, separated temporarily within the

FIG. 1-3. Proposed "copy-splice" mechanism for production of immunoglobulin light chains, for membrane-bound receptor molecules, and for other specific differentiated systems that perform recognition function in organisms higher than bacteria. The process is depicted as a conservative copying, involving two different stretches of double-stranded DNA. The specificity strand (*left*, in *a* and *b*) contains many individual variable (specificity) genes separated by "program code" sequences of DNA; the other strand (*right*, in *a* and *b*) contains the unique common region gene, plus its particular program code DNA.

(a) *Base recognition at splice region:* Anticodons that recognize and pair with program code words on DNA strands are contained in two adapters of the replisome and bring variable and common genes into correct alignment. The recognition process here is exclusive to genes and adapters although not held to be obligatory. Thus, a variable gene adapter in position at the start of gene No. 497 (after finishing with No. 496) acts as program reader to enable variable genes to be expressed in an orderly sequence.

(b) *Copying of variable gene to commit progeny cell to a particular receptor molecule (light chain, membrane-bound receptor, etc.):* The strand containing the common gene has been severed immediately after triplet 108, and the distal ends have been temporarily attached to the replisome. The remainder of the strand here is stationary during the copying process, a probable event with membrane-bound replisomes. The free ends of the common gene then act as growing points for the addition of nucleotides, and a copy of the variable gene is built up onto it, working back toward the first triplet. Some of the free energy of reaction is used to drive the DNA strands through the replisome. As the strands emerge they take up the characteristic double-helix structure, producing coils and supercoils and turning the DNA in the direction shown. When the copy is complete, the ends of the common gene strand are spliced to remake a continuous stretch of chromosomal DNA. The net result is a common gene chromosome that contains a stretch of DNA coding for a specific, intact subunit; thus, the program for the production of a recognition unit (light chain, heavy chain, membrane-bound receptor, etc.) has progressed one more step.

Asymmetric cell division is assumed. Alteration of program control regions may occur as they are read, thus aiding in subsequent control events following cell division.

The drawing, although basically similar to the system for incorporation of λ phage into an *Escherichia coli* chromosome, differs in not invoking large numbers of free episomes to explain differentiation. The rearrangements of DNA, although resembling mechanisms in microbial systems, differ in higher organisms by calling for the presence of large families of closely related V-genes and for far greater numbers of program control words. (From Dreyer, 1970.)

replisome from that spliced portion involved in copying, would then splice back into the common gene chromosome at the end of the growth of the nucleotide copy. The code for one particular light chain sequence is then transmitted to progeny cells, but the clone is now committed to that particular sequence.

The Smithies (1967) hypothesis supposes that light chain production is controlled by a gene pair consisting of a master gene and a scrambler gene that is similar to but not identical to the master. During somatic recombination a recombinant master could be produced (as well as a complementary recombinant scrambler) that could specify any one of 2^{20} different arrangements out of an original master and scrambler that differed only in 20. Instead of multiple genes in the germ line to account for diversity only two would be needed. Another somatic recombination model (Gally, 1967; Edelman and Gally, 1967) has also been proposed as a variant, but it still basically tries to limit the required number of V genes to just a bare few.

Genetic translocation (Edelman and Gall, 1969) proposes that variable and constant regions are specified by separate genes and that very simply one of the genes is translocated to form a single complete VC gene capable of being transcribed. The process would take place within the somatic differentiating stem cells of the lymphoid line, and the V genes would provide the necessary start signals. The proposal finds difficulty in explaining the fact that κ-chains have variable regions with one set of subgroups, whereas λ-chains have variable regions with a different set of subgroups and that the two never mix. Thus, while compatible with data for heavy chain variable regions as outlined in the next chapter, translocation struggles with the requirements for the light chains. It places no limit on the number of variable genes, hence, does not necessarily rise or fall with any particular pauci- or multigene hypothesis.

Hood and Talmage (1970) have provided the most comprehensive evolutionary scheme for the development of a multigene system,

FIG. 1-4. "Phylogenetic" tree constructed from the amino terminal 20 residues of 41 κ and 223 λ proteins by the method of Fitch and Margoliash (1967) which reduces the number of mutations to a minimum. The 64 proteins are indicated by *closed rectangles*. Deletions are indicated by *triangles* and mutations by *numbers*. The letters a, b, or c indicate which nucleotide is changed according to the genetic code. *Closed circles* indicate major classes and subclasses. *Dotted circles* indicate subdivisions of the subclasses, or highly improbable identical somatic mutations occurring in two different individuals. (From Hood and Talmage, 1970.)

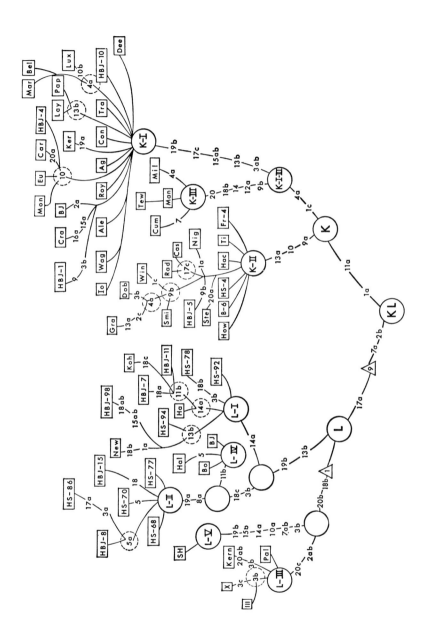

and have certainly removed any doubts that 20,000 variable genes could be conveniently encoded in the human genome. One variable region of 107 amino acids would require control by 321 base pairs per variable gene; 20,000 variable genes would involve 6.4×10^6 base pairs; on the basis of 3.7×10^9 base pairs per cell the variable genes would utilize only 0.2% of the total available pool of genetic material in a human haploid cell. Given 1,600 different variable genes upon which to build, as many as 12 different common genes could be accomodated.

Accepting the premise that a germ line for each variable region specificity is commensurate with rational evolution, Hood and Talmage then went on to construct a phylogenetic tree from the N-terminal didecapeptide sequence data of 41 κ- and 23 λ-chains (Fig. 1–4). The method of Fitch and Margoliash (1967) was used to minimize mutations. Additonal genealogies were constructed by Smith, Hood, and Fitch (1971), and out of them arose a strong case for a germline theory, marred only (but significantly) by a lack of reconciliation with rabbit heavy-chain allotype data.

REFERENCES

Appella, E., and Ein, D. (1967). Two types of λ-polypeptide chains in human immunoglobulin based on an amino acid substitution at position 190. Proc. Natl. Acad. Sci. 57: 1449–1454.

Appella, E., Mage, R. G., Dubiski, S., and Reisfeld, R. A. (1968). Chemical and immunochemical evidence for different classes of rabbit light polypeptide chains. Proc. Natl. Acad. Sci. 60: 975–981.

Apella, E., and Perham, R. N. (1967). The structure of immunoglobulin light chains. Symp. Quant. Biol. 32: 37–44.

Baczko, K., Braun, D. G., Hess, M., and Hilschmann, N. (1970). Die Primärstruktur einer monoklonalen Immunoglobulin L-Kette der Subgruppe IV vom λ-Typ (Bence-Jones Protein Bau): Untergruppen innerhalf der Subgruppen. Hoppe-Seylers Z. Physiol. Chem. 351: 763–767.

Baglioni, C., Zonta, L. A., Cioli, D., and Carbonara, A. (1966). Allelic antigenic factor Inv(a) of the light chains of human immunoglobulins: chemical basis. Science 152: 1517–1519.

Baynes-Jones, S., and Wilson, D. W. (1921). Specific immunological reactions of Bence-Jones proteins. Proc. Soc. Exp. Biol. Med. 18: 220–222.

Berggard, I. (1961). On a γ-globulin of low molecular weight in normal human plasma and urine. Clin. Chim. Acta 6: 545–549.

Bigelow, C. C. (1967). On the average hydrophobicity of proteins and the relation between it and protein structure. J. Theor. Biol. 16: 187–211.

Brenner, S., and Milstein, C. (1966). Origin of antibody variation. Nature 211: 242–243.

Cohen, S., and Milstein, C. (1967a). Structure of antibody molecules. Nature 214: 449–452, 540–541.

Cohen, S., and Milstein, C. (1967b). Structure and biological properties of immunoglobulins. Adv. Immunol. *7:* 1–89.

Cunningham, B. A., Gottlieb, P. D., Konigsberg, W. H., and Edelman, G. M. (1968). The covalent structure of human γG-immunoglobulin. V. Partial amino acid sequence of the light chain. Biochemistry *7:* 1983–1995.

Cunningham, B. A., Pflumm, M. N., Rutishauser, V., and Edelman, G. M. (1969). Subgroups of amino acid sequences in the variable regions of immunoglobulin heavy chains. Proc. Natl. Acad. Sci. *64:* 997–1003.

Dalrymple, (1848). Dublin Quart. J. *2:* 85, as referred to by Geshickter and Copeland (1928).

Dayhoff, M. O. (1969). *Atlas of Protein Sequence and Structure,* Vol. 4., National Biomedical Research Foundation (Silver Spring, Md., xxvi + 109 text pp. + 252 data pp.).

Deutsch, H. F. (1963). Crystalline low molecular weight γ-globulin from a human urine. Science *141:* 435–436.

Deutsch, H. F., Kratochvil, C. H., and Reif, A. G. (1955). Immunochemical relation of Bence-Jones proteins to normal serum proteins. J. Biol. Chem. *216:* 103–111.

Doolittle, R. F., and Astrin, K. H. (1967). Light chains of rabbit immunoglobulin: Assignment to the κ class. Science *156:* 1755–1757.

Dray, S. (1962). Effect of maternal isoantibodies on the quantitative expression of two allelic genes controlling the γ-globulin allotype specificities. Nature *195:* 677–680.

Dray, S., and Young, G. O. (1958). Differences in the antigenic components of sera of individual rabbits as shown by induced isoprecipitins. J. Immunol. *81:* 142–149.

Dray, S., Young, G. O., and Gerald, L. (1963). Immunochemical identification and genetics of rabbit γ-globulin allotypes. J. Immunol. *91:* 403–415.

Dreyer, W. J. (1970). A proposed new and general chromosomal control mechanism for commitment of specific lines during development. In *Developmental Aspects of Antibody Formation and Structure,* Sterzl, J., and Riha, I., eds., Academia Publishing House of the Czechoslovak Academy of Sciences (Prague pp. 919–932).

Dreyer, W. J., and Bennett, J. C. (1965). The molecular basis of antibody formation: a paradox. Proc. Natl. Acad. Sci. *54:* 864–869.

Dreyer, W. J., Gray, W. R., and Hood, L. (1967). The genetic, molecular, and cellular basis of antibody formation: some facts and a unifying hypothesis. Symp. Quant. Biol. *32:* 353–367.

Dubiski, S. (1967). Synthesis of allotypically defined immunoglobulins in rabbits. Symp. Quant. Biol. *32:* 311–316.

Dubiski, S., Dubiska, A., Skalba, D., and Kelus, A. (1961). Antigenic structure of rabbit γ-globulin. Immunology *4:* 236–243.

Dubiski, S., Dudziak, Z., Skalba, D., and Dubiska, A. (1959). Serum groups in rabbits. Immunology *2:* 89–92.

Edelman, G. M. (1959). Dissociation of γ-globulin. J. Am. Chem. Soc. *81:* 3155–3156.

Edelman, G. M., and Gall, W. E. (1969). The antibody problem. Annu. Rev. Biochem. *38:* 415–466.

Edelman, G. M., and Gally, J. A. (1962). The nature of Bence-Jones proteins. Chemical similarities to polypeptide chains of myeloma globulins and normal γ-globulins. J. Exp. Med. *116:* 207–227.

Edelman, G. M., and Gally, J. A. (1967). Somatic recombination of duplicated genes: an hypothesis on the origin of antibody diversity. Proc. Natl. Acad. Sci. *57:* 353–358.

Edelman, G. M., Heremans, J. F., Heremans, M.-T., and Kunkel, H. G. (1960). Immunological studies of human γ-globulin. Relation of the precipitin lines of whole γ-globulin to those of the fragments produced by papain. J. Exp. Med. *112:* 203–223.

Ein, D. (1968). Nonallelic behavior of the Oz groups in human λ immunoglobulin chains. Proc. Natl. Acad. Sci. *60:* 982–985.

Ein, D., and Fahey, J. L. (1967). Two types of λ-polypeptide chains in human immunoglobulins. Science *156:* 947–948.

Fahey, J. L. (1963). Two types of 6.6S γ-globulins, β2A-globulins, and 18S γ 1-macroglobulins in normal serum and γ-microglobulins in normal urine. J. Immunol. *91:* 438–447.

Feinstein, A., Gell, P. G. H. and Kelus, A. S. (1963). Immunochemical analysis of rabbit γ-globulin allotypes. Nature *200:* 653–654.

Fitch, W. M., and Margoliash, E. (1967). Construction of phylogenetic trees. Science *155:* 279–284.

Fleischman, J. B., Porter, R. R., and Press, E. M. (1963). The arrangement of the peptide chains in γ-globulin. Biochem. J. *88:* 220–228.

Frangione, B. (1969). Correlation of the C-terminal sequence of rabbit light chains with allotypes. Fed. Eur. Biochem. Soc. Letters *3:* 341–342.

Franklin, E. C., and Stanworth, D. R. (1961). Antigenic relationships between immune globulins and certain related paraproteins in man. J. Exp. Med. *114:* 521–533.

Fudenberg, J., and Franklin, E. C. (1963). Genetic control and its relation to disease. Ann. Intern. Med. *58:* 171–180.

Gally, J. A. (1967). Discussion following O. Smithies' paper. Symp. Quant. Biol. *32:* 166–168.

Geshickter, C. F., and Copeland, M. M. (1928). Multiple myeloma. Arch. Surg. *16:* 807–863.

Gilman, A. M., Nisonoff, A., and Dray, S. (1964). Symmetrical distribution of genetic markers in individual rabbit γ-globulin molecules. Immunochemistry *1:* 109–120.

Gilman-Sachs, A., Mage, R. G., Young, G. O., Alexander, C., and Dray, S. (1969). Identification and genetic control of two rabbit immunoglobulin allotypes at a second light chain locus, the c locus. J. Immunol. *103:* 1159–1167.

Gottlieb, P. D., Cunningham, B. A., Rutishauser, U., and Edelman, G. M. (1970). The covalent structure of a human γG-immunoglobulin. VI. Amino acid sequence of the light chain. Biochemistry *9:* 3155–3160.

Gray, W. R., Dreyer, W. J., and Hood, L. E. (1967). Mechanism of antibody synthesis: size differences between mouse κ-chains. Science *155:* 465–467.

Gutman, A. B. (1948). The plasma proteins in disease. Adv. Protein Chem. *4:* 155–250.

Hektoen, L. (1921). Specific precipitin for Bence-Jones protein. J. A. M. A. *76:* 929–930.

Hektoen, L., and Welker, W. H. (1940). Immunological differences of crystalline Bence-Jones proteins. Biochem. J. *34:* 487–489.

Hess, M., and Hilschmann, N. (1970). Genetischer Polymorphismus in konstanten Teil von humanen Immunoglobulin-L-Ketten vom L-Typ. Hoppe-Seylers Z. Physiol. Chem. *135:* 67–73.

Hilschmann, N. (1967). Die vollstandige Aminosäuresequenz des Bence-Jones-Proteins Cum. (κ-Typ). Hoppe-Seylers Z. Physiol. Chem. *348:* 1718–1722.

Hilschmann, N., and Craig, L. C. (1965). Amino acid sequence studies with Bence-Jones proteins. Proc. Natl. Acad. Sci. *53:* 1403–1409.

Hilschmann, N., Ponstingl, H., Baczko, K., Braun, D., Hess, M., Suter, L., Barnikol, H. V., and Watanabe, S. (1969). Antibodies and genes. Behringwerk-Mitteil. *49:* 66–68.

Hood, L., Gray, W. R., Sanders, B. G., and Dreyer, W. J. (1967). Light chain evolution. Symp. Quant. Biol. *32:* 133–146.

Hood, L. E., and Talmage, D. W. (1970). Mechanism of antibody diversity: germ line basis for variability. Science *168:* 325–334.

Jones, H. Bence. (1847). Papers on chemical pathology, Lecture III. Lancet *2:* 88–92.

Korngold, L., and Lipari, R. (1955). Immunological studies of Bence-Jones proteins. Proc. Am. Assoc. Cancer Res. *2:* 29–30.

Korngold, L., and Lipari, R. (1956). Multiple-myeloma proteins. I. Immunological studies. Cancer *9:* 183–192.

Laskowski, N. (1846). Ueber die Proteintheorie. J. Liebigs Ann. Chem. *58:* 129–166.

Lawler, S. D., and Cohen, S. (1965). Distribution of allotypic specificities on the peptide chains of human γ-globulin. Immunology *8:* 206–212.

Lederberg, J. (1959). Genes and antibodies. Science *129:* 1649–1653.

Lennox, E. S., Knopf, P. M., Munro, A. J., and Parkhouse, R. M. E. (1967). A search for biosynthetic subunits of light and heavy chains of immunoglobulins. Symp. Quant. Biol. *32:* 249–254.

Leskowitz, S. (1963). Immunochemical study or rabbit γ-globulin allotypes. J. Immunol. *90:* 98–106.

Litwin, S. D., and Kunkel, H. G. (1965). Relationships between Inv (a) and Inv (l) genetic factors obtained from studies of myeloma and Bence-Jones protein. Clin. Res. *13:* 544 incl.

Litwin, S. D., and Kunkel, H. G. (1967). The relationship between the Inv (1) and (2) genetic antigens of κ human light chains. J. Immunol. *99:* 603–609.

Mage, R. G. (1967). Quantitative studies on the regulation of expression of genes for immunoglobulin allotypes in heterozygous rabbits. Symp. Quant. Biol. *32:* 203–210.

Mage, R. G., Young, G. O., and Reisfeld, R. A. (1968). The association of the c7 allotype of rabbits with some light polypeptide chains which lack b locus allotypy. J. Immunol. *101:* 617–620.

Mannik, M., and Kunkel, H. G. (1962). Classification of myeloma proteins, Bence Jones proteins, and macroglobulins into two groups on the basis of common antigenic characters. J. Exp. Med. *116:* 859–877.

Mannik, M., and Kunkel, H. G. (1963). Two major types of normal 7Sγ-globulin. J. Exp. Med. *117:* 213–230.

Marrack, J. R., Richards, C. B., and Kelus, A. (1961). Antigenic specificity of hydrolysis products of γ-globulins. Protides Biol. Fluids *8:* 200–206.

McIntyre (1850). Med.-Chim Tr. *33:* 211, as referred to by Geshickter and Copeland (1928).

Milstein, C. (1964). Disulphide bridges and dimers of Bence-Jones protein. J. Mol. Biol. *9:* 836–838.

Milstein, C. (1966a). Variations in amino-acid sequence near the disulphide bridges of Bence-Jones proteins. Nature *209:* 370–373.

Milstein, C. (1966b). The disulphide bridges of immunoglobulin κ-chains. Biochem. J. *101:* 338–351.

Milstein, C. (1966c). Chemical structure of light chains. Proc. Roy. Soc. Lond. *166:* 138–146.

Milstein, C. (1966d). Variations in amino-acid sequence near the disulphide bridges of Bence-Jones proteins. Nature *209:* 370–373.

Milstein, C. (1967). Linked groups of residues in immunoglobulin κ chains. Nature *216:* 330–332.

Milstein, C., Frangione, B., and Pink, J. R. L. (1967). Studies on the variability of immunoglobulin sequence. Symp. Quant. Biol. *32:* 31–36.

Moore, D. H., Kabat, E. A., and Gutman, A. B. (1943). Bence-Jones proteinemia in multiple myeloma. J. Clin. Invest. *22:* 67–75.

Moulton, F. R., ed. (1942). Liebig and After Liebig. *A Century of Progress in Agricultural Chemistry.* Symposium. AAAS Publication No. 16, Washington, D.C.

Mulder, G. W. (1838). Zusammensetzung von Fibrin, Albumin, Leimzucker, Leucin, u.s.w. J. Liebigs Ann. Chem. *28:* 73–82.

Niall, H. D., and Edman, P. (1967). Two structurally distinct classes of κ-chains in human immunoglobulins. Nature *216:* 262–263.

Ouchterlony, O. (1953). Antigen-antibody reactions in gels. IV. Types of reactions in co-ordinated systems of diffusion. Acta Pathol. Microbiol. Scand. *32:* 231–240.

Oudin, J. (1956). Réaction de précipitation spécifique entre des sérums d'animaux de même espèce. C. R. Acad. Sci. *242:* 2489–2490.

Oudin, J. (1960). Allotypes of rabbit serum proteins. I. Immunochemical analysis leading to the individualization of seven main allotypes. J. Exp. Med. *112:* 107–124.

Perham, R., Appella, E., and Potter, M. (1966). Light chains of mouse myeloma proteins: partial amino acid sequence. Science *154:* 391–393.

Perlzweig, W. A., Delrue, G., Geshickter, C. (1928). Hyperproteinemia associated with multiple myelomas. J. A. M. A. *90:* 755–757.

Polmar, S. H., and Steinberg, A. G. (1967). The effect of the interaction of heavy and light chains of IgG on the Gm and Inv antigens. Biochem. Genet. *1:* 117–130.

Ponstingl, H., Hess, M., and Hilschmann, N. (1968). Die vollständige Aminosäure-sequenz des Bence-Jones-Proteins Kern eine neue Untergruppe der Immunglobulin-L-Ketten vom λ-Typ. Hoppe-Seylers Z. Physiol. Chem. *349:* 867–871.

Porter, R. R. (1959). The hydrolysis of rabbit γ-globulin and antibodies with crystalline papain. Biochem. J. *73:* 119–126.

Poulik, M. D., and Edelman, G. M. (1961). Comparison of reduced alkylated derivatives of some myeloma globulins and Bence-Jones proteins. Nature *191:* 1274–1276.

Press, E. M., and Hogg, N. M. (1969). Comparative study of two immunoglobulin G Fd-fragments. Nature *223:* 807–810.

Putnam, F. W. (1962). Structural relationships among normal human γ-globulin, myeloma globulins, and Bence-Jones proteins. Biochim. Biophys. Acta *63:* 539–541.

Putnam, F. W., Easley, C. W., Lynn, L. T., Ritchie, A. E., and Phelps, R. A. (1959). The heat precipitations of Bence-Jones proteins. I. Optimum conditions. Arch. Biochem. Biophys. *83:* 115–130.

Putnam, F. W., and Hardy, S. (1955). Proteins in multiple myeloma. III. Origin of Bence-Jones protein. J. Biol. Chem. *212:* 361–369.

Putnam, F. W., and Stelos, P. (1953). Proteins in multiple myeloma. II. Bence-Jones proteins. J. Biol. Chem. *203:* 347–358.

Putnam, F. W., Tan, M., Lynn, L. T., Easley, C. W., and Migita, S. (1962). The cleavage of rabbit γ-globulin by papain. J. Biol. Chem. 237: 717–726.

Putnam, F. W., Titani, K., and Whitley, E., Jr. (1966). Chemical structure of light chains: amino acid sequence of type K Bence-Jones proteins. Proc. Roy. Soc. Lond. 166: 124–137.

Putnam, F. W., Titani, K., Wikler, M., and Shinoda, T. (1967). Structure and evolution of κ and λ light chains. Symp. Quant. Biol. 32: 9–29.

Putnam, F. W., and Udin, B. (1953). Proteins in multiple myeloma. I. Physicochemical study of serum proteins. J. Biol. Chem. 202: 727–743.

Reisfeld, R. A., Dray, S., and Nisonoff, A. (1965). Differences in amino acid composition of rabbit γG-immunoglobulin. Light polypeptide chains controlled by allelic genes. Immunochemistry 2: 155–167.

Rejnek, J., Mage, R. G., and Reisfeld, R. A. (1969). Rabbit light chains lacking b-allotypic specificities. I. Isolation and characterization of light chains from normal and allotype-suppressed homozygotes. J. Immunol. 102: 638–646.

Ropartz, C., Lenoir, J., and Rivat, L. (1961). A new inheritable property of human sera: the InV factor. Nature 189: 586 incl.

Ruffili, A., Compere, A., and Baglioni, C. (1970). Repression of the synthesis of immunoglobulins in newborn mice by antibodies directed against the variable region of light chains. J. Immunol. 104: 1511–1522.

Schwartz, J. H., and Edelman, G. M. (1963). Comparisons of Bence-Jones proteins and L polypeptide chains of myeloma globulins after hydrolysis with trypsin. J. Exp. Med. 118: 41–53.

Smith, G. P., Hood, L., and Fitch, W. M. (1971). Antibody diversity. Annu. Rev. Biochem. 40: 969–1012.

Smithies, O. (1963). γ-Globulin variability: a genetic hypothesis. Nature 199: 1231–1236.

Smithies, O. (1967). The genetic basis of antibody variability. Symp. Quant. Biol. 32: 161–166.

Solomon, A., McLaughlin, C. L., and Steinberg, A. G. (1970). Bence-Jones proteins and light chains of immunoglobulins. III. Inv antigenicity: a genetic expression with serologic dependency on the intact κ-light chain molecule. Immunochemistry 7: 709–714.

Stemke, G. W. (1964). Allotypic specificities of A- and B-chains of rabbit γ-globulin. Science 145: 403–405.

Tanford, C. (1962). Contribution of hydrophobic interactions to the stability of the globular conformation of proteins. J. Am. Chem. Soc. 84: 4240–4247.

Tischendorf, F. W. (1969). Subtypes of human λ-chains and the amino acid substitution at position 190: structural and genetic implications. Behringwerk-Mitteil. 49: 100–104.

Titani, K., and Putnam, F. W. (1965). Immunoglobulin structure: amino- and carboxyl-terminal peptides of type I Bence-Jones protein. Science 147: 1304–1305.

Vice, J. L., Hunt, W. L., and Dray, S. (1970). Contribution of the b and c light chain loci to the composition of rabbit γG-immunoglobulins. J. Immunol. 104: 38–44.

Webb, T., Rose, B., and Sehon, A. H. (1958). Biocolloids in normal human urine. II. Physicochemical and immunochemical characteristics. Can. J. Biochem. Physiol. 36: 1167–1175.

Welscher, H. D. (1969). Correlations between the amino acid sequence and conformation of immunoglobulin polypeptide chains. Behringwerk-Mitteil. *49:* 133–142.

WHO. (1969). An extension of the nomenclature for immunoglobulins. Asofski, R., Binaghi, R. A., Edelman, G. M., Goodman, H. C., Heremans, J. F., Hood, L., Kabat, E. A., Rejnek, J., Rowe, D. S., Small, P. A., Jr., and Trnka, Z. Bull. W.H.O. *41:* 975–978.

Wikler, M., Titani, K., Shinoda, T., and Putnam, F. W. (1967). The complete amino acid sequence of a λ-type Bence-Jones protein. J. Biol. Chem. *242:* 1668–1670.

Wu, T. T., and Kabat, E. A. (1970). An analysis of the sequences of the variable regions of Bence-Jones proteins and myeloma light chains and their implications for antibody complementarity. J. Exp. Med. *132:* 211–250.

2

THE HEAVY CHAINS OF IMMUNOGLOBULINS

1. Evolution of the heavy chain

The initial difficulties in the sequencing of Bence-Jones proteins and light chains were enormous, but relatively slight in comparison to the heavy chain problem; nevertheless, Hill, Delaney, Lebovitz, and Fellows by 1966 were able to publish the sequence for the C-terminal quarter of pooled normal rabbit γG-heavy chain, a stretch of 105 residues (Hill *et al.*, 1966b). The occasion was the same conference at which Putnam reported the first complete sequence of a human Bence-Jones light chain. The report of the sequence would have generated enough interest in itself, but Hill, Delaney, Fellows and Lebovitz (1966a), on the basis of their and Putnam's sequence studies, went on to make an even more startling disclosure: the hypothesis that light chains and heavy chains were derived from the same ancestor gene which originally had controlled the synthesis of a 110 residue long peptide chain. The chain was based upon homology studies between sequences of the C-terminal quarter of rabbit γ-chain and the C-terminal halves of human Bence-Jones proteins. At about the same time Singer and Doolittle (1966) likewise made a similar pronouncement. At the time there were far fewer sequences from which to make firm alignments and the announcement was bold. Now there are many published sequences, all of which are supportive. In Table 2-1 the original sequence of Hill *et al.* is aligned according to Dayhoff (1969) and compared with a few representative light chain sequences of different origin including C_κ from mouse 41 and human Roy, New, and Eu.

When Edelman, Cunningham, Gall, Gottlieb, Rutishauser, and Waxdal (1969)* had finished the monumental task of completely

---

* See also: Edelman, Gall, Waxdal, and Konigsberg (1968); Waxdal, Konigsberg, Henley, and Edelman (1968); Waxdal, Konigsberg, and Edelman (1968); Gall, Cunningham, Waxdal, Konigsberg, and Edelman (1968); Cunningham, Gottlieb, Konigsberg, and Edelman (1968); Gottlieb, Cunningham, Rutishauser, and Edelman (1970); Cun-

TABLE 2-1

Alignment of Rabbit Heavy Chain C_H3 with Various Human κ- and λ-Chains

Chain*	Residue Sequence								Residue Positions
γ Rabbit			PL–	EPKVY	TMGPP	REQLS	SRSVS	LT	343–366H
λ New			PKA	APSVT	LFPPS	SEELQ	ANKAT	LV	109–133L
κ Roy			TVA	APSVF	IFPPS	DEQLK	SGTAS	VV	109–133L
κ #41			ABA	APTVS	IFPPS	SEQLT	GGSAS	VV	109–133L
κ Eu			TVA	APSVF	IFPPS	DEQLK	SGTAS	VV	109–133L
γ Rabbit	CMIDG	FYPSD	ISVGW	EKDGK	--AED	DYKTT	P		367–395H
λ New	CLISD	FYPGA	VTVAW	KADSS	PVKAG	V-ETT	T		134–162L
κ Roy	CLLNN	FYPRE	AKVQW	KVDNA	LQSGN	SQESV	T		134–162L
κ #41	CFLNN	FYPKD	INVKW	KIDGS	ERQBG	VLZSB	T		134–162L
κ Eu	CLLNN	FYPRE	AKVQW	KVDNA	LQSGN	SQESV	T		134–162L
γ Rabbit	AVLDS	DGSWF	LYSKL	SVPTS	EWQRG	DVFTC			396–425H
λ New	PSKQS	NNKYA	ASSYL	SLTPE	QWKSH	RSYSC			163–194L
κ Roy	QQDSK	DSTYS	LSSTL	TLSKA	DYEKH	KLYAC			163–194L
κ #41	BWDSK	DSTYS	MSSTL	TLTKB	ZYZRH	BSYTC			163–194L
κ Eu	EQDSK	DSTYS	LSSTL	TLSKA	DYEKH	KVYAC			163–194L
γ Rabbit	SVMHE	ALHNH	YTQKS	ISRSP	G-				426–446H
λ New	QVTHE	GST--	V-EKT	VAPTE	CS				192–214L
κ Roy	EVTHQ	GLSSP	V-TKS	FNRGE	C-				195–214L
κ #41	ZATHK	TSTSP	I-VKS	FNRNE	C-				195–214L
κ Eu	EVTHQ	GLSSP	V-TKS	FNRGE	C-				195–214L

* Rabbit C_H3: Hill, Delaney, Lebovitz, and Fellows (1966b); New C_λ: Langer, Steinmetz-Kayne, and Hilschman (1968); Roy C_κ: Hilschmann (1967); Mouse #41 C_κ: Dreyer, Gray, and Hood (1967); Dayhoff (1969); and Eu C_κ: Gottlieb, Cunningham, Rutishauser, and Edelman (1970).

Alignments according to Dayhoff (1969, p. D-224).

sequencing the human γG-immunoglobulin, *Eu,* (Table 2-2), there was no longer any question about the Vγ-Cγ1-Cγ2-Cγ3 formulation of the heavy chain. They had already sequenced enough of another γG, *He,* to know that whereas the first 114 residues of the two proteins were highly variable, the remaining 332 residues were identical. Moreover, the sequences given by Piggot and Press (1966) for the C-terminal octadecapeptide and by Press and Hogg (1969) for the Fd region of *Daw* were homologous with Eu except for two interchanges. Finally, Hill, Lebovitz, Fellows and Delaney (1967) were able to furnish sequences for Cγ2 of rabbit γG and Fruchter, Jackson, Mole, and Porter (1970) were able to continue the sequences through Cγ1 of rabbit γG. A remarkably high degree of homology, 69%, was obtained in all three constant regions (Table 2-2).

But were Cγ1, Cγ2, and Cγ3 homologous enough with each other and with Cκ to indicate a common ancestry from the primordial C_O of Hill *et al.* and of Singer and Doolittle? The tests were made for

ningham, Rutishauser, Gall, Gottlieb, Waxdal, and Edelman (1970); Rutishauser, Cunningham, Bennett, Konigsberg, and Edelman (1970); Bennett, Konigsberg, and Edelman (1970); Gall and Edelman (1970); and Edelman (1970).

TABLE 2-2

Complete Heavy Chain Sequence of Human γG1 Eu and Comparison with Rabbit γG, Human γG1 Daw, and Human γM Ou

Chain Region*	Source†	Sequence of Portion							Residue Positions (Eu Numbering)
(a)	Rabbit	Z-SLE	ESGGR	LVTPT	PGLTL	T–			1–21
	Eu	ZVQLV	QSGAE	VKKPG	SSVKV	S–			
	Daw	ZVTLR	ESGPA	LVRPT	QTLTL	T–			
	Ou	ZVTLT	ESGPA	LVKPK	QPLTL	T–			
(b1)	Rabbit	CTASG	FSLSS	YAM	.....	.....	.....	.....	22–58
	Eu	CKASG	GTFSR	––SAI	IWVRQ	APGQG	LEWMG	GIVPM	FGPP
	Daw	CTFSG	FSLSG	ETMCV	AWIRQ	PPGEA	LEWLA	WDILN	DDK–
	Ou	CTFSG	FSLST	SRMRV	SWIRR	PPGKA	LEWLA	RIBBB	DKF–
(b2)	Rabbit	.....	.....	.....	.....	.....	ITSPT	QDTAT	YFC	59–96
	Eu	NYAQK	FQGRV	TITAD	ESTNT	AYMEL	SSLRS	EDTAF	YFC
	Daw	YYGAS	LETRL	AVSKD	TSKNQ	VVLSM	NTVGP	GDTAT	YYC
	Ou	YWSTS	LRTRL	SISKN	DSKNQ	VVLIM	INVNP	VDTAT	YYC
(c)	Rabbit	AR···	.....	.....	BL	GGLVT	V		97–114
	Eu	AGGYG	I––––	––––Y	SPEEY	NGGLV	T		
	Daw	ARSCG	SQ–––	––––Y	FDYWG	QGILV	T		
	Ou	ARVVN	SVMAG	YYYYY	MDVWG	KGTTV	T		
(d)	Rabbit	SZPSG	TKAPS	VFPLA	PCCGD	TPSST	VTLG		115–143
	Eu	VSSAS	TKGPS	VFPLA	PSSKS	TSGGT	AALG		
	Daw	VSSAS	TKGPS	VFPLA	PSSKS	TSGGT	AALG		
	Ou	VSSGS	ASAPT	LFPLV	SCENS	BPSST	VAVG		
(e1)	Rabbit	CLVKG	YLPEP	VTVTW	––NSG	TLTDG	VRTFP		144–171
	Eu	CLVKD	YFPEP	VTVSW	––NSG	ALTSG	VHTFP		
	Daw	CLVKD	YFPEP	VTVSW	––NSG	ALTSG	VHTFP		
	Ou	CLAZB	FLPDS	ITFSW	KYBBS	BKISS	TRGFP		
(e2)	Rabbit	SVRQS	SGLYS	VPSTV	SVSZP	PST--	-----	–C	172–200
	Eu	AVLQS	SGLYS	LSSVV	TVPSS	SLGTQ	TYI--	–C	
	Daw	AVLQS	SGLYS	LSSVV	TVPSS	–LGTQ	TYI--	–C	
	Ou	SVLR–	GGKYA	ATSZV	LLPSK	–DVMQ	GTDEH	VC	
(f)	Rabbit	BVAHA	–TBTK	VDKTV	APSTC	SKP-$_M^T$	CPP--	–PE	201–233
	Eu	NVNHK	PSNTK	VDKRV	EPKSC	DKTHT	CPPCP	APE	
	Daw	NVNHK	PSNTK	VDKKV	QPKSC	DKTHT	CPPCP	APE	
	Ou	-----	----K	VDHRG	LTFQZ	BASSM	CVP--	–DE	

* (a) Variable N-terminal subgroup peptide, residues 1–21, Eu numbering.
  (b) Variable loop peptide, residues 22–96, Eu numbering.
  (c) Variable pivot and switch peptide residues 97–120, Eu numbering.
  (d) Cγ1 N-terminal peptide residues 121–143, Eu numbering.
  (e) Cγ1 loop peptide, residues 144–200, Eu numbering.
  (f) Cγ1-Cγ2 (Fd-Fc) hinge peptide, residues 201–234, Eu numbering.
  (g) Cγ2 N-terminal peptide, residues 235–260, Eu numbering.
  (h) Cγ2 loop peptide, residues 261–321, Eu numbering.
  (i) Cγ2-Cγ3 switch peptide, residues 322–344, Eu numbering.
  (j) Cγ3 N-terminal peptide, residues 345–366, Eu numbering.
  (k) Cγ3 loop peptide, residues 367–425, Eu numbering.
  (l) Cγ3 carboxy-terminal peptide, residues 426–446, Eu numbering.
  † Rabbit residues 1–30: Wilkinson (1967); rabbit residues 84–252: Fruchter, Jackson, Mole, and Porter (1970); rabbit residues 232–446: Hill, Lebovitz, Fellows, and Delaney (1967); Eu residues 1–446: Edelman (1970); Daw residues 1–224: Press and Hogg (1969); Daw residues 225–252: Fruchter, Jackson, Mole, and Porter (1970); and Ou residues 1–258, 380–465: Shimizu, Paul, Köhler, Shinoda, and Putnam (1971). (Ou is actually about 600 residues long, but only 465 based upon an extension of Eu numbering.)

(Continued on page 48.)

TABLE 2-2—(*Continued*)

Chain Region*	Source†	Sequence of Portion								Residue Positions (Eu Numbering)
(g)	Rabbit	LLGGP	SVFIF	KPPPK	DTLMI	SRTPE	VE			234–260
	Eu	LLGGP	SVFLF	PPKPK	DTLMI	SRTPE	VT			
	Daw	LLGGP	SVFLF	PPKPK	DTLM	.....	.....			
	Ou	DTAIR	–VFAI	PPSFA	SIFTL	KSTKL	.....			
(h1)	Rabbit	CVVVD	VSYED	PEVEF	DWYID	DEEVR	TARPP			261–290
	Eu	CVVVD	VSHED	PQVKF	NWYVD	GVQVH	NAKTK			
	Daw	.....	.....	.....	.....	.....	.....			
	Ou	.....	.....	.....	.....	.....	.....			
(h2)	Rabbit	LREQQ	FBSTI	RVVST	LPIAH	EDWLR	GKEFK	C		291–321
	Eu	PREQQ	YBSTY	RVVSV	LTVLH	QNWLD	GKEYK	C		
	Daw	.....	.....	.....	.....	.....	.....	.		
	Ou	.....	.....	.....	.....	.....	.....	.		
(i)	Rabbit	KVHDK	ALP–A	PIEKT	ISKAR	GE				322–342
	Eu	KVSNK	ALP–A	PIEKT	ISKAK	GQ				
	Daw	.....	.....	.....	.....	..				
	Ou	.....	.....	.....	.....	..				
(j)	Rabbit	PLEPK	VYTMG	PPREQ	LSSRS	VSLT				343–366
	Eu	PREPQ	VYTLP	PSREQ	MTKNQ	VSLT				
	Daw	.....	.....	.....	.....	.....				
	Ou	.....	.....	.....	.....	.....				
(k1)	Rabbit	CMIDG	FYPSD	ISVGW	EKDGK	AEDDY	KTTP–	–		367–395
	Eu	CLVKG	FYPSD	IAVEW	ESNDG	EPENY	KTTP–	–		
	Daw	.....	.....	.....	.....	.....	.....	.		
	Ou	.....	.....	···MQ	RGEPL	SPQKY	VTSAP	M		
(k2)	Rabbit	AVLDS	DGSWF	LYSKL	SVPTS	EWQRG	DVFTC			396–425
	Eu	PVLDS	DGSFF	LYSKL	TVDKS	RWQEG	NVFSC			
	Daw	.....	.....	.....	.....	.....	.....			
	Ou	PEPQA	PGRYF	AHSIL	TVSEE	EWNTG	QTYTC			
(l)	Rabbit	SVMHE	ALHNH	YTQKS	ISRSP	G				426–446
	Eu	SVMHE	ALHNH	YTQKS	LSLSP	G				
	Daw	.....	.....	.....	.....					
	Ou	VVAHE	ALPBR	VTERT	VDKST	GKPTL	YBVSL	VMSDT	AGTCY	

internal homology (Rutishauser, Cunningham, Bennett, Konigsberg and Edelman, 1968, 1970) with the finding that 30% of the individual C regions of *Eu* were vestiges of a common ancestry (Table 2-3). Tests were made between C_K and C_γ of *Eu* (Edelman, 1970) with the same result, 30% (Table 2-3). Meanwhile, Wikler, Köhler, Shinoda, and Putnam (1969) established that enough homology existed between μ- and γ-heavy chains to support their common ancestry and relation to light chains.

Shimizu, Paul, Köhler, Shinoda, and Putnam (1971), after determining the sequence of the complete variable region of Ou heavy chain as well as $C\gamma1$, a part of $C\gamma2$, and the 88 residue carboxy-

TABLE 2-3

Comparison of Constant Regions of Eu

Constant Region	Residue Sequence	Residues Involved
EuC$_L$	TVAAP SVFIF PPSDE Q--LK SGTAS VV	109–133L
EuC$_H$1	STKGP SVFPL APSSK S--TS GGTAA LG	119–143H
EuC$_H$2	LLGGP SVFLF PPKPK DTLMI SRTPE VT	234–260H
EuC$_H$3	QPREP QVYTL PPSRE Q—MT KNQVS LT	342–366H
EuC$_L$	CLLNN FYPRE AKV-- QWKVD NALQS GNSQE S	134–162L
EuC$_H$1	CLVKD YFPEP VTV-- SWNS- GALTS G-VHT F	144–170H
EuC$_H$2	CVVVD VSHED PQVKF NWYVD G-VQV HNAKT K	261–290H
EuC$_H$3	CLVKG FYPSD IAV-- EWESN D-GEP ENYKT T	367–394H
EuC$_L$	VTEQD SKDST YSLSS TLTLS KADYE KHKVY AC	163–194L
EuC$_H$1	PAVLQ S-SGL YSLSS VVTVP SSSLG TQ-TY IC	171–200H
EuC$_H$2	PREQQ Y-BST YRVVS VLTVL HQNWL DGKEY KC	291–321H
EuC$_H$3	PPVLD S-DGS FFLYS KLTVD KSRWQ EGNVF SC	395–425H
EuC$_L$	EVTHQ GLSSP VT-KS F--NR GEC	195–214L
EuC$_H$1	NVNHK PSNTK V-DKR V--EP KSCDK THTCP PCPAP E	201–233H
EuC$_H$2	KVSNK ALPAP I-EKT ISKAK G	322–341H
EuC$_H$3	SVMHE ALHNH YTQKS LSLSP G	426–446H

Alignment according to Edelman, Cunningham, Gall, Gottlieb, Rutishauser, and Waxdal (1969).

terminal peptide (as presented in Table 2-2), calculated, however, that there is less homology between the human Ou and the human Eu constant regions than there is between the rabbit γG and the human Eu constant regions: in the former, 35% or less; in the latter, 65%. Although there had been indications prior to this work, it was now clear that "the constant regions of the μ- and the γ1-heavy chains diverged during evolution almost as early as did the light and heavy chains." In contrast the V$_H$ region of Ou, in keeping with the mechanism described below, carried with it a completely separate ancestry from that of the constant regions. Its first 100 residues possessed a sequence 75% homologous to Daw, but only 30% homologous to Eu, thus supporting the concept of variable region subgroups and the separate-gene concept of V$_H$ and C$_H$ codes.

Hill and his colleagues (1966) visualized that a primordial sequence of about 110 residues had doubled at some point in early evolution, had diverged to light and double light (heavy) families, had formed their respective isotypic classes (κ, λ and γ, μ, α, etc.), and had then become organized into the familiar multichain globulins that we know today (Fig. 2-1). The statement was a remarkable intellectual achievement and of great import to immunochemistry. For the first time there was a recognizable common ancestral bond between light and heavy chains.

The assumption of doubling and double-doubling to form light and heavy chains was made at a time when adequate sequence informa-

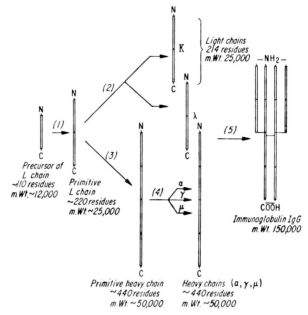

FIG. 2-1. Tentative scheme for the genetic origins of the immunoglobulins. (From Hill, Delaney, Fellows, and Lebovitz 1966a.)

tion on $C\gamma1$ and $C\gamma2$ was unavailable. With the proof of the V-C-C-C arrangement it was necessary to replace the double-doubling hypothesis of heavy chain formation with a $C\gamma$-triplication mechanism, leaving the V chain at its original length of about 110 residues. One such proposal (Dayhoff, 1969) is shown in Figure 2-2, but now that scheme must be replaced also because of recent findings.

Wang, Pink, Fudenberg, and Ohms (1970) have proved that a given heavy chain variable region may be shared by all classes of immunoglobulin. Just as subgroups of light chain variable regions had been typed so now heavy chain subgroups were becoming known based upon N-terminal peptide sequence analyses. Wang et al. utilized three of these V_H subgroups in their experiments. The results were in marked contrast to the V_L properties of light chains. Whereas the variable region subgroups of κ-chains had always been found in association with κ-chains and never with λ and, whereas the variable region subgroups of λ-chains had always been found in association with λ-chains and never with κ, each of the three V_H subgroups was found in association with a variety of γ-, μ-, and α-heavy chain isotypes. The fusion of V_H and C_H-C_H-C_H genes through a splicing step, to make the production of a single 446 residue long chain possible must therefore have occurred at a much later time in evolution than

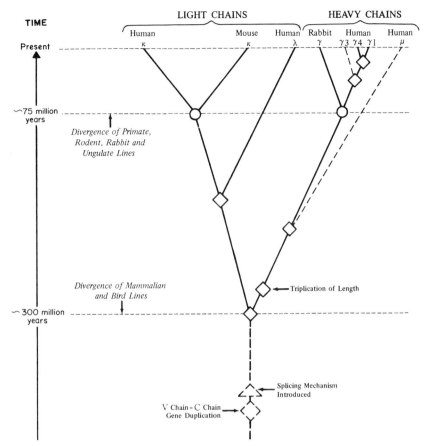

Fig. 2-2. Summary of the evolutionary course of events in the C gene of immuno-globulins. The tree is derived from inferences made from amino acid sequence data presently available and from fossil evidence which gives the times of species divergence. A chromosomal duplication took place roughly 300 million years ago, giving rise to the ancestral genes for heavy and light chains. The light chain gene duplicated again about 170 million years ago, giving rise to the ancestral gene for the κ- and λ-chains. The heavy chain gene underwent triplication in length soon after the gene duplication which led to the light chain lines. Following this triplication, a duplication occurred which led to the ancestral genes for a μ-chain and for a γ-chain. In the human, a separate gene duplication, which took place after the species divergence of primate, rodent, rabbit, and ungulate lines, led to the genes for γ1, γ2, γ3, and γ4. The special splicing mechanism must have originated *before* the light-heavy divergence, but could not have preceded the duplication giving rise to distinct V and C genes (see text). These developments are indicated on the trunk of the tree leading from the ancestral gene. The species divergence between mammals and birds most probably occurred after the heavy-light chain divergence. The heavy chains of the two lines would then be homologous, as would the light chains. The κ- and λ-light chain divergence may have occurred only in the mammalian line. Because of the evolutionary distances involved, the immunolobulin heavy and light chains found in sharks may have arisen by an independent gene duplication in the shark line. However, the striking correspondence of chain types in the shark and human lines suggests a common origin for each kind of chain. (From Dayhoff, 1969, p. 28)

51

indicated in Figure 2-2. As in the case of light chains, however, the fusion is in genetic material since the entire 446 residue heavy chain is encoded for in a 300S polyribosome and synthesized as a single unit (Askonas and Williamson, 1966).

To change the scheme in Figure 2-2, even in the most conservative manner, one is still obliged to draw a separate line of descent for the V chain after V chain-C chain gene duplication and to insert the V-C splicing mechanism at a later time in V chain evolution. One such arrangement is shown in Figure 2-3 in which the primordial unit diverges into variable and constant orders before the latter diverges further into C_L and $(C_H)_3$ families.

The up-to-date drawing would suggest that the primordial gene was a variable chain gene, V_O, whose selective advantage in evolution was to produce diverse variable chains from the very beginning, that one particular V gene, C_O, formed a clone whose selective advantage was to produce stable chains probably of transport and other effector functions. Still later a splicing gene developed that would be capable of fusing V and C genes. Selective advantage was still diversity but

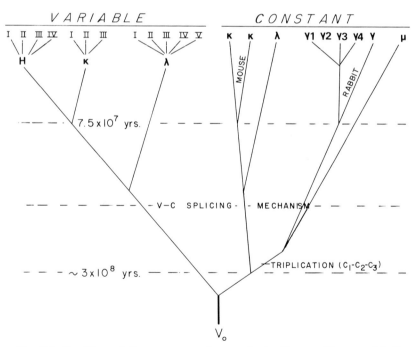

FIG. 2-3. Possible evolutionary course of events in the V gene of immunoglobulins which diverges into unrestricted (variable) and restricted (constant) orders before the formation of variable and constant families.

was restricted because of the association of V with stable C_L and $(C_H)_3$. Meanwhile, V_X continued to evolve into greater diversity, limited only by ability to fuse with certain types of C_L and any type of $(C_H)_3$ before actual cell commitment. Evolvement of the three V_H subgroups, the three V_K subgroups, and the five V_λ subgroups indicates restriction but this is clearly not geared to $(C_H)_3$ isotypes. It may have something to do with light chain accommodation. Indeed Wang, Wilson, Hopper, Fudenberg, and Nisonoff (1970) in their investigation of a patient, *Til*, whose multiple myeloma give rise to two serum paraproteins (Wang, Wang, McCormick, and Fudenberg, 1969) found that identical $V_L C_L$ and identical V_H chains were associated with the two different tricentapeptides $(C\gamma)_3$ and $(C\mu)_3$. Thus, at least in this case, the same particular V_L, C_L, and V_H genes were associated regardless of the C_H gene.

In the manner of Wu and Kabat (1970) we should remember that the evolutionary development of the structural genes of the variable regions, whether light or heavy, is not necessarily a valid description of the development of complementarity-determining regions, and that the "insertion model," for example, is independent of and apart from any theory that describes the generation of overall structural diversity. On the other hand, whatever may be the genetic answer to the development of complementarity *per se*, its heterogeneous message is carried within the structure of the variable chain, and expressed by the novel genetic process which Wang *et al.* call "reciprocal sharing." By this process, for example, as few as 10 different V_H genes and 10 different C_H genes can control 100 different structures. The superimposition of the insertion episome hypothesis of Wu and Kabat upon reciprocal sharing provides in a very conservative way an extensive system of diversity.

2. Allotypy in human heavy chains

The Gm (for γ) allotypes discovered in 1956 by Grubb (1970) were found associated with the Fc-fragment of IgG, were specific for γ-heavy chains, and therefore did not appear in IgA or IgM (Franklin, Fudenberg, Meltzer, and Stanworth, 1962; Harboe, Osterland, and Kunkel, 1962; Martensson, 1961; Fahey and Lawler, 1961). The naturally occurring fragments found in the first reports of heavy-chain disease (Franklin, Lowenstein, Bigelow, and Meltzer, 1964; Osserman and Takatsuki, 1964) were found to contain Gm determinants and therefore could be classified as γ-chain fragments. There are now over 25 known and accepted factors at the Gm locus (Fudenberg and Warner, 1970; Grubb, 1970), and a new notation replaces the unsatisfactory original system (Table 2-4).

TABLE 2-4
Notation for Factors at the Gm Locus

New	Old	New	Old	New	Old	New	Old	New	Old
1	a	6	c	11	bβ	16	t	21	g
2	x	7	r	12	bγ	17	z-Rockefeller	22	y
3	bʷ and B²	8	e	13	b³	18	Rouen 2	23	n
4	f	9	p	14	b⁴	19	Rouen 3	24*	m
5	b and b'	10	bα	15	s	20	z-San Francisco	25*	c³
								26*	c⁵

* Not necessarily fixed.
(From Fudenberg and Warner, 1970.)

The first of these, Gm(1), was found by Thorpe and Deutsch (1966) to be represented by aspartic acid and leucine, linked by glutamic acid, in the midst of an isolated undecapeptide whereas the same comparable triad in Gm(–1) γ-chains contained two glutamic acid residues and methionine. Frangione, Franklin, Fudenberg, and Koshland (1966) observed the same amino acid differences in a variety of Gm(1) and Gm(–1) types, and also noted that the "non-1" types, regardless of other Gm types [e.g., Gm(4) Gm(5)], were uniform in the Gm(–1) region. When the sequence of Eu, which was Gm(–1), began to be disclosed (Waxdal, Konigsberg, and Edelman, 1968) it became clear that the Gm(–1) sequence was E-E-M in positions 356-357-358 in the middle of the N-terminal peptide of Cγ3 and that Gm(1) was D-E-L in the same triad. Frangione, Milstein, and Pink (1969) and Burton and Deutsch (1970) confirmed the arrangement for both the positive and the negative types of Gm(1) allotypic protein. Because of the great variety of other Gm allotypes, their sequence positions have remained obscure in spite of intensive work. Harrington, Hood, and Terry (1970), for example, analyzed the complete C-terminal octadecapeptides of several Gm(1)(–3), Gm(–1)(3), Gm(23), and Gm(–23) γ-chains from both γ1 and γ2 isotypes without finding any differences. And Natvig and Turner (1970) could exclude only Gm(5) and Gm(21) from the pFc' subfragment region. In the γ4 isotype a replacement of leucine for proline at position 445 was obtained but could not be related to any allotype since all γ4-chains available contained the interchange. On the other hand, γ3-chains did show evidence of possible allotypy (Prahl, 1967) as well as isotypic specificity in their C-terminal octadecapeptides with arginine at position 435 as a γ marker and with phenylalanine at 436 in a Gm(5) and tyrosine at 436 in a Gm(21) allotype.

The allotypes Gm(1, 2, 4, 8, 9, 17, 18, 22) are associated with γG1-heavy chain; Gm(8, 23) with γG2; and Gm(5, 6, 10, 11, 14, 15, 16,

21) with γG3. Yet a whole phenogroup such as Gm(4, 5, 8, 10, 11) among Caucasians may be inherited together (Ropartz and Rivat, 1969). Within a γ isotype there are mutually exclusive alleles: γG1 may have Gm(1) and (17) or Gm(4) and (22) but not both; γG3 may have Gm(5) or Gm(21) but not both (Natvig, Kunkel, and Litwin, 1967). Among isotypic subclasses of γ-chain in a given individual there are high frequencies of association of alleles—among many Caucasians Gm(4) and (5) and Gm(−4) and (−5) segregate as pairs; among many Africans Gm(−4) and (+5) are common (Martensson, 1964). In the γG4 isotype in which no Gm allelic forms have been identified, there are still indications of linkage to Gm systems: there is a genetic γG4a variant that shares specificities only with γG1 and γG3 isotypes but not γG2; another variant, γG4b, that shares selectively with γG2 (Kunkel, Joslin, Penn, and Natvig, 1970). This seems to raise the possibility that γG4 preceded the development of the other γG classes in evolution. All of the subclasses including γG4 are of relatively recent origin on the basis of species comparisons (Pink, Buttery, DeVries, and Milstein, 1970).

The Gm locus is not confined to man but controls the type of antigenic determinants on the heavy chains of γG in apes and certain Old World monkeys. It excludes Prosimians, New World monkeys, and some Old World monkeys from its control (Litwin, 1967; van Loghem, Shuster, and Fudenberg, 1968). The first real indication that Gm may not have evolved in association with particular γ isotypes came with the study of the gibbon (Shuster, Wang, and Fudenberg, 1970). Even though γG3 was not a detectable isotype in the Gibbon, Gm specificities (11), (15), and (26) were easily measured. Another clue concerning the possible separation of Gm evolution from γ isotype evolutions is offered by Wang and Fudenberg (1969): although Gm(1) peptides appear only with γG1, identical peptides for Gm(−1) can be found in γG1, γG2, and γG3.

It will be remembered that Gm(1) is the only type that has a specific sequence associated with it. The question has been raised, however, that since Gm(1) and (17) are always present together or absent together, the sequence may not have been due to Gm(1) but perhaps to (17) or both. Shuster, Wang, and Fudenberg (1970), having found that baboon γG1 is Gm(−1, +17), went on to show that the particular peptide previously associated with Gm(1) was indeed absent from the peptide map of baboon γG. The sequence was therefore shown not to be under Gm(17) control and therefore obviously under Gm(1) control.

Although two serologically distinguishable subclasses of μ-chain of human macroglobulins have been disclosed (Franklin and Frangione, 1967, 1968) they are definitely isotypic in nature and not separable as allotypes by simple Mendelian inheritance. Moreover, one of the two classes appears to predominate while the minor class remains restricted and exhibits a preference for one particular minor subgroup of κ-chains (Cooper, Chavin, and Franklin, 1970).

Two isotypic subclasses of α-chains, α_1 and α_2, have also been found (Vaerman and Heremans, 1966; Kunkel and Prendergast, 1966; Feinstein and Franklin, 1966) and are represented by the myeloma proteins He and Le. In γA_2 a genetic marker, $Am(1)$, has been discovered which is inherited as a Mendelian dominant trait in strict allotypic fashion (Vyas and Fudenberg, 1969), but its structural expression has not yet been uncovered.

3. Allotypy in rabbit heavy chains

As described in the previous chapter allelism had been found in the Fab fragment of rabbit γG in six forms (Gilman, Nisonoff, and Dray, 1964), three of which were expressed in the light chain and three in the Fd portion of the heavy chain. These latter—a1, a2, and a3—involve several amino acid residues per type in the same manner as had been described for b4, b5, and b6. The differences are so distinct that peptide maps appear controlled by them (Small, Reisfeld, and Dray, 1966). Koshland (1967) has shown the difference between a1 and a3 through amino acid analysis of specific antibody γG from rabbits homozygous for A1 and A3 and immunized against two different non-cross-reacting antigens (Table 2-5). Alanine, glutamic acid, and phenylalanine are decreased in a1, compared to a3, whereas isoleucine, proline, arginine, threonine, and valine are increased. The analysis is essentially the same regardless of the antigen used to raise the antibodies and therefore eliminates any possible selectivity due to antigen. Koshland concludes that "the allotypic residues are not restricted to the C-terminal half of Fd but if anything are concentrated in the 40 amino-terminal amino acids known to be of mixed sequence." She also pointed out that the specificity residues of antibody sites and the allotypic residues could not help but overlap and that such overlaps "put new limits and raise new questions for possible mechanisms of antibody synthesis."

Micheli, Mage, and Reisfeld (1968) isolated Fd, solubilized the fragment by polyalanylation, and used it directly to demonstrate in a quantitative way the presence of a1, a2, and a3 specificities.

Wilkinson (1969) began a study of the variation in N-terminal sequences of rabbit V_γ of different allotypes, and discovered that allotype a3, for example, might have limited variation (cf. Table 2-2, positions 1–30):

TABLE 2-5

Amino Acid Analysis of Fd of Purified Rabbit Anti-Rp and Anti-Lac Antibodies (γG) of a1 and a3 Allotypes

Amino Acid	Residues/25,000 MW				Differences	
	a1		a3		a1–a3	a1–a3
	Rp	Lac	Rp	Lac	Rp	Lac
A	11.8	11.8	14.5	13.8	−**2.7**	−**2.0**
C	7.2	7.0	7.2	7.4	0.0	−0.4
D	12.4	12.5	12.1	12.4	0.3	0.1
E	13.2	13.2	13.9	13.9	−**0.7**	−**0.7**
F	7.3	7.2	8.0	8.2	−**0.7**	−**1.0**
G	20.1	19.7	19.7	19.5	0.4	0.2
H	1.5	1.6	1.5	1.5	0.0	0.1
I	5.8	5.6	4.9	5.0	**0.9**	**0.6**
K	10.3	10.1	10.2	10.1	0.1	0.0
L	17.0	17.0	17.0	17.0	0.0	0.0
M	1.1	1.2	1.4	1.3	−0.3	−0.1
P	21.8	20.7	20.5	19.7	**1.3**	**1.0**
R	7.0	6.9	6.1	6.1	**0.9**	**0.8**
S	27.5	25.2	26.7	25.0	0.8	0.2
T	29.8	29.1	27.6	26.8	**2.2**	**2.3**
V	20.8	20.2	19.6	19.1	**1.2**	**1.1**
Y	8.3	6.4	8.3	6.7	0.0	−0.3

Rp and Lac antigens, used for raising and purifying antibodies, are described in Chapter 6.

(From Koshland, 1967.)

$$Z^S_{EQ}LEESGG^D_VLV^K_XPG^A_XSLTLTCTASGFN^G_ASS^F_YY-$$

Previous N-terminal sequences in pooled rabbit γG γ-chains (Wilkinson, Press, and Porter, 1966) had revealed that about 50% of the chains began with Z-S-V-E-E-S-G-G-R-; 20% with Z-S-L-E; and 20% with Z-Q-. After his attempts met with only limited success to correlate any particular amino acid sequence with rabbit immunoglobulin a1 and a3 allotypes of either α- and γ-chains, which he attributed to so many amino acids in a single allotypic pair, Wilkinson (1970) was also led to declare that "it would therefore seem that the amino acid sequence differences responsible for the a-group specificities are present in the variable region" of both α- and γ-chains.

It not only remains a curiosity but also continues to be a matter of considerable theoretical import that the Aa locus is expressed in V_H. The interest is heightened because it is known that γM (Todd, 1963), γA (Feinstein, 1963), and γE (Kindt and Todd, 1969) share the locus with γG. This is in contrast to other allotypes which are specific for immunoglobulin isotypes: A8 for γG2 (Hamers and Hamers-

Casterman, 1967); Ac' for γA (Masuda, Kuribayashi, and Hanaoka, 1969); Ae14 and Ae15 on γG (Dubiski, 1969a, b), and Af with its five specificities f71–f75 for γA (Lichter, Conway, Gilman-Sachs, and Dray, 1970). It would clearly appear as if the Aa_1 gene were indeed controlling the allotypic expression of V_H quite independent of heavy chain *per se*. There are two other constant region allotypes, however, which have some type of association with the Aa_1 gene and which therefore prevent such a strong conclusion from being made without further study. These are the A11 and A12 allotypes of the hinge peptide.

4. Hinge peptide

The structure that forms the link between Fc and Fd in rabbit γG contains the following sequence (cf. Table 2-2) beginning with cysteine at position 220 (Eu numbers):

```
2              2 2 2 2              2                 2                      2
2              2 2 3 3              4                 5                      6
0 1 2 3  5 6 7 8 2 3 4 5 6 7 8 9 0 1 2 3  4 5 6 7  8 9 0 1  2 3 4 5 6 7 8 9 0 1
                  T
-C S K P  M C P P P E L L G G P S V F I F K P P P K D T L M I S R T P E V E C-
```

Smyth and Utsumi (1967) among others refer to the first third of this sequence as the "hinge" region and call attention to the three prolines in a row, unique among known protein structures. Such a figure is repeated in the latter half, as we can see from the sequence provided by Fruchter, Jackson, Mole, and Porter (1970). Between these two sterically ultrastable halves is a double glycine peptide at 236–237 of the type described by Wu and Kabat (1970) as helpful in chain flexibility. An extra loop peptide (cf. Paragraph 7 below) is terminated at the crysteine at position 220; the inter H—H chain disulfide bond occurs at position 226; and the Cγ3 loop peptide begins at position 261. The function of the "hinge" will become apparent later in discussion of the Y configuration of intact globulin, but at present it is useful because it locates the markers for allotypes A11 and A12. Prahl and Porter (1968) had observed that an extra methionine in the Fd-Fc area seemed to be associated with a1-a3 allotypic specificity and that it apparently had replaced threonine. The molecular determinants were established by Prahl, Mandy, and Todd (1969) as involving the threonine-methionine interchange at position 225, A11 with methionine and A12 with threonine. Although the specificities could be measured by routine agglutination-inhibition techniques (Mandy and Todd, 1969, 1970), cyanogen bromide cleavage was found to be a unique way of determining specificity (Kindt, Mandy, and Todd, 1970b). In both types the methionine residue at position 252 was cleaved by CNBr but, in addition, the methionine residue in A11 was cleaved while the A12 specificity remained intact. When γG was reacted with CNBr an intact 5S (Fab')₂ was formed in the case of A12, two 3.5S Fab' fragments with A11 (Fig. 2-4). That the inheritance of these constant region allotypes, A11 and A12, is linked to the inheritance of the Aa allotypes has been established by Kindt, Mandy, and Todd (1970a) which requires at the very least that separate genes controlling the Aa and the A11-A12 allotypic specificities on the variable and constant regions of the heavy γ-chain must be on the chromosome of one parent. One wonders, of course, whether the hinge peptide itself really belongs to the constant region. As seen in Table 2-3 it lies completely outside the internal homology regions of *Eu* immunoglobulin as an extra peptide insertion. The A11-A12 linkage to Aa almost makes one believe that the hinge is actually encoded in the variable gene itself.

5. Alloytpes in mouse heavy chains

In one study Potter and Lieberman (1967) have listed 14 allotypic

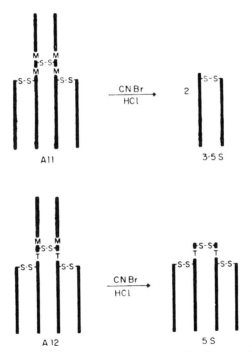

Fig. 2-4. Action of CNBr on IgG molecules bearing the allotypic determinants A11 and A12. *M* represents methionine and *T* represents threonine in the amino acid sequence at position 225, Eu numbering. (From Kindt, Mandy, and Todd, 1970b.)

antigens in 7 prototype and 31 other strains of mice; in another, Herzenberg and Warner (1969) have provided a separate compilation of 19 allotypes without attempting to match them all with previous reports. Fudenberg and Warner (1970) have updated this information. Structural information is scant even though genetic data are in rich supply, but eventually the allotype story in the mouse should be our most completely understood. Even the wild mice of Kitty Hawk, North Carolina, and Kyosho, Japan, have been investigated with the finding of 2 new heavy chain linkage groups and a new heavy chain allotype (Lieberman and Potter, 1969).

Interestingly enough, in spite of the ample number of allotypes for each of the isotypic subclasses γG_{2a}, γG_{2b}, and γA, polymorphism has yet to be demonstrated in γG_1 and in γM or in mouse light chains. That such genetic factors must be at play at least in γG_1, however, is suspected because of heterogeneous electrophoretic mobilities therein that can be segregated (Minna, Iverson, and Herzenberg, 1967).

6. N-terminal amino acids of the heavy chain

Prior to 1965, according to Putnam (1965), "the single most frustrating obstacle to establishing a coherent model for the structure of the γ-globulins of various species has been the inability to obtain consistent stoichiometric values for the N-terminal groups." The

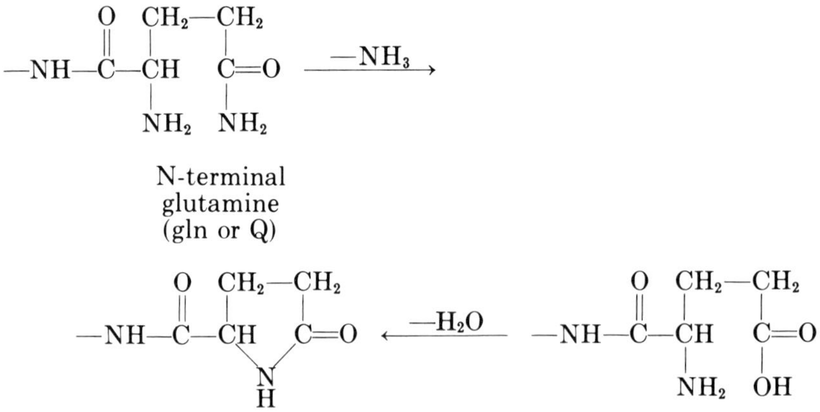

N-terminal
glutamine
(gln or Q)

N-terminal
pyrrolid-2-one-5-carboxylic acid
(PCA or Z)

N-terminal
glutamic acid
(glu or E)

problem was not entirely the fault of heterogeneity, for even among the homogeneous myelomas difficulty was often encountered. Porter and Press (1965) and Press, Piggot, and Porter (1966) finally solved the mystery, aided greatly in their work by the availability of a homogeneous myeloma protein, *Daw*, that contained no free N-terminal amino acids and by a personal communication from a graduate student (then), J. M. Wilkinson (1967), that normal rabbit γG contained N-terminal pyrrolidone carboxylic acid (PCA). The appearance of PCA as the N-terminal residue of a protein chain had been noted as early as 1949 by Dekker, Stone, and Fruton in a tripeptide from *Pelvetia fastigiata*: L-pyrrolidonyl-α-L-glutaminyl-L-glutamic acid. Anastasi and Erspamer (1963) had found it in eledoisin and had referred to it as a pyroglutamic acid residue. And Gregory, Hardy, Jones, Kenner, and Sheppard (1964) had discovered it in gastrin. Yet its appearance in immunoglobulins came as some surprise since it had never been encountered in the more usual biological proteins. The structure of glutamine (α-aminoglutaramide) can be seen to lend itself readily to ring formation by loss of an ammonia group and to form pyrrolid-2-one-5-carboxylic acid; thus, it really comes within the category of an encoded amino acid, glutamine or glutamic acid, that has undergone condensation. Moav and Harris (1967) showed that ^{14}C-PCA was not incorporated into γG at a later stage and that it must therefore have been bound to transfer RNA in the immunoglobulin-producing cells.

Although as many as an estimated 90% of heavy chains probably contain PCA as the first residue and therefore have no unbound amino groups (Wilkinson, Press and Porter, 1966; Bennett, 1968; Wikler, Köhler, Shinoda, and Putnam, 1969), the term amino-terminal or "N-terminal" has persisted in the nomenclature. PCA itself has become so important that a search was made for specific method to remove it. Finally, Doolittle and Armetrout (1968) found a pyrrolidonyl peptidase from *Pseudomonas fluorescens* which had the specificity of selective removal of the pyroglutamyl derivative from polypeptides.

The appearance of PCA relatively early in evolution is witnessed by its appearance as a blocked N-terminal residue in a large proportion of leopard shark γ-chains (Goodman, Klaus, Nitecki, and Wang, 1970). Previously Suran and Papermaster (1967) had found unblocked E-I-V-L-T-Q-. A comparison between the N-terminal hexapeptide of human μ-chains and the most probable sequence of the blocked N-terminal hexapeptide of leopard shark γ-chains shows remarkable agreement, particularly since the two nonhomologous residues can be related through single point mutations.

		1 5	
Human	V_μ, Ou	Z-V-T-L-T-E-S-G-	Wikler *et al.* (1969).
Human	V_μ, Dos	Z-S-V-A-D-	Bennett (1968).
Human	V_μ, Bus	Z-S-V-L-D-	Bennett (1968).
Human	V_μ, Bal	Z-S-V-A-E-	Bennett (1968).
Leopard Shark	V_γ	Z-V-G-P-D-E-	Goodman *et al.* (1970).

Another witness of early evolution is the persistence of PCA as the first residue of three of the five subgroups of λ-light chains (cf. Table 1-10):

$V_{\lambda I}$ Z-S-V-L-T-Q-P-P-

$V_{\lambda II}$ Z-S-A-L-T-Q-P-A-

$V_{\lambda IV}$ Z-S-A-L-T-Q-P-P-

The κ-chains are remarkable in contrast and have no PCA; in fact, $V_{\kappa II}$ begins with an unblocked N-terminal glutamic acid residue:

$$V_{\kappa II} \quad E-I-V-L-T-Q-S-P-$$

When Wang, Goodman, and Fudenberg (1969) found PCA present in three of five different human α-chains, their suspicions were reinforced that heavy chain genes must have been derived from a common ancestor gene, one, in fact, that may have been closer to the λ-light chain gene than to the κ gene. That V_α could not be correlated with any of the $(C_\alpha)_3$ isotypic subclasses or the Am(1) allotype gave support to the growing belief that V_H may very very well have had an evolution all its own with subclasses based at least in part upon the presence or absence of PCA.

The alignment among the N-terminal V_H sequences of the macroglobulin *Ou* (Wikler, Köhler, Shinoda, and Putnam, 1969), the γG1-γ-globulins *Daw* and *Cor* (Press, 1967; Press and Piggot, 1967; Press and Hogg, 1969), and the γA1-globulin *He* (Cunningham, Pflumm, Rutishauser, and Edelman, 1969) suggests that they all belong to a single subgroup of V_H. (This has been assigned subgroup number II by WHO.) The alignment between the N-terminal $V_{\gamma 1}$ sequence of *Eu* (Edelman, 1970) and N-terminal $V_{\gamma 1}$ sequence of *Ca* (Pitcher and Konigsberg, 1970) suggests a second subgroup of V_H (called subgroup I by WHO). And the alignment among six additional N-terminal sequences—$V_{\gamma 4}$ of the γG4-globulin *Vin* (Pink and Milstein, 1969), $V_{\gamma 2}$ and V_μ of the γG2- and γM-globulins *Til* (Wang, Pink, Fudenberg, and Ohms, 1970), $V_{\alpha 1}$ of the γA1-globulin *For*, $V_{\gamma 2}$ of the γG2-globulin *Wat* (Wang, Pink, Fudenberg, and Ohms, 1970) and V_ϵ of the γE-globulin *Sha* (Terry, Ogawa, and Kochwa, 1970) suggests a third subgroup of V_H (to be called subgroup III by WHO) (Table 2-6). The signatories of WHO will no doubt continue to follow the practice of numbering the subgroups in order of frequency and designating prototype sequences for each group and may rearrange the subgroup designations later on on the basis of up-to-date frequencies. The *Eu, Daw,* and *Vin* will remain the prototypes for three of the subgroups.

The extension of the number of subgroups from two (Cunningham *et al.*, 1969; Porter, 1969; Press and Hogg, 1970) to three was made convincing after Wang, Pink, Fudenberg, and Ohms (1970) pub-

TABLE 2-6

Subgroup Homologies Among N-terminal Peptides of Heavy Chains

			1 5	10	15	20	25	30	35
Human	V_{HI}	Eu γ1	ZVQLV	QSGAE	VKKPG	SSVKV	SCKAS	GGTFS	RSAII
		Ca γ1	ZVQLV	QSGAE	VRKPG	ASVKI	SCKTS	GYTFS	HYAM
Human	V_{HII}	Daw γ1	ZVTLR	ESGPA	LVRPT	QTLTL	TCTFS	GFSLS	GETMC
		Ou μ	ZVTLT	ESGPA	LVKPK	QPLTL	TCTFS	GFSLS	TSRMR
		Cor γ1*	ZVTLR	ESGPA	LVKPT	QTLTL	TCTFS	GFSLS	SSTGM
		He γ	ZVTLK	ENGPT	LVKPT	QTLTL	TC		
Human	V_{HIV}	Dos	ZSVAD						
		Bus, Dan	ZSVLD						
		Bal	ZSVAE						
Human	V_{HIII}	Vin γ4	EVQLV	ESGGG	LIQPG	GSLRL	SCAAS	GFTVS	TNYMA
		Til γ2	EVQLL	ESGGG	LVQPG	GSLRL	SCAAS	GF	
		Til μ	EVQLL	ESGGG	LVQPG	GSLRL	SCAAS	GF	
		For α1	EIQLV	ESGGG	LVKGG	GSLRL	SCAAS	GF	
		Wat γ2	EVQLV	ESGGG	LVQPG	GSLRL	SCAAS	GF	
		Sha ε	EVQLM	ESGGG	VVKPG	GSLRL	S		
Rabbit	V_{HII}		Z–SLE	ESGGR	LVTPT	PGLTL	T		
Leopard shark	V_{HII}		ZVGPD	E					
	V_{HIII}		EIVLT	Q					
Paddlefish†	$V_{H\mu}$		DIVIT						
	V_L		DIVIT						
Human	V_λ	λI	ZSVLT						
		λII	ZSALT						
		λIV	ZSALT						
Human	V_κ	κII	EIVLT						
		κIII	DIVMT						

* The sequence is taken from Press and Hogg (1970). Although Metzger (1970) in his review designates subgroups III and IV differently, Smith, Hood, and Fitch (1971) in their review reverse the subgroups so that Vin is now III. Since Kaplan, Hood, Terry, and Metzger (1971) also designate Vin as III and Dos as IV, the latter nomenclature would appear to be settled.

lished their definitive article. Terry, Ogawa, and Kochwa (1970) proposed that *Sha* be in a group IV but it probably will be included in III. It would appear, however, that a fourth subgroup is in evidence (called V_{HIV} by WHO), that it is the one most closely related to light chain $V_{\lambda I}$, and found in the four N-terminal V_{μ} penta-peptides found by Bennett (1968), as well as in similar V_{μ} penta-peptides of the leopard shark (Goodman *et al.*, 1970). Sequences for the entire N-terminal di- or tridecapeptides are needed to confirm this possibility. The identity between the other leopard shark N-terminal pentapeptide (Suran and Papermaster, 1967) and the κ-chain subgroup variable region, V_{KII}, cannot escape notice, nor can the identity of the light and heavy chain N-terminal pentapeptides of the paddlefish (Pollara, Suran, Finstad, and Good, 1968) and their obvious relationship to the κ subgroup V_{KIII}. More extensive sequencing is needed to make a firm hypothesis possible, but for now it would continue to appear that the variable half of the light chain V_L actually evolved separately from C_L. Subgroups apparently became restrictive only in terms of accommodation to light chain isotypes C_κ and C_λ but not to heavy chain isotypes $C_\mu 1$, $C_{\gamma 1} 1$, $C_{\gamma 2} 1$, $C_{\gamma 4} 1$, $C_{\alpha} 1$, or presumably any other $C_H 1$. Hopefully the advent of the protein sequenator technique (Edman and Begg, 1967) and the commercial availability of automatic sequenators will provide the proper impetus for the data needed to explore this area of biochemical evolution.

7. Intrachain disulfide bonds and resultant loop peptides in heavy chains

We have already seen how the light chain in each of its two halves supports a loop peptide formed by the disulfide bridging between two very conservative and evolutionarily ancient cysteine residues. In keeping with the theory of heavy chain derivation from the same primordial V_o structure that was responsible for light chains, the same loop peptides are preserved in all known heavy chains. The complete sequence of *Eu* and extensive sequences of other heavy chains in Table 2-2 show the location of the cysteine residues responsible for the closing of the loops. In *Eu* numbering they are 22–96 in V, 144–200 in $C_\gamma 1$, 261–321 in $C_\gamma 2$, and 367–425 in $C_\gamma 3$. Frangione, Milstein, and Pink (1969), in discussing the loop structures which they located, described these intrachain bridges as "an extremely stable feature of the heavy chains" and that as in the light so in the heavy they "are essentially invariant within each chain type and allotype."

There are variants upon a theme, however, even in loop formation

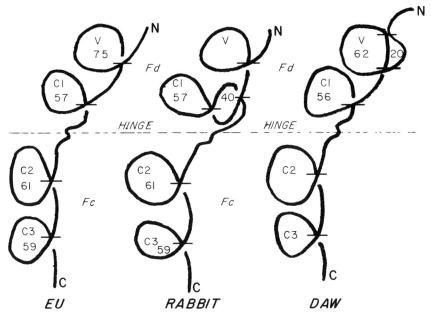

Fig. 2-5. Intrachain disulfide bonds (—) and resultant loop peptides in heavy chains. *Left*, human protein Eu, the traditional form; *middle*, rabbit γG with a double loop in C1; *right*, human protein *Daw* with a double loop in V. Numbers within loops indicate the number of residues involved.

(Fig. 2-5). For example, in rabbit γG-heavy chains there are not only the traditional four intrachain disulfide bridges but also a fifth bridge between positions 132 and 226 (*Eu* numbering) (O'Donell, Frangione, and Porter, 1970). In the human myeloma protein, *Daw*, there are also five disulfide bridges but in this case the extra pair is located in the variable region between positions 35 and 101 (Press and Hogg, 1969). The analog *Cor* has cysteine at 35 but not 101, thus does not defy tradition. It is not known whether Cor_{35} remains free as a sulfhydryl group or is involved in light chain binding. The latter would almost preclude its lack of an open binding site. Other subtle arrangements should not be unexpected even in the limited heterogeneity allowed for intrachain looping.

REFERENCES

Anastasi, A., and Erspamer, V. (1963). The isolation and amino acid sequence of Eledoisin, the active endecapeptide of the posterior salivary glands of *Eledone*. Arch. Biochem. Biophys. *101:* 56–65.

Askonas, B. A., and Williamson, A. R. (1966). Biosynthesis of immunoglobulins on polyribosomes and assembly of the IgG molecule. Proc. Roy. Soc. Lond. *166:* 232–243.

Bennett, C., Konigsberg, W. H., and Edelman, G. M. (1970). The covalent structure of a human γG-immunoglobulin. IX. Assignment of asparaginyl and glutaminyl residues. Biochemestry 9: 3181–3187.

Bennett, J. C. (1968). The amino terminal sequence of the heavy chain of human immunoglobulin M. Biochemistry 7: 3340–3344.

Burton, R. M., and Deutsch, H. F. (1970). Structure of peptides of Fc fragments from γG-globulins of known allotypic specificity. Immunochemistry 7: 145–156.

Cooper, A. G., Chavin, S. I., and Franklin, E. C. (1970). Predominance of a single μ chain subclass in cold agglutinin heavy chains. Immunochemistry 7: 479–484.

Cunningham, B. A., Gottlieb, P. D., Konigsberg, W., and Edelman, G. M. (1968). The covalent structure of a human γG-immunoglobulin. V. Partial amino acid sequence of the light chain. Biochemistry 7: 1983–1995.

Cunningham, B. A., Pflumm, M. N., Rutishauser, U., and Edelman, G. M. (1969). Subgroups of amino acid sequences in the variable regions of immunoglobulin heavy chains. Proc. Natl. Acad. Sci. 64: 997–1003.

Cunningham, B. A., Rutishauser, U., Gall, W. E., Gottlieb, P. D., Waxdal, M. J., and Edelman, G. M. (1970). The covalent structure of a human γG-immunoglobulin. VII. Amino acid sequence of heavy-chain cyanogen bromide fragments H₁–H₄. Biochemistry 9: 3161–3170.

Dayhoff, M. O. (1969). Atlas of Protein Sequence and Structure, Vol 4, National Biomedical Research Foundation (Silver Spring, Md., xxvi + 109 text pp. + 252 data pp.).

Dekker, C. A., Stone, G., and Fruton, J. S. (1949). A peptide from a marine alga. J. Biol. Chem. 181: 719–729.

Doolittle, R. F., and Armetrout, R. W. (1968). Pyrrolidonyl peptidase. An enzyme for selective removal of pyrrolidonecarboxylic acid residues from polypeptides. Biochemistry 7: 516–521.

Dreyer, W. J., Gray, W. R., and Hood, L. (1967). The genetic, molecular, and cellular basis of antibody formation: some facts and a unifying hypothesis. Symp. Quant. Biol. 32: 353–367.

Dubiski, S. (1969a). Immunochemistry and genetics of a "new" allotypic specificity Aₑ¹⁴ of rabbit γG immunoglobulins: recombination in somatic cells. J. Immunol. 103: 120–128.

Dubiski, S. (1969b). Does antibody synthesis involve somatic recombination? Protides Biol. Fluids 17: 117–124.

Edelman, G. M. (1970). The covalent structure of a human γG-immunoglobulin. XI. Functional implications. Biochemistry 9: 3197–3204.

Edelman, G. M., Cunningham, B. A., Gall, W. E., Gottlieb, P. D., Rutishauser, U., and Waxdal, M. J. (1969). The covalent structure of an entire γG immunoglobulin molecule. Proc. Natl. Acad. Sci. 63: 78–85.

Edelman, G. M., Gall, W. E., Waxdal, M. J., and Konigsberg, W. H. (1968). The covalent structure of a human γG-immunoglobulin. I. Isolation and characterization of the whole molecule, the polypeptide chains, and the tryptic fragments. Biochemistry 7: 1950–1958.

Edman, P., and Begg, G. (1967). A protein sequenator. Eur. J. Biochem. 1: 80–91.

Fahey, J. L., and Lawler, S. D. (1961). Gm factors in normal γ-globulin fraction, myeloma proteins, and macroglobulins. J. Natl. Cancer Inst. 27: 973–981.

Feinstein, A. (1963). Character and allotype of an immune globulin in rabbit colostrum. Nature 199: 1197–1199.

Feinstein, D., and Franklin, E. C. (1966). Two antigenically distinguishable subclasses of human A myeloma proteins differing in their heavy chains. Nature 212: 1496–1498.

Fisher, C. E., Palm, W. H., and Press, E. M. (1969). The N-terminal sequence of a human γ1 chain of allotype Gm (A⁻f⁺). Fed. Eur. Biochem. Soc. Letters 5: 20–22.

Frangione, B., Franklin, E. C., Fudenberg, H. H., and Koshland, M. E. (1966). Structural studies of human γG-myeloma proteins of different antigenic subgroups and genetic specificities. J. Exp. Med. 124: 715–732.

Frangione, B., Milstein, C., and Pink, J. R. L. (1969). Structural studies of immuno-golublin G. Nature 221: 145–148.

Franklin, E. C., and Frangione, B. (1967). Two serologically distinguishable subclasses of μ-chains of human macroglobulins. J. Immunol. 99: 810–814.

Franklin, E. C., and Frangione, B. (1968). Structural differences between macro-globulins belonging to two serologically distinguishable subclasses. Biochemistry 7: 4203–4211.

Franklin, E. C., Fudenberg, H., Meltzer, M., and Stanworth, D. R. (1962). The structural basis for genetic variations of normal human γ-globulins. Proc. Natl. Acad Sci. 48: 914–922.

Franklin, E. C., Lowenstein, J., Bigelow, B., and Meltzer, M. (1964). Heavy chain disease—a new disorder of serum γ-globulins: Report of the first case. Am. J. Med. 37: 332–350.

Fruchter, R. G., Jackson, S. A., Mole, L. E., and Porter, R. R. (1970). Sequence studies of the Fd section of the heavy chain of rabbit immunoglobulin G. Biochem. J. 116: 249–259.

Fudenberg, H. H., and Warner, N. L. (1970). Genetics of immunoglobulins. Adv. Hum. Genet. 1: 131–209.

Gall, W. E., Cunningham, B. A., Waxdal, M. J., Konigsberg, W. H., and Edelman, G. M. (1968). The covalent structure of a human γG-immunoglobulin. IV. The interchain disulfide bonds. Biochemistry 7: 1973–1982.

Gall, W. E., and Edelman, G. M. (1970). The covalent structure of a human γG-immunoglobulin. X. Intrachain disulfide bonds. Biochemistry 9: 3188–3196.

Gilman, A. M., Nisonoff, A., and Dray, S. (1964). Symmetrical distribution of genetic markers in individual rabbit γ-globulin molecules. Immunochemistry 1: 109–120.

Goodman, J. W., Klaus, G. G., Nitecki, D. E., and Wang, A.-C. (1970). Pyrrolidone-carboxylic acid at the N-terminal positions of polypeptide chains from leopard shark immunoglobulins. J. Immunol. 104: 260–262.

Gottlieb, P. D., Cunningham, B. A., Rutishauser, U., and Edelman, G. M. (1970). The covalent structure of a human γG-immunoglobulin. VI. Amino acid sequence of the light chain. Biochemistry 9: 3155–3160.

Gottlieb, P. D., Cunningham, B. A., Waxdal, M. J., Konigsberg, W. H., and Edelman, G. M. (1968). Variable regions of heavy and light polypeptide chains of the same γG-immunoglobulin molecule. Proc. Natl. Acad. Sci. 61: 168–175.

Gregory, H., Hardy, P. M., Jones, D. S., Kenner, G. W., and Sheppard, R. C. (1964). The antral hormone gastrin. Nature 204: 931–933.

Grubb, R. (1970). The Genetic Markers of Human Immunoglobulins. (Mol. Biol. Biochem. Biophys., Vol. 9). Springer-Verlag (New York, 168 pp.).

Hamers, R., and Hamers-Casterman, C. (1967). Evidence for the presence of the Fc allotypic marker As8 and the Fd allotypic marker As1 in the same molecule of rabbit IgG. Symp. Quant. Biol. 32: 129–132.

Harboe, M., Osterland, C. K., and Kunkel, H. G. (1962). Localization of two genetic factors to different areas of γ-globulin molecules. Science 136: 979–980.

Harrington, J. T., Hood, L. E., and Terry, W. D. (1970). C-terminal peptides from human γ-chains of the differing subclass and allotype. Immunochemistry 7: 393–399.

Herzenberg, L. A., and Warner, N. L. (1969). Genetic control of mouse immunoglobulins. In *Regulation of the Antibody Response*, Cinader, B., ed., Charles C Thomas (Springfield, Ill., 400 pp.), pp. 322–348.

Hill, R. L., Delaney, R., Fellows, R. E., Jr., and Lebovitz, H. (1966a). The evolutionary origins of the immunoglobulins. Proc. Natl. Acad. Sci. *56:* 1762–1769.

Hill, R. L., Delaney, R., Lebovitz, H. E., and Fellows, R. E., Jr. (1966b). Studies on the amino acid sequence of heavy chains from rabbit immunoglobulin G. Proc. Roy. Soc. Lond. *166:* 159–175.

Hill, R. L., Lebovitz, H. E., Fellows, R. E., Jr., and Delaney, R. (1967). The evolution of immunoglobulins as reflected by the amino acid sequence studies of rabbit Fc fragment. In *Gamma Globulins: Structure and Control of Biosynthesis*, Nobel Symposium 3, Killander, J., ed. Interscience (New York, 643 pp.), pp. 109–127.

Hilschmann, N. (1967). Die chemische Struktur von zwei Bence-Jones-Proteinen (Roy and Cum.) vom κ-Typ. Hoppe-Seylers Z. Physiol. Chem. *348:* 1077–1080.

Kaplan, A. P., Hood, L. E., Terry, W. D., and Metzger, H. (1971). Amino terminal sequences of human immunoglobulin heavy chains. Immunochemistry *8:* 801–811.

Kindt, T. J., Mandy, W. J., and Todd, C. W. (1970a). Association of allotypic specificities of group a with allotypic specificities A11 and A12 in rabbit immunoglobulin. Biochemistry *9:* 2028–2032.

Kindt, T. J., Mandy, W. J., and Todd, C. W. (1970b). The action of cyanogen bromide on rabbit IgG molecules of allotypes A11 and A12. Immunochemistry *7:* 467–477.

Kindt, T. J., and Todd, C. W. (1969). Heavy and light chain allotypic markers on rabbit homocytotropic antibody. J. Exp. Med. *130:* 859–866.

Koshland, M. E. (1967). Location of specificity and allotypic amino acid residues in antibody Fd fragments. Symp. Quant. Biol. *32:* 119–127.

Kunkel, H. G., Joslin, F. G., Penn, G. M., and Natvig, J. B. (1970). Genetic variants of γG4 globulin. A unique relationship to other classes of γG globulin. J. Exp. Med. *132:* 508–520.

Kunkel, H. G., and Prendergast, R. A. (1966). Subgroups of γA immune globulins. Proc. Soc. Exp. Biol. Med. *122:* 910–913.

Langer, v. B., Steinmetz-Kayne, M., and Hilschmann, N. (1968). Die vollstandige Aminosäuresequenz des Bence-Jones-Proteins New (λ-Typ) Subgruppen im Variablen Teil bei Immunoglobulin-L-Ketten-vom λ-Typ. Hoppe-Seylers Z. Physiol. Chem. *349:* 945–951.

Lichter, E. A., Conway, T. P., Gilman-Sachs, A., and Dray, S. (1970). Presence of allotypic specificities of three loci a, b, and f on individual molecules of rabbit colostral γA immunoglobulin. J. Immunol. *105:* 70–74.

Lieberman, R., and Potter, M. (1969). Crossing over between genes in the immunoglobulin heavy chain linkage group of the mouse. J. Exp. Med. *130:* 519–541.

Litwin, S. D. (1967). Phylogenetic differences among the Gm factors of non-human primates. Nature *216:* 268–269.

Mandy, W. J., and Todd, C. W. (1969). Characterization of allotype A11 in rabbits: a specificity detected by agglutination. Immunochemistry *6:* 811–823.

Mandy, W. J., and Todd, C. W. (1970). Rabbit immunoglobulin allotype A12: A new agglutinating specificity. Biochem. Genet. *4:* 59–71.

Martenson, L. (1961). Gm characters of m-components. Acta Med. Scand. Suppl. *367:* 87–93.

Martensson, L. (1964). On the relationships between the γ-globulin genes of the Gm system. A study of Gm gene products in sera, myeloma globulins, and specific antibodies with special reference to the gene Gm f. J. Exp. Med. *120:* 1169–1188.

Masuda, T., Kuribayashi, K., and Hanaoka, M. (1969). A new allotypic antigen of rabbit colostral γA immunoglobulin. J. Immunol. *102:* 1156–1162.

Metzger, H. (1970). The antigen receptor problem. Annu. Rev. Biochem. *39:* 889–928.

Micheli, A., Mage, R. G., and Reisfeld, R. A. (1968). Direct demonstration and quantitation of Aa1, Aa2, and Aa3 allotypic specificities on Fd-fragments of rabbit immunoglobulin G. J. Immunol. *100:* 604–611.

Minna, J. D., Iverson, G. M., and Herzenberg, L. A. (1967). Identification of a gene locus for γ-G-1 immunoglobulin H chains and its linkage to the H-chain chromosome region in the mouse. Proc. Natl. Acad. Sci. *58:* 188–194.

Moav, B., and Harris, T. N. (1967). Pyrrolid-2-one-5-carboxylic acid involvement in the biosynthesis of rabbit immunoglobulin. Biochem. Biophys. Res. Commun. *29:* 773–776.

Natvig, J. B., Kunkel, H. G., and Litwin, S. D. (1967). Genetic markers of the heavy chain subgroups of human γG globulin. Symp. Quant. Biol. *32:* 173–180.

Natvig, J. B., and Turner, M. W. (1970). Rheumatoid anti-Gm factors with specificity of the pFc′ subfragment of human immunoglobulin G. Nature *225:* 855–857.

O'Donnell, I. J., Frangione, B., and Porter, R. R. (1970). The disulfide bonds of the heavy chain of rabbit immunoglobulin G. Biochem. J. *116:* 261–268.

Osserman, E. F., and Takatsuki, K. (1964). Clinical and immunochemical studies of four cases of heavy (H-γ2) chain disease. Am. J. Med. *37:* 351–373.

Piggot, P. J., and Press, E. M.(1966). C-terminal peptide of the heavy chain of normal human immunoglobulin. Biochem. J. *99:* 16P–17P.

Pink, J. R. L., Buttery, S. H., DeVries, G. M., and Milstein, C. (1970). Human immunoglobulin subclasses. Partial amino acid sequence of the constant region of a γ4 chain. Biochem. J. *117:* 33–47.

Pink, J. R. L., and Milstein, C. (1969). Sequence studies on a γ4 immunoglobulin chain. Fed. Eur. Biochem. Soc. Proc. *15:* 177–182.

Pitcher, S. E., and Konigsberg, W. (1970). The sequence of the NH₂-terminal cyanogen bromide fragment from the heavy chain of a γG1 myeloma protein. J. Biol. Chem. *245:* 1267–1295.

Pollara, B., Suran, A., Finstad, J., and Good, R. A. (1968). N-terminal amino acid sequences of immunoglobulin chains on *Polyodon spathula*. Proc. Natl. Acad. Sci. *59:* 1307–1312.

Porter, R. R. (1969). Sequence studies of the heavy chains of human myeloma immunoglobulins. Behringwerk-Mitteil. *49:* 56–59.

Porter, R. R., and Press, E. M. (1965). N-terminal peptide of the heavy chain of immunoglobulin IgG. Biochem. J. *97:* 32P–33P.

Potter, M., and Lieberman, R. (1967). Genetic studies of immunoglobulins in mice. Symp. Quant. Biol. *32:* 187–202.

Prahl, J. W. (1967). The C-terminal sequences of the heavy chains of human immunoglobulin G myeloma proteins of differing isotypes and allotypes. Biochem. J. *105:* 1019–1028.

Prahl, J. W., Mandy, W. J., and Todd, C. W. (1969). The molecular determinants of the A11 and A12 allotypic specificities in rabbit immunoglobulin. Biochemistry *8:* 4935–4940.

Prahl, J. W., and Porter, R. R. (1968). Allotype-related sequence-variation of the heavy chain of rabbit immunoglobulin G. Biochem. J. *107:* 753–763.

Press, E. M. (1967). The amino acid sequence of the N-terminal 84 residues of a human heavy chain of immunoglobulin G (Daw). Biochem. J. *104:* 30c–33c.

Press, E. M., and Hogg, N. M. (1969). Comparative study of two immunoglobulin G Fd-fragments. Nature *223:* 807–810.

Press, E. M., and Hogg, N. M. (1970). Amino acid sequences of the Fd fragments of two human γ1 heavy chains. Biochem. J. *117:* 641–660.

Press, E. M., and Piggot, P. H. (1967). The chemical structure of the heavy chains of human immunoglobulin G. Symp. Quant. Biol. *32:* 45–51.

Press, E. M., Piggot, P. J., and Porter, R. R. (1966). The N- and C-terminal amino acid sequences of the heavy chain from a pathological human immunoglobulin IgG. Biochem. J. *99:* 356–366.

Putnam, F. W. (1965). Structure and function of the plasma proteins. In *The Proteins*, 2nd ed., vol. III, Neurath, H., ed., Academic Press (New York, pp. 153–267), p. 234

Ropartz, C., and Rivat, L. (1969). Allotypy of human immunoglobulins and hypogammaglobulinemia. Behringwerk-Mitteil. *49:* 85–91.

Rutishauser, U., Cunningham, B. A., Bennett, C., Konigsberg, W. H., and Edelman, G. (1968). Amino acid sequence of the Fc region of a human γG-immunoglobulin. Proc. Natl. Acad. Sci. *61:* 1414–1421.

Rutishauser, U., Cunningham, B. A., Bennett, C., Konigsberg, W. H., and Edelman, G. M. (1970). The covalent structure of a human γG-immunoglobulin. VIII. Amino acid sequence of heavy-chain cyanogen bromide fragments H_5–H_7. Biochemistry *9:* 3171–3180.

Shimizu, A., Paul, C., Köhler, H., Shinoda, T., and Putnam, F. W. (1971). Variation and homology in the mu and gamma heavy chains of human immunoglobulins. Science *173:* 629–632.

Shuster, J., Wang, A.-C., and Fudenberg, H. H. (1970). Evolutionary dissociation of allotypes and other antigenic determinants of immunoglobulins in nonhuman primates. Immunochemistry *7:* 91–97.

Singer, S. J., and Doolittle, R. F. (1966). Antibody active sites and immunoglobulin molecules. Science *153:* 13–25.

Small, P. A., Jr., Reisfeld, R. A., and Dray, S. (1966). Peptide maps of rabbit γG-immunoglobulin heavy chains controlled by allelic genes. J. Mol. Biol. *16:* 328–333.

Smith, G. P., Hood, L., and Fitch, W. M. (1971). Antibody diversity. Annu. Rev. Biochem. *40:* 969–1012.

Smyth, D. S., and Utsumi, S. (1967). Structure at the hinge region in rabbit immunoglobulin G. Nature *216:* 332–335.

Suran, A. A., and Papermaster, B. W. (1967). N-terminal sequences of heavy and light chains of leopard shark immunoglobulins: evolutionary implications. Proc. Natl. Acad. Sci. *58:* 1619–1623.

Terry, W. D., Ogawa, M., and Kochwa, S. (1970). Structural studies of immunoglobulin E. II. Amino terminal sequence of the heavy chain. J. Immunol. *105:* 783–785.

Thorpe, N. O., and Deutsch, H. F. (1966). Studies on papain produced subunits of human γG-globulins. II. Structures of peptides related to the genetic Gm activity of γG-globulin Fc-fragments. Immunochemistry *3:* 329–337.

Todd, C. W. (1963). Allotypy in rabbit 19S protein. Biochem. Biophys. Res. Commun. *11:* 170–175.

Vaerman, J.-P., and Heremans, J. F. (1966). Subclasses of human immunoglobulin A based on differences in the α-polypeptide chains. Science *153:* 647–649.

van Loghem, E., Shuster, J., and Fudenberg, H. H. (1968). Gm factors in nonhuman primates. Vox Sang. *14:* 81–94.

Vyas, G. N., and Fudenberg, H. H. (1969). *Am (1)*, the first genetic marker of human immunoglobulin A. Proc. Natl. Acad. Sci. *64:* 1211–1216.

Wang, A.-C., and Fudenberg, H. H. (1969). Genetic control of α-chain synthesis: a chemical and evolutionary study of the Gm(a) factor of immunoglobulins. J. Mol. Biol. *44:* 493–500.

Wang, A.-C., Goodman, J. W., and Fudenberg, H. H. (1969). N-terminal residues of heavy chains of human IgA myeloma proteins. J. Immunol. *103:* 1149–1151.

Wang, A.-C., Pink, J. R. L., Fudenberg, H. H., and Ohms, J. (1970). A variable region subclass of heavy chains common to immunoglobulins G, A, and M and characterized by an unblocked amino-terminal residue. Proc. Natl. Acad. Sci. 66: 657–663.

Wang, A.-C., Wang, I. Y. F., McCormick, J. N., and Fudenberg, H. H. (1969). The identity of light chains of monoclonal IgG and monoclonal IgM in one patient. Immunochemistry 6: 451–459.

Wang, A.-C., Wilson, S. K., Hopper, J. E., Fudenberg, H. H., and Nisonoff, A. (1970). Evidence for control of synthesis of the variable regions of the heavy chains of immunoglobulins G and M by the same gene. Proc. Natl. Acad. Sci. 66: 337–343.

Waxdal, M. J., Konigsberg, W. H., and Edelman, G. M. (1968). The covalent structure of a human γG-immunoglobulin. III. Arrangement of the cyanogen bromide fragments. Biochemistry 7: 1967–1972.

Waxdal, M. J., Konigsberg, W. H., Henley, W. L., and Edelman, G. M. (1968). The covalent structure of a human γG-immunoglobulin. II. Isolation and characterization of the cyanogen bromide fragments. Biochemistry 7: 1959–1966.

Wikler, M., Köhler, H., Shinoda, T., and Putnam, F. W. (1969). Macroglobulin structure:homology of μ and γ-heavy chains of human immunoglobulins. Science 163: 75–78.

Wilkinson, J. M. (1967). The chemical structure of rabbit immunoglobulin. Ph.D. Thesis. University of London.

Wilkinson, J. M. (1969). Variation in the N-terminal sequence of heavy chains of immunoglobulin G from rabbits of different allotype. Biochem. J. 112: 173–185.

Wilkinson, J. M. (1970). Genetic markers of rabbit immunoglobulins. Biochem. J. 117: 3P–4P.

Wilkinson, J. M., Press, E. M., and Porter, R. R. (1966). The N-terminal sequence of the heavy chain of rabbit immunoglobulin IgG. Biochem. J. 100: 303–308.

Wu, T. T., and Kabat, E. A. (1970). An analysis of the sequences of the variable regions of Bence-Jones proteins and myeloma light chains and their implications for antibody complementarity. J. Exp. Med. 132: 211–250.

3

THE SIZES AND SHAPES OF
IMMUNOGLOBULINS

1. The early model of γ G

The frustrations in the Fifties of trying to determine the number of chains in an immunoglobulin molecule by N-terminal amino acid identification led to the alternative of trying to isolate the chains themselves by some method. There were some who were beginning to believe that an immunoglobulin must not be just one long polypeptide chain, compactly folded, but rather constructed in multichain fashion. Edelman (1959), hypothesizing that there were indeed chains held together by disulfide bonds but that unfolding of the protein molecule was necessary to expose them, subjected human IgG to the double treatment of unfolding in 6 M urea and reduction of disulfide linkages with mercaptoethanol. Fragments with an average molecular weight of 50,000 were obtained and Putnam's conclusion was thereby supported. In quick order a variety of human and animal immunoglobulins were treated with chemical cleavage reagents with similar results (Franek, 1961; Edelman and Poulik, 1961; Phelps, Neet, Lynn, and Putnam, 1961). The final result was the isolation of pairs of light and heavy polypeptide chains of which the light, as described above, had a community of properties in common with Bence-Jones proteins.

A problem to be resolved was the number of disulfide bridges connecting the various chains. After complete reductions of all S—S bonds in rabbit IgG, for example, a total of 44 sulfhydryl groups were found (Porter, 1959; Markus, Grossberg, and Pressman, 1962), which would make possible as many as $44!/22!\ 2^{22}$ or 5.6×10^{26} different disulfide linkages if these were random. For rabbit IgG, Palmer, Nisonoff, and Van Holde (1963) were able to cleave the molecule into only two subunits of equal size. Reduction was accomplished with 0.1 M 2-mercaptoethylamine and separation was maintained by lowering the pH to 2.5 in 0.1 M NaCl. The agreement between weight- and number-average molecular weights of the subunit preparation, its homogeneity in the ultracentrifuge, and a very low yield of light chains all strongly indicated that dissociation into half-molecules had been accomplished. Of even greater importance was the fact that when the reduced, acidified preparation was returned to neutral pH, and recombinations of the subunits through restoration of disulfide were thus accomplished, the recombination obviously did not take place randomly. The major product in the restored preparation had physicochemical characteristics of the untreated native protein. If recombination had been random there would not have been such remarkable renaturation. When an antihapten antibody was subjected to this treatment, it retained its specific combining capacity, again reinforcing the concept that half-molecule recombination into whole molecules involved a very specific type of disulfide bond.

Palmer and Nisonoff (1964) investigated this type of dissociation in greater detail and discovered that within the normal IgG of individual rabbits about one-half to two-thirds of the molecules could be split in half after the reduction of only one very labile disulfide bond. The remaining molecules could be split in half only by further reduction, an indication of heterogeneity in intrachain disulfide bridging. The amino acid content of the split products was identical to that of the whole protein and was also consistent with the concept that each half-molecule was composed of a light and heavy chain. Furthermore, the work substantiated a former concept that the single labile disulfide bond (as well as each of the less easily reduced multiple bridges in some of the molecules) was a link between two heavy chains.

Further resolution of the problem of disulfide bridging between the multiple chains of immunoglobulins is found in reports concerning the effect of reduction upon subunits obtained by limited enzymatic digestion rather than chemical processes. Historically, the treatment of immunoglobulins with proteolytic enzymes preceded treatment with reducing agents by a number of years. The results were highly varied and the reports conflicting (Marrack, 1938). Retention of antibody function was the only measurable quantity that was generally assayed; however, one important conclusion was drawn from the early work—that a relatively short and limited exposure to an enzyme such as pepsin could result in partial digestion without loss of antibody combining capacity. This idea was incorporated into Parfentjev's (1936) patented pepsin process for preparing a horse diphtheria antitoxin that would still be potent but would, by loss of certain protein parts, be less antigenic in humans in whom it was administered. Pope (1938, 1939a, b), who developed a similar process, incorporated not only short-term pepsin digestion but also selective heat denaturation of the cleaved products at an acid pH in the presence of ammonium sulfate. He observed that two types of protein were obtained, one nonantitoxic and easily heat-coagulable, the other antitoxic and heat-stable. By 1942 Northrop had obtained a crystalline *trypsin* derivative of diphtheria antitoxin with full toxin combining power.

Porter (1950) obtained a fragment of rabbit antibody against egg albumin by papain digestion which, although it had lost precipitating activity, would bind with egg albumin and block precipitation of the albumin by whole antibody. The fragment had an average molecular weight of 40,000. With the advent of crystalline papain and the improvement in fractionation procedures Porter returned to this system in 1958 and found that he could now control the splitting process, separate the fragments, and analyze the products (Porter, 1958, 1959).

He prepared rabbit γG from several different antisera, digested the proteins with papain (using cysteine as an enzyme activator), and separated the fragments via carboxymethyl (CM)-cellulose ion-exchange chromatography. The profile of the effluent from the ion-exchange column revealed three sharp peaks which were designated I, II, and III in order of their appearance. Immunological reactivity was confined to I and II as shown by inhibition of precipitation of antigens. Dialysis of the fragments against distilled water at 2°C resulted in a crystalline precipitate of fraction III. Molecular weight studies showed that fragment I was about 50,000; II, 53,000; III, 80,000; and the intact γG, 188,000.

Confirmation of this significant work came quickly (Nisonoff and Woernley, 1959) followed, shortly thereafter, by an explanation of mode of action (Nisonoff, Wissler, Lipman, and Woernley, 1960). In Porter's (1950) hands only papain had the property of yielding split products with retention of precipitin-blocking activity. Nisonoff, noting that cysteine was generally used in conjuction with papain as activator, turned to the action of pepsin upon antibody and found that he could produce a 5S bivalent antibody fragment, and that the 5S fragment would in turn split into two univalent 3.5S fragments upon the application of cysteine. The 5S fragment, although reduced in molecular weight from the natural state to 100,000, retained its capacity to precipitate antigen (which, as will be shown later, depends on two combining sites). The 3.5S fragments, like those of Porter's fractions I and II, would block but not precipitate, and represented fragments with single combining sites. The univalent fragments would also recombine to give a bivalent product (Nisonoff, Wissler, and Lipman, 1960).

It was clear from a study of this work and that of Palmer and Nisonoff (1964) cited above that the single labile disulfide bond that joined the two halves of rabbit γG was also the bond that joined the two univalent fragments. Since reductions alone (and subsequent dissociation in acid) resulted in two symmetrical fragments that were univalent with respect to antibody activity whereas enzyme cleavage alone resulted in two asymmetrical fragments, one of which retained full bivalency, and since, further, the bivalent fragment could be symmetrically cleaved into two small univalent fragments, a structural model could be constructed in which the plane of symmetry of chemical cleavage was sectioned by a plane of asymmetrical enzyme cleavage.

Although at first it was felt that fragments I and II were not antigenic and that fragment III carried the antigenic determinants that made possible the immunization of one species with γG from another, Putnam, Tan, Lynn, Easley, and Migita (1962) showed that each fragment carried partial determinants of the whole. Fleischman, Porter, and Press (1963) finally discovered the actual relationship between the enzyme fragments (I and II) and the light chains of γG found originally by Edelman. This required obtaining light chains that would be soluble in aqueous solution rather than those obtained in urea, which were insoluble when urea was removed. By reducing γG in urea-free solutions and separating the resultant chains on Sephadex-75 in the presence of weak acids (1 N acetic or propionic), Fleischman et al., (1963) obtained in nearly 100% yield two fractions representing light and heavy chains. This same system, when applied to fragments I and II, gave rise to intact light chains and only a fragment of heavy chain material. The linkage of the light chain to the heavy chain was shown to be that of a single disulfide bond.

From these data a preliminary chain model of IgG structure was constructed by Fleischman et al. (1963) and modified by Nisonoff and Thorbecke (1964). The early model (Fig. 3-1) shows two heavy chains joined by one labile disulfide bond and further bound by noncovalent forces as well as, in some instances, by additional S—S bonds. The labile S—S bond lies to one side of the plane of enzymatic cleavage whereas the other bonds lie on the other. Bound to each heavy chain by a single S—S bond is a light chain whose point of attachment is somewhere near the S—S bond joining the two heavy chains and on the same side of the plane of enzymatic cleavage.

The initial findings of the two fragments, I and II, in Porter's

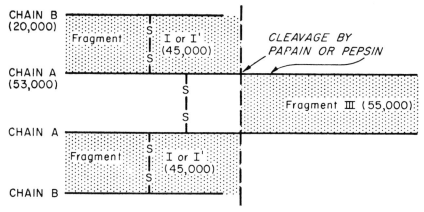

FIG. 3-1. Early model of multichain structure of rabbit IgG. (From Nisonoff and Thorbecke, 1964.)

papain digest could have been interpreted two ways: either I and II appeared in the same naturally occurring molecule or they came from separate molecules as pairs of one or the other. The work of Amiraian and Leikhim (1961), which was confirmed by Palmer, Mandy, and Nisonoff (1962), indicated that the latter was true and that I and II resulted from heterogeneous populations of globulin molecules.

With regard to N-terminal amino acids, alanine and aspartic acid in rabbit γG were found associated with the light chains (Fleischman et al., 1963). The carbohydrate moiety, on the other hand, was found joined to the heavy chains and principally in fragment III.

2. Current model of γG—disulfide bonds

With the knowledge gained from amino acid sequencing the positions of cysteine residues in the light and heavy chains became clear and, ultimately, the positions of the particular cysteine pairs involved in interchain disulfide bridging (Frangione, Milstein, and Pink, 1969). The conservative cysteine in the ultimate C-terminal position of κ-light chains and in the penultimate C-terminal position of λ-light chains was found to bridge almost universally with heavy chains, but the position of the particular heavy chain cysteines, with which the light chain cysteine would pair was found to vary widely. In human γG1 proteins such as *Daw* and *Eu* the L-H bridge occurs at position 220 (Eu numbering) just in advance of the hinge peptide connecting Fd and Fc (Fig. 3-2a). In rabbit γG (O'Donnell, Frangione, and Porter, 1970), with its intrachain doubly bridged loop peptide involved in the structure of $C\gamma2$, the L-H bridge occurs at position 131 (Eu numbering). As one can see in Figure 3-2b the L-H bridge in

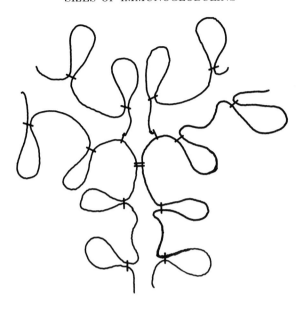

YG1

(a)

FIG. 3-2. Immunoglobulin models (pp. 77–82): (a) human γG1, (b) rabbit γG, (c) human γG2, (d) human γG3, (e) human γG4, (f) human γA2 and BALB/c mouse γA. Inter- and intrachain disulfide bond arrangements (—) are emphasized.

rabbit γG approaches the hinge peptide since the doubly bridged loop structure brings position 131 to within only two residues' distance from position 221. The L-H arrangement in human γG2, γG3, and γG4 is actually more like rabbit γG than human γG1 (Fig. 3-2c–e). The L-H bridge occurs before the Cγ2 loop structure rather than after.

In six out of six mouse myeloma γA proteins light chains were not covalently bound to heavy chains by disulfide bonds (Abel and Grey, 1968); instead, the two light chains formed L-L dimers in much the same fashion as urinary Bence-Jones proteins. In spite of this lack of covalent bridging the traditional light-heavy arrangement necessary for binding was preserved (Grey, Sher, and Shalitin, 1970). This latter group also found that normal γA from BALB/c strain mice uniformly lacked the L-H bridge and learned from N. Warner that NZB strain mice routinely preserved the bond. In the human Grey, Abel, Yount, and Kunkel (1968) discovered that the isotypic γA2 subclass also lacked interchain L-H disulfide bridges and related this property to a genetic variant. Structural studies have yet to

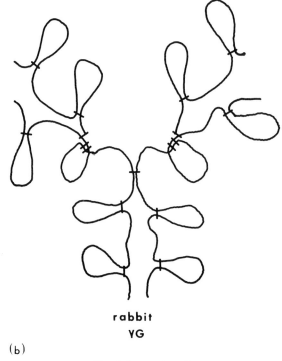

rabbit
γG

(b)

Fig. 3-2—*continued*

determine whether the absence of L-H bridges is due to a missing cysteine in the heavy chain or to one involved in doubly bridged loop structures, but suspicions favor the former since partial reduction releases only five SH groups per mole of γA2-heavy chain vs. seven per mole of γA1 (Jerry, Kunkel, and Grey, 1970). A schematic structure of the γA2 variant of light-heavy chain arrangements is shown in Figure 3-2*f*.

Grey (1969) asked the question whether the maintenance of overall structure in γA2 without the aid of L-H bond formation could be reproduced in other immunoglobulins. He prepared γG-light chains that were reduced but *not* alkylated, thus preventing L-H bond formation but allowing L-L dimerization. When he reconstituted the mixture he found that a protein with all the characteristics of whole γG was formed but with 65% of the light chains in the form of dimers. It was thus clear that H-L bond formation was not absolutely necessary for tertiary structure although it was energetically favored over L-L bonds.

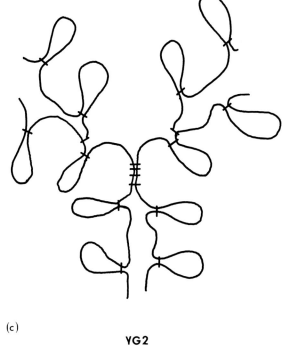

(c)

γG2

Fig. 3-2—*continued*

Heterogeneity exists not only in L-H bond positioning but also in the number and position of the interchain H-H bonds. In pooled rabbit γG, as mentioned above, Palmer and Nisonoff (1964) learned that as much as one-half to two-thirds could be halved by reduction of only a single labile disulfide bridge. Later sequences showed that this bond formed between heavy chains at position 226 (Eu numbering) of the γ-chain immediately after the A11-A12 allotypic residue, and also explained why cyanogen bromide cleavage of the A11 methionine residue caused the formation of 2 Fab fragments (cf. Chapter 2). This H-H bond seems to be most conservative one in multichain construction, and, together with a second H-H bond at position 229 (Eu numbering), forms a double H-H bridge in human γG1 and γG4. In γG2 and γG3 a third H-H bridge forms at position 220 (Eu numbering) since the L-H bridge is moved back, a fourth appears in γG2 a few residues earlier still, and a fourth and fifth are likely to exist in γG3 at undesignated positions in the C-terminal portion of C_H2 (Milstein, 1969).

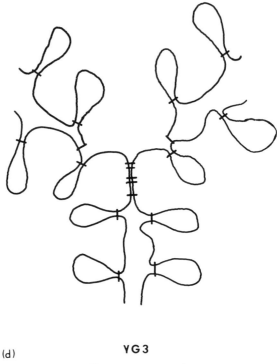

(d)   **YG3**

Fig. 3-2—*continued*

3. Bioassembly of immunoglobulins

By whatever mechanism the VC gene complex operates to produce heavy and light chains, the biosynthesis of each type of chain occurs in separate ribosomes, 200S for light and 300S for heavy (Askonas and Williamson, 1966) and involves synthesis from a single growing point (Fleischman, 1967a, b). The chain can also be synthesized by isolated polyribosomes in a cell-free system (Nezlin and Rokhlin, 1969; Mach, Koblet, and Gros, 1967; and Ralph, Becker, and Rich, 1967). There are three patterns of assembly (Zolla, Buxbaum, Franklin, and Scharff, 1970): unbalanced with the production of light chains only; unbalanced with the production of intact 4-chain immunoglobulin and excess light chains; and balanced with the production of heavy and light chains in equimolar concentrations. Through pulse-chase studies of a γG myeloma protein it has been established that the final assembly is through interaction of half-molecule intermediates. By capitalizing upon four different transplantable mouse myelomas that had lost ability to produce immunoglobulins (Schubert and

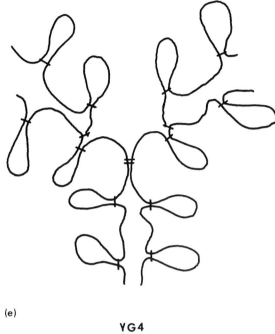

(e)

YG4

Fig. 3-2—*continued*

Horibata, 1968), and building upon the model of Shapiro, Scharff, Maizel, and Uhr (1966), Schubert and Cohn (1968) were able to reconstruct some normal cellular events and some that might lead to blocks in defective synthesis:*

(a) Heavy and light chains are made on separate classes of polysomes, but

(b) light chains are released from polysomes at twice the rate of heavy chains and enter a cellular pool of light chain monomers.

(c) The light chains complement with nascent heavy chains to form HL intermediates on the heavy chain polysomes and the excess uncomplemented light chains are ordinarily destroyed rather than secreted.

(d) As the HL intermediates dimerize either on the H polysome or immediately thereafter,

(e) the $(HL)_2$-bearing polysomes become fixed in the endoplasmic reticulum, triggered by a signal from light chain deter-

* See also: Askonas and Williamson (1967a, b); Kern and Swenson (1967); Scharff, Shapiro, and Ginsburg (1967); and Fahey and Finegold (1967).

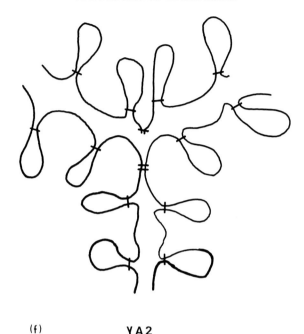

(f)   **Y A 2**

FIG. 3-2—*continued*

minants and held by a special transport protein.

(f) The immunoglublin is then transported through the ER to the cisternal space by a specialized step that uniquely accounts for immunoglobulin secretion.

(g) Carbohydrate is added in the cisternal space by means of membrane-bound enzymes, and

(h) the assembled immunoglobulin is passed to the outside of the cell.

In the mutant myelomas some failed to form HL intermediates even though biosynthesis was normal; in one there was blockage in the first step.

The suggestion in step (c) that excess light chains are destroyed rather than secreted certainly does not always apply, as Matsuoka, Yagi, Moore, and Pressman (1969a) demonstrated with an established cell line of human myeloma cell origin. The cultured cells secreted λ-chains into the culture medium, but no heavy chains. Likewise, the suggestion in step (c) that assembly begins between a complete light chain and a nascent heavy chain does not hold in the case of rabbit lymph node cells (Moav and Harris, 1970a). Assembly of rabbit IgG does not begin until both chains are complete. Differences in mode of assembly were noted by Sutherland, Zimmerman, and Kern (1970) who compared the intermediates formed in cultures of rabbit lymph node cells with those of a mouse myeloma. In rabbit cells LHHL and HL were formed but not HHL or HH; in the mouse cells LHHL, HHL, HH, and L were obtained but no HL! Thus, in the one case the first disulfide bond to form was between heavy and light chains as suggested in step (c), while in the other the first inter-chain disulfide bond was made between two heavy chains in complete violation of the Schubert-Cohn dogma. And in rabbit lymph node cells Moav and Harris (1970b) observed H-H bonds forming before L-H bonds. The HH dimer and the HHL intermediate which had been found earlier by Askonas and Williamson (1967a, b) and which had puzzled various investigators (Baglioni, 1969) were therefore explained.

4. Defective bioassembly and heavy chain disease

Heavy chain disease was discovered in 1964 in the human (Franklin, Lowenstein, Bigelow, and Meltzer, 1964; Osserman and Takatsuki, 1964; Franklin, 1964). In the same year a similar condition was reported in the newborn normal piglet (Franek and Riha, 1964). Almost from the moment that the condition was observed it was recognized that the heavy chains involved were abnormal and defective. In every case, however, the disease was characterized by the appearance of polypeptide chains containing heavy chain determinants with no light chains attached (Buxbaum, Franklin, and Scharff, 1970). Franklin's first extensive report on protein Cr described a disulfide-linked dimer somewhat larger than Fc. The best characterized heavy chain disease proteins are Zuc as reported by Milstein and Frangione (1969) and Hi by Terry and Ohms (1970). Sequences and structural alignments with other heavy chains are available. Zuc heavy chain belongs to the isotypic subclass of γG3-globulins and contains an N-terminal portion of 18 amino acids that belongs to variable region subgroup V_{HI}; however, it contains an internal deletion of 200 residues, including the first two loop peptides; the attachment site for light chains; and two of the five H-H disulfide linkages. The result is a dimer with three disulfide bonds consisting of Fc, hinge peptide, and N-terminal octadecapeptide. The comparison with intact γG3 is shown in Figure 3-3. The protein Hi contains 34 residues of the N-terminal subgroup V_{HIV}, suffers an internal deletion of about 100 residues (including the V_H loop) and begins the sequences of the constant region just a few residues removed from the beginning of the C_H1 loop peptide. According to Woods, Blumenschein, and Terry (1970)

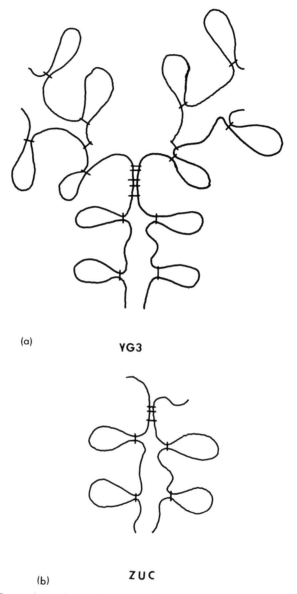

(a)   **ɣG3**

(b)   **ZUC**

Fɪɢ. 3-3. Comparison of normal human ɣG3 (a) and protein Zuc (b). Zuc has suffered an internal deletion of 200 residues including the first two loop peptides, the
attachment site for light chains, and two of the five H-H disulfide linkages. The N-
terminal portion of 18 amino acids is intact (subclass V_{HI}) and the C_H3-C_H4 portion
(isotype ɣG3) is also complete.

the chains in the dimers of *Hi* are noncovalently linked and contain the allotypic specificity Gm(8). The protein therefore belongs either to isotypic subclass γG1 or γG2. One would imagine that γG1 with its fewer number of interchain disulfide bridges to account for might be the more likely, but even there cysteines 22 and 200 would be free and would have to be accounted for along with cysteines 226 and 229 in intrachain disulfide bridging. Regardless of the final mechanism to account for heavy chain disease the fact remains that the Schubert-Cohn dogma for chain assembly has once again been violated. As Ein and Waldmann (1969) pointed out heavy chain disease must arise from excessive synthesis rather than defective catabolism.

Terry and Ohms (1970), in assessing the effect of their findings upon genetic mechanisms for immunoglobulin chain coding, have noted that in the original translocation hypothesis the physical joining of variable region information to the common region could have been proposed equally well for deoxyribonucleic acid (DNA) or for messenger ribonucleic acid (RNA). The hypothesis did not distinguish between these forms because three pathways were open:

(a) V-region DNA could translocate and integrate permanently into C-region DNA to give a stable V-C gene.

(b) V-region DNA could translocate and integrate temporarily into C-region DNA, then, after transcription, dissociate and translocate again at the time of the next transcription.

(c) V-region messenger RNA could translocate and integrate into C-region *m*-RNA with integrated RNA carrying out the actual translation, a process repeated with each transcription.

Terry and Ohms realized that whichever translocation process was utilized, recognition sites must be present in the nucleotide sequences to permit accurate joining of the V-C regional information. Their analysis of the shortened, internally deleted heavy chains in heavy chain disease suggested to them that DNA rather than RNA would have to be involved in translocation and that the integration would have to be considered permanent. It would be much more likely that translocation occurs before deletion since this would require only a single translocation event in cell differentiation. Their conclusion: V-region DNA is translocated to C-region DNA and permanently integrated to form a V-C gene. In heavy chain disease the synthesizing cells encounter a subsequent genetic event leading to a larger internal deletion.

5. Defects in light chain synthesis

Through the years a variety of reports accumulated concerning the secretion of light chain components smaller in size than the usual V-C monomer. A few were characterized and found to correspond to V-region portions (Solomon, Killander, Grey, and Kunkel, 1966; Baglioni et al., 1967). A case in point was a 1.2S urinary component that was homologous to the V-region of a Bence-Jones protein with which it was mixed (Van Eyk and Myszkowska, 1967). Karlsson, Peterson, and Berggard (1969) questioned whether these light chain fragments were formed de novo or were degraded from intact light chains. By carrying out limited proteolysis of light chains they were able to establish, at least, that there were limited regions between the V and C regions that were particularly susceptible to proteolysis and that the finding of V-region peptides in urine might be attributed to degradation. On the other hand, observations of light chain secretions by established cell lines have shown that V-region-like peptides can be produced de novo (Matsuoka, Yagi, Moore, and Pressman, 1969b). Evidence for internal deletions has not been forthcoming in the case of light chains so that a choice between the two possibilities posed by Karlsson et al. cannot be immediately made.

6. Carbohydrate moieties of immunoglobulins and their rôle in secretion

The Schubert-Cohn studies on nonsecreting myeloma cells provided an explanation for some of the more unusual myelomas that had been observed from time to time—typical flaming plasma cells but no secretions (Forssman and Nilsson, 1967); clinical symptoms without secretory aspects (DiGuglielmo, 1966); and an extensive monoclonal cellular myeloma without serum or urinary symptoms (Hurez, Preud'Homme, and Seligmann, 1970). Carbohydrate must be added or no secretion would be forthcoming from the cells.

Whatever the reason for defective secretion it was already fairly well established by 1967 that carbohydrate was a prerequisite for transport of protein out of cells and secretion into the milieu (Melchers and Knopf, 1967). Thus, inability to add carbohydrate could in itself prevent secretion. Nearly all plasma proteins, including the albumins and globulins, had long been known to contain residues of carbohydrate, so much so that Schultze (1962) had reclassified them according to their relative carbohydrate content and their solubility in 0.6 M perchloric acid. The categories of carbohydrate in human immunoglobulins per se had been used to distinguish between the three major classes, γG, γA, and γM (Table 3-1) in spite of the known heterogeneity within each class.

With the advent of sequencing came the opportunity to examine

TABLE 3-1

Carbohydrate in Human Immunoglobulins

Carbohydrate	IgG	IgA	IgM
	%	%	%
Hexose	1.2	4.8	6.2
Fucose	0.3	0.2	0.7
Hexosamine	1.1	3.8	3.3
Sialic acid	0.2	1.7	2.0
Total	2.8	10.5	12.2

(From Cohen and Porter, 1964, Table V. See reference for additional data and sources.)

the mode of carbohydrate attachment and its biosynthesis. One of the myths to be exploded early was the belief that only the heavy chains contained carbohydrate residues. Melchers and Knopf (1967), for example, showed that cells from the mouse plasmacytoma MOPC 46 produced a light chain with carbohydrate attached at an asparaginyl residue, and Melchers (1969a) established the exact point as position 28. In terms of weight the CHO represented 12% of the entire light chain glycopeptide. As reported by Dayhoff (1969), Melchers (1969b) also found analogous sites in mouse heavy chains.

Although the Schubert-Cohn scheme (1968) relegated carbohydrate assembly to the responsibility of membrane-bound enzymes in the cisternal space, the experiments of Moroz and Uhr (1967), among others, presented a more complex picture. Glucosamine incorporation required polyribosomal guidance whereas mannose and galactose became attached after completion and release of polypeptide chains from the polyribosomes. Melchers (1969c) observed that among the subcellular particles of cells from MOPC 46, the rough endoplasmic reticulum membranes engineered glucosamine incorporation primarily while smooth ER and cytoplasmic supernatant could also bring about mannose and galactose attachments to light chains. Thus, the carbohydrate moiety was thought to build up in stepwise fashion as the immunoglobulin moved from rough to smooth ER and then into the cytoplasm. By so doing it was envisioned as effecting the transport and secretion of the immunoglobulins through and out of the plasma cells.

Sox and Hood (1970) reported that whereas oligosaccharides find attachment in only 15% of the light chains from known myelomas, they are covalently bound to the constant region of all known heavy chains. A catalog of the sequences involved revealed that the common denominator often was an aparaginyl residue once removed from a serine-threonine residue couple and that those light chains that contained the triplet also had CHO attached. An enzyme to catalyze such a reaction would be an N-acetylglucosamine-asparagine trans-glycosylase. This was not the first time that such an observation nor the idea of transferases was advanced. In the human heavy chain *Eu*, for example, polysaccharide is attached at aspargine 297, which in-volves the sequence,

$$-Q-Q-Y-\underset{|}{\overset{297}{N}}-S-T-Y$$
$$CHO$$

Edelman (1970) in commenting upon this finding, also made note of the unique sequential arrangement in *Eu* as well as in other glyco-proteins.

In the experiments which Melchers (1969c) conducted on sub-cellular particulate activity, fucose incorporation could not be de-tected at any point, but in a cell-freee system of lymph node cells D'Amico and Kern (1970) did observe sialic acid incorporation. The usual carbohydrate is about 14 residues long, but the demands of heterogeneity make it impossible to pinpoint specific structures at this time. Even the heavy chain disease protein, *Zuc*, contained a carbohydrate—interestingly enough at the point where the internal deletion occurred. One would presume that any internal genetic deletions that left out CHO attachment points would result in es-sence in nonsecreting cells.

7. Systematic cleavage of immunoglobulins in the laboratory

Although the degradation of immunoglobulins is not considered to be as important a process for production of natural fragments as is defective or excessive biosynthesis, yet from the point of view of laboratory investigators the artificial techniques are most valuable. We have already learned how effective reductive and enzymatic proc-esses were in the initial unfolding of the immunoglobulin story. They have applied so universally to the complete phylogenetic and iso-typic varieties of immunoglobulins that the very classification of the proteins has developed in accordance with the fragments they pro-duce. A review of fragment nomenclature, therefore, seems appro-priate, at this juncture.

The 7S 4-chain immunoglobulin that forms most rabbit γG can be cleaved through the hinge region with papain to produce two 3.5S fragments, *Fab*, and one 3.5S fragment, *Fc*. Fab contains one light chain and an approximate N-terminal half of one heavy chain, *Fd*, joined by a disulfide bridge. The papain cleavage point is on the N-terminal side of the interchain disulfide bridges of this immunoglobulin; thus the 7S protein easily falls into the three parts. Note, however, that some differences do exist even between soluble papain cleavage and that by insoluble papain.

Pepsin cleaves on the C-terminal side of the interchain disulfide bridges and forms the 5S (Fab')$_2$ fragment plus a number of oligopeptides of Fc origin. Reduction of the 5S fragment forms two Fab' fragments with slightly longer Fd chains.

Mild reduction and aminoethylation followed by trypsin produces two 3.5S (Fab)$_t$ fragments and (Fc)$_t$ all of which are similar in size to papain-produced fragments.

Cyanogen bromide cleavage in weak acid gives rise to a 5S (Fab'')$_2$ fragment, the methionine at position 252 (Eu numbering) being affected, and reductive cleavage forms two 3.5S Fab'' fragments somewhat larger in heavy chain than either Fab or Fab'. Further reduction produces light chains and a very stable form of Fd which laboratories find more useful than the enzymatically derived products. Utsumi and Karush (1967) in summing up the order of size of the H-chain in Fab subunits in cleaved rabbit γG gave the following order:

CNBr > pepsin > water-insoluble papain > soluble papain

In their study of a new serum factor in rabbits that reacted with buried determinants of rabbit γG, Richie, Woolsey, and Mandy (1970) proceeded stepwise along the entire hinge region cleaving first with CNBr at the C-terminus of Fab'', then with pepsin at the C-terminus of Fab', and then with papain at the C-terminus of Fab, exposing all the while additional determinants normally covered by polypeptide folding. Watanabe and Kitagawa (1970) also were able to distinguish the subtle difference between (Fab)$_t$ and Fab and their difference from Fab' and Fab '' through the use of another naturally occurring rabbit serum homoreactant.

What happens when papain fragments are made of an immunoglobulin that is known to have polypeptide chains shorter than those of typical γG? Such a protein was *Sac* (Connell, Dorrington, Lewis, and Parr, 1970), which was not the usual heavy-chain disease protein since it had intact light chains, but which was definitely smaller than normal. Papain digestion produced a very normal Fc fragment, but cysteine reduction produced an Fab with only half the usual molecular weight and with an atypical optical rotatory dispersion spectrum.

Globulins vary widely in their susceptibility to cleavage. For example, papain sensitivity among 50 γG myeloma proteins was measured by Gergely, Fudenberg, and van Loghem (1970) with the finding that 3/14 γG1, 4/4 γG2, and 3/3 γG3 proteins were very sensitive. Jefferis, Weston, Stanworth, and Clamp (1968) had previously found the same distinction between papain-resistant γG2 and γG4 vs. papain-sensitive γG1 and γG3. They did not find any correlation with carbohydrate content as had previously been supposed.

The papain-resistant class of human γG can be rendered susceptible by cysteine (Gergely, Stanworth, Jefferis, Normansell, Henney, and Pardoe, 1967), but the mechanism appears to be an elusive one. However, in the case of rabbit γG, which requires a two-stage process of cleavage by soluble papain and reducing agents, Zappacosta, Nisonoff, and Mandy (1968) found an answer: After gel filtration to separate the globulin from papain and the addition of iodacetamide to inactivate any enzyme traces, the subsequent addition of cysteine caused cleavage seemingly in the absence of papain; however, it was found that soluble papain adheres to γG in appreciable quantity during gel filtration and that the adsorbed enzyme is resistant to inactivation. The action of the cysteine at the second step was, therefore, to activate the adsorbed enzyme, not to split some S—S bridge that was ostensibly holding Fc and (Fab)$_2$ together.

Not only Fab but also Fc differences have been noted by the different methods of cleavage at the hinge region. Utsumi (1969) in carrying out stepwise cleavage of rabbit γG by papain was able to isolate four types of Fc fragment. Since the days when Porter first obtained crystals from the constant half after papain cleavage (hence the abbreviation Fc for crystalline fragment) it was observed that most of the forces binding the C-terminal halves of the two heavy chain portions together were noncovalent, but in one of these four Utsumi obtained a portion of the hinge region including a disulfide bridge. Three kinds of Fc crystals were obtained (Fig. 3-4). In the case of chicken γG, Kubo and Benedict (1969) found that one type of Fc crystal formed at 37°C, another type at 4°C (Fig. 3-5).

8. Molecular weight of γG and "7S" subunits

It was the practice well into the Sixties to accept a molecular weight of 160,000 for γG and for the 7S subunit of γA and γM. This is reflected in Table 3-2 which lists some of the physicochemical properties of the three major classes of immunoglobulins as given in Putnam's review of 1965. The values were only suggestive and were expected to vary operationally from one preparation to the next. Another prac-

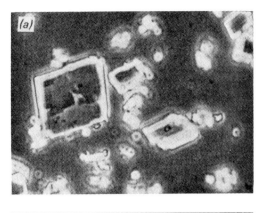

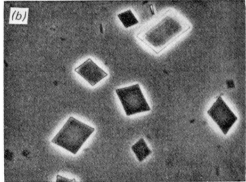

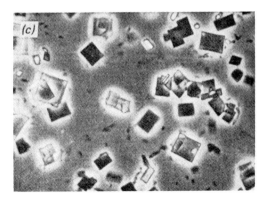

FIG. 3-4. Three kinds of Fc crystals obtained by stepwise papain cleavage of rabbit γG. (From Utsumi, 1969.)

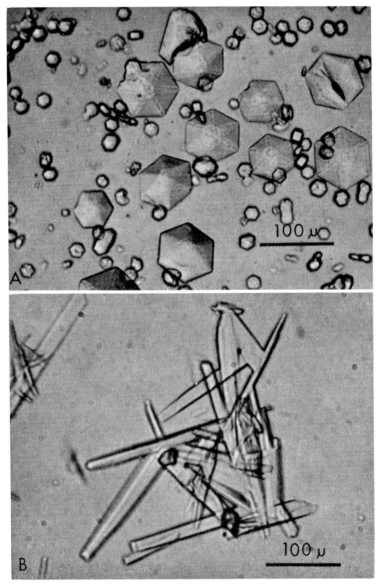

FIG. 3-5. Crystals of chicken Fc. (*A*) Crystals formed at 37°C (× 200); (*B*) crystals formed at 4°C (× 200). (From Kubo and Benedict, 1969.)

tice was to accept a molecular weight of 20,000 for light chains and 50,000 for heavy chains, the 7S 4-chain subunit then becoming 140,000. This was in keeping with the values of 22–23,000 and 53,000, that Small and Lamm (1966) had obtained for light and heavy chains, respectively. Allowing another 10,000 for CHO and H_2O the accepted molecular weight became revised to 150,000, a current oft-quoted value. It was felt that even if an individual preparation were analyzed with extreme precision [such as the 137,000 given for the molecular weight of rabbit γG by Cammack (1962)], slightly different values might result for exacting analyses of other individual preparations, and that all would be well within the established limits of heterogeneity. Thus, 5 years later (Metzger, 1970), one finds a revised listing (Table 3-3).

Perhaps the most searching study of the molecular weight of rabbit antibody has been that of Mamet-Bratley (1970) who obtained a value of 135,000 ± 5,000 for the γG 6.55S monomer, a molecular weight very close to that previously quoted from Cammack (1962). The study was made in accordance with the recommendations of Schachman (1963) and Steinberg and Schachman (1966), and involved the use of Rayleigh optics under sedimentation equilibrium

TABLE 3-2
Physicochemical Properties of Human Immunoglobulin

Properties	IgG	IgA	IgM
f/f_0	1.38	1.38	1.73
Molecular weight	160,000	$(160,000)_{1,2,4}$	$(160,000)_{6,8,\ldots}$
s_{20}^0	6.6	6.6, 10, 13	19, 26, 32, …
s_{20} in mercaptoethanol	6.6	6.6	6.6
μ, pH 8.6, $\Gamma/2 = 0.1$	1.1*	1.2–3.6	0.5–2.3
pI	6.2–8.5	4.8–6.5	5.5–7.4
In normal serum (gm%)	1.2	0.1–0.4	0.1

* Average value.
(From Putnam, 1965, p. 231. See reference for additional data and original sources.)

TABLE 3-3 ·
Approximate Molecular Weight of Immunoglobulins

Heavy Chains		Light Chains		Whole Molecule			
Class	Mol. wt.	Class	Mol wt.	Formula	%CHO	$S_{20\ w}^0$	Mol. wt.
γ	5.3×10^4	κ	2.2–2.3×10^4	$\kappa_2\gamma_2$	2.9	6.7	$\sim 1.5 \times 10^5$
α	$\sim 6 \times 10^4$	λ	2.2–2.3×10^4	$(\kappa_2\alpha_2)_1$	7.5	7	1.6×10^5
μ	6–7×10^4			$(\kappa_2\mu_2)_5$	7.7–10.7	18–20	9–10×10^5
δ	$\sim 6 \times 10^4$			$\kappa_2\delta_2$	12	6.6	1.7–1.8×10^5
ϵ	$\sim 7.5 \times 10^4$			$\kappa_2\epsilon_2$	10.7	7.9	$\sim 2 \times 10^5$

(From Metzger, 1970. See reference for additional data and original sources.)

conditions. Care was taken to account for any possible association since rabbit antibody exhibited a weak tendency to dimerize at pH 7.4 and 20°C. Typical results in abbreviated form are shown in Table 3-4 where it can be seen that rabbit γG dimers contribute significantly to and account for the usual accepted values of 150–160,000 that had in the past been accepted for the average molecular weight of 7S γG.

To investigate the individuality in molecular weights among immunoglobulins perhaps the best way is to compare individual homogeneous myeloma proteins. Hansson, Laurell, and Bachmann (1966) obtained sedimentation coefficients—one parameter of molecular weight—for 7 γG and 3 γD myeloma proteins, and compared them with 11 individual samples of so-called normal γG, obviously a heterogeneous mixture (Table 3-5). Recognizing that such values do not take into account the problem of association one can still observe the range of individual values that may be expected.

TABLE 3-4

Molecular Weight of Rabbit γG Antibody as Function of Protein Concentration at Sedimentation Equilibrium

At the Meniscus (Monomer)		At the Bottom (Dimer Present)		Overall	
Concentration (fringes)*	Mol. wt. (wt. av.)	Concentration (fringes)	Mol. wt. (wt. av.)	Concentration (fringes)	Mol. wt. (wt. av.)
6.06	129,000	20.11	170,000	13.10	147,000
9.70	132,000	28.68	174,000	19.51	150,000
15.68	139,000	41.05	181,000	28.45	156,000
22.56	145,000	51.22	186,000	37.14	166,000

* In these experiments 10.0 mg/ml were equivalent to 42.0 fringes.
(From Mamet-Bratley, 1970.)

TABLE 3-5

Sedimentation Constants of Individual Immunoglobulins

Normal Globulins	Myeloma Globulins
γG 7.04 ± 0.8	γG 6.81 ± 0.4
γG 6.91 ± 0.6	γG 6.77 ± 0.6
γG 6.88 ± 1.0	γG 6.46 ± 0.6
γG 6.89 ± 0.6	γG 6.91 ± 0.4
γG 6.90 ± 0.5	γG 6.72 ± 0.4
γG 6.79 ± 0.5	γG 6.82 ± 0.5
γG 6.78 ± 0.3	γG 6.78 ± 1.0
γG 6.77 ± 0.7	
γG 6.76 ± 0.6	γD 6.76 ± 0.8
γG 6.81 ± 0.6	γD 6.19 ± 1.0
γG 6.83 ± 0.7	γD 6.54 ± 0.9

(From Hansson, Laurell, and Bachmann, 1966.)

Among the subclasses of human γA-globulins there is a distinct molecular weight difference (Dorrington and Rockey, 1970) in the heavy chains (Table 3-6) which makes a difference of about 8,000 in every 7S subunit.* For the rabbit α-chain, meanwhile we have a value of 64,000 ± 3,000 (Cebra and Small, 1967).

The molecular size of the heavy μ-chain varies widely also. Lamm and Small (1966) had obtained 70,000 for rabbit μ-chain; Suzuki and Deutsch (1967), 66,000 for human μ-chain; Habeeb, Schrohenloher, and Bennett (1970), 75,000 for human μ-chain. Filitti-Wurmser, Tempete-Gaillourdet, and Hartmann (1970) in a study of heavy chains from three monoclonal γM myeloma immunoglobulins obtained three different values for the three chains—49,000, 59,000, and 72,000—while obtaining a single value of 23,000 for the κ-light chains from all three. One cannot safely estimate a molecular weight of an assembled subunit since the chain makeup does not always follow the rule of the H_2L_2 formula. Suzuki and Deutsch (1967) obtained 8S subunits of 200,000 molecular weight with a formula perhaps of H_2L_3 as well as a 7S subunit of 160,000 molecular weight with a formula perhaps of H_2L. Filitti-Wurmser *et al.* (1970) obtained one subunit with a formula H_2L_4 and a molecular weight of 190,000. Its heavy chain had the 49,000 molecular weight. Another subunit did have a formula of H_2L_2, a molecular weight of 164,000, and a heavy chain of 59,000 molecular weight. Two subunits were obtained from the 72,000 molecular weight μ-chain: pure heavy chain dimer, H_2, with a molecular weight of 144,000 and H_2L_4 with a molecular weight of 235,000. Lamm and Small (1966) did obtain an H_2L_2 subunit from

TABLE 3-6
Molecular Sizes of γA1 and γA2 Globulins

Immunoglobulin Subunit	Molecular Weight (wt. av.)	
	γA1	γA2
H chain monomer	56,300	52,000
L chain monomer	22,700	22,800
H chain dimer	—	104,600
L chain dimer	—	45,400
L_2H_2 subunit*	158,000	150,000

* Calculated.
(Data from Dorrington and Rockey, 1970.)

---

* A difference of about 36 residues per heavy chain was estimated by the authors, and attributed by them to a deletion in α_2-chains. One could just as easily attribute the difference to an insertion in the α_1-chain.

rabbit γM, however, with a molecular weight of approximately 180,000.

Studies on human γD (Rowe, Dolder, and Welscher, 1969) gave rise to two close values: 184,000 for a $6.14S^0_{20, w}$ protein and 183,000 for $6.19S^0_{20, w}$ protein. Human γG that was measured in the same way at the same time gave a value of 161,000 for a $6.64S^0_{20, w}$ protein. Thus, in view of Mamet-Bratley's results one would tend to consider the value for γD monomer perhaps 15% too high if weak dimerization were a problem there also. On the other hand, Saha, Chowdhury, Sambury, Behelak, Heimer, and Rose (1970) obtained a weight-average value of 200,000 $\pm$ 2,000 for two different human γD that was based upon precise sedimentation equilibrium values through use of a photoelectric ultraviolet scanner. These results would tend to confirm the values of Rowe *et al.* and, if anything, make them minimal.

The value of 200,000 for human γE antibody seems to be a well established central value (Ishizaka, 1970) for an 8.2S 4-chain structure containing 10.7% carbohydrate. The equivalent immunoglobulin in rabbits, with the same homocytotropic biological function (and presumably a γE only on that basis), has a lower molecular weight of 141,500 (McVeigh and Voss, 1969).

Among avian species the molecular weight of γG tends to be greater than in rabbits or humans. Orlans, Rose, and Marrack (1961) had reported a value of 178–179,000 for chicken γG which was confirmed by Gallagher and Voss (1969) by two different methods: 182,750 using the Svedberg-Pedersen method and 174,920 using the Uphantis technique. Once again, however, one is not sure of association effects, for Hersh, Kubo, Leslie, and Benedict (1969) obtained only 168,000 for chicken γG by a technique that gave 150,000 for rabbit γG. Quail and pheasant γG were also measured and found to have molecular weights of 170,000 by the same technique.

9. Structure and molecular weights of γA

γG has only a very weak tendency to associate into dimers at neutral pH and when it does form stable complexes such as the 13S immunoglobulin reported by Heimer, Martinez, and Abruzzo (1970) there are always unusual and unique conditions or denaturation responsible for the aggregation. Secretory γA, however, is assembled as a dimer by the cells that produce it.

Salivary and colostral γA from the rabbit were found by Tomasi, Tan, Solomon, and Prendergast (1965) to have the characteristics of an 11S polymer and were believed to be produced locally in the interstitial tissues rather than transported there from the serum as a 7S subunit. In 5 M guanidine two 7S subunits could be obtained plus a polypeptide chain (called secretory piece or SP by Tomasi but now more frequently referred to as SC or secretory component), and each 7S subunit produced a pair of α-chains and a pair of light chains (Cebra and Robbins, 1966; Cebra and Small, 1967). Similar secretory 11S γA was found in the human but the SC-chains were more tightly bound (Hong, Pollara, and Good, 1966). The proposed model by Hong *et al.* (1966) contained a trimer of γA molecules radiating outward from the S-piece, but it is now known that the trimer arrangement is erroneous. Svehag and Bloth (1970) have suggested a molecular model, based upon ultrastructural considerations (Fig. 3-6), which pictures two Y-shaped γA monomers, 125 $\times$ 140A, superimposed on each other in a closely packed state and held together by an SC-chain embedded in the constant region of the α-chains. Only in this way can they account for the measured molecular weight of 350,000 within the measured electron micrograph (EM) dimensions. Biosynthetic evidence also points very clearly to the local exocrine synthesis of dimers by plasma cells. Local synthesis of SC-chain is provided by other cells, and the association of dimers and SC-chain to form the 11S complex takes place in the same local intercellular milieu before transport into the surrounding intercellular fluids (Lawton, Asofsky, and Mage, 1970a, b; Bienenstock and Strauss, 1970). An earlier report that the dimers were mixed γA molecules (Costea, Yakulis, Schmale, and Heller, 1968) can be discounted. The allotypic symmetry in the dimers studied by Lawton and Mage

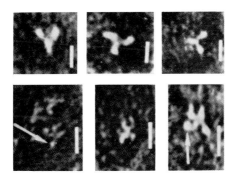

Fig. 3-6. Electron micrographs of purified human and rabbit γA molecules. (*Top*) Variable forms of Y-shaped, single *secretory* 11S γA molecules which have a molecular weight of more than 350,000 and which must, therefore, within the dimensions shown, contain two γA monomers, superimposed upon each other in a closely packed state with the SC-chain inserted in the constant region of the four α-chains. (*Bottom*) Single human high-polymer *serum* γA molecules, each with four visible appendages. One appendage is indicated by *arrows*. The scale lines represent 10 nm. (From Svehag and Bloth, 1970.)

(1969) could not be obtained except on the basis of single cell synthesis.

The molecular weight of the SC-chain has been reported to be as high as 76,000 (Newcomb, Normansell, and Stanworth, 1968) in human colostrum and as low as 58,500 (Tomasi and Bienenstock, 1968) in rabbit while Cebra and Small (1967) and O'Daly and Cebra (1968) believe it to be a dimer of two chains of 43,200 molecular weight held together by disulfide bridges. Free SC-chain has been found in all normal urines investigated (Bienenstock and Tomasi, 1968) and in the ovine and caprine species (Pahud and Mach, 1970).

The molecular weight of the $(\gamma A)_2$-SC complex appears to be about 390,000 for both rabbit and human: 385,000 for rabbit colostral γA (Cebra and Small, 1967) and 393,000 for human colostral γA (Newcomb et al. 1968). In the dog the exocrine γA appears to be the same size as the human although the serum 7S γA component seems to be larger (Vaerman and Heremans, 1969). The same is true for the pig colostrum (Vaerman and Heremans, 1970) with a 10S dimer appearing in the serum. Sheep colostrum reportedly contains three principle components: a dimeric 10.8S $\gamma A1$ with no secretory piece, a dimeric 15S $\gamma A2$ with SC-chain, and a monomeric 6.5S $\gamma G1$ protein (Heimer, Jones, and Maurer, 1969).

The quaternary structure of the complex is tight and well stabilized by both noncovalent and covalent forces such that some antigenic determinants of the SC-chain are inaccessible before unfolding (Bradtzaeg, 1970), and there is even evidence of a hidden light chain under atypical conditions (Hashimoto, Chandor, Mandy, and Yokoyama, 1970). Antigenic specificity of γA polymers has been distinguished from γA monomers which also indicates conformational changes in the complex (Apicella and Allen, 1970). As revealed by Svehag and Bloth's ultrastructural views, however, there are four Fab arms, each 55–75 by 25–30 A, that are extending outward from two monomers joined at an EM contrast-rich center. The complete span of the 11S or 13S dimer is 100–110 A. The implication is that the binding sites are free.

Secretory γA not only contains two moles of γA monomer and one mole of SC, but also a mole of another protein chain with a molecular weight of 23,000. Because of its fast migration when free, this chain is called the F-component by O'Daly and Cebra (1971), but is more likely to be known as the J-chain after Halpern and Koshland (1970). Unlike SC, the J-chain may also be found in γM (Mestecky, Zikán, and Butler, 1971) to provide another unit for cross-reactivity between the two isotypes. The original small molecular weight T-chain (Cebra and Robbins, 1966) is now known to be J-chain rather than SC (O'Daly and Cebra, 1971).

10. Structure and molecular weights of γM

The ultrastructural view of an intact human IgM molecule (Svehag, Chesebro, and Bloth, 1967, 1968; Svehag, 1969) suggests a structural model with a spiderlike complex of five legs of varying length that are joined to a central ring. After papain digestion (Mihaesco and Seligmann, 1968) the central ring structure remains intact and can be shown to contain the C-terminal ends of μ-chains. (Fab)$_2$ μ-fragments constitute 75% of the appendages while Fc μ-fragments comprise the ring Svehag, Bloth, and Seligmann, 1969). The outer diameter of the ring is 85 Å, the inner diameter is 40 Å, and the protrusions are 20–30 Å.

In another electron microscope investigation Parkhouse, Askonas, and Dourmashkin (1970) showed that γM formed by a mouse plasmacytoma also displayed a central core from which five and sometimes 6 protrusions radiated outward. Each subunit was Y-shaped, the point of branching occurring 100–110Å from the center and the branches extending 60–80Å further. Partial reduction with dithiothreitol produced subunits which became reconstituted after removal of this sulfhydryl reagent. The model thus confirmed and extended the one presented by Svehag and colleagues.

Beale and Feinstein (1970) meanwhile have provided a structural view based upon investigations of the disulfide bridges involved in γM. Doolittle, Singer, and Metzger (1966) as well as Abel and Grey (1967) had previously suggested that inter-subunit disulfide bridges might form from the cysteines next to the C-terminal tyrosines of the μ-chains. Beale and Feinstein, however, discovered that the penultimate C-terminal cysteines were involved in intra-subunit bridging and that the intersubunit bridges were formed further up the chain (Fig. 3-7).

The pentameric structure of γM macroglobulin was deduced by Miller and Metzger (1965a, b; 1966) by reduction and alkylation studies following the lead of Deutsch and Morton (1957), and was confirmed many times over by such work as that of Onoue, Kishimoto, and Yamamura (1967) and of Chen, Reichlin, and Tomasi (1969), but the ultrastructural view and the disulfide-bridge fixation were needed to establish the model with certainty.

As we have already seen, however, the model is not all inclusive, for many subunit variations apparently can occur. In fact, Filitti-Wurmser, Tempete-Gaillourdet, and Hartmann (1970) obtained some evidence from thorough ultracentrifugal studies that the oligomers of γM appeared to contain 4, 6, and 8 subunits much more often than 5 subunits. The γM obtained from four normal individuals (Filitti-Wurmser, Gentou, and Hartmann, 1966) was found to be a mixture of three quaternary structures that became separable in the ultracentrifuge (Table 3-7). It is as yet unknown what the quaternary structures of higher molecular weight γM species may be, but the existence of such units as 32S γM are actually not too infrequent. As for the more frequent 18-19S variety, one frequently encounters molecular weight data in the literature that assign 900,000 for γM

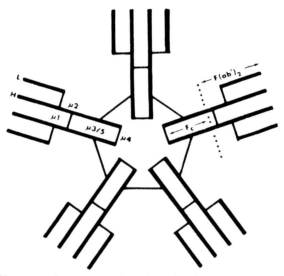

FIG. 3-7. Diagrammatic representation of a molecule of IgM made up of 5 4-chain subunits. *H*, heavy chain; *L*, light chain. *Thick lines* indicate polypeptide chains and *thin lines* represent interchain disulfide bridges. μ1, μ2, μ3/5, and μ4 indicate the approximate positions of peptides associated with the interchain bridges. The *dotted line* indicates the position where a subunit can be enzymatically cleaved into F(ab')$_2$ and Fc fragments. (From Beale and Feinstein, 1970.)

TABLE 3-7
Molecular Weights of Four Normal γM Preparations

Individual	γM$_1$	γM$_2$	γM$_3$
1	618,000	2,053,000	—
2	874,000	1,905,000	5,114,000
3	966,000	2,103,000	8,096,000
4	1,107,000*	4,015,000	18,714,000

* Probable γM-γG complex according to authors.
(From Filitti-Wurmser *et al.*, 1966.)

and 70,000 for μ-chain and that conclude with the statement that such data are consistent with γM structure involving 5 subunits, each containing 2 heavy and 2 light chains. This is no more true than that the data are also consistent with other subunit structures, and is therefore not really supportive of the current pentameric dogma.

Another aspect of the γM problem is that not all circulating "macroglobulin" is oligomeric. The finding was not unexpected in patients with diseases associated with immunoglobulin abnormalities after Rothfield, Frangione, and Franklin (1965) had found a slowly sedimenting mercaptoethanol-resistant subunit separate from related γM in patients with systemic lupus erythematosus. For example, Stobo and Tomasi (1967) found γM subunits in patients with ataxia telangiectasia, Waldenstrom's macroglobulinemia, and disseminated lupus; and Solomon and Kunkel (1967) obtained a monoclonal type of low molecular weight γM subunit from macroglobulinemic serum. Damacco, Giustino, and Bonomo (1970) recorded the frequency of 7S γM subunits in the sera of patients with Waldenstrom's macroglobulinemia and with rheumatoid arthritis—44.4% in the former and 27.9% in the latter—and asked the question whether such subunits might actually represent a separate class of immunoglobulin independent of though antigenically related to 19S γM.

The finding of 7S γM subunits in normal human serum came as somewhat of a surprise, but the phenomenon was established beyond all doubt when Bush, Swedlund, and Gleich (1967) and Klein, Mattern, Radema, and van Zwet (1967) came to the same conclusion independently of each other in the same year. Solomon (1969) in his extensive study of 7S protein with γM determinants found that the relative proportions of 7S to 19S varied widely in normal and patient serum (Table 3-8).

Solomon and McLaughlin (1970) found that culture fluids of bone-marrow cells from patients whose serum contained both 7S and 19S

TABLE 3-8

Serum Levels of 7S and 19S Proteins with γM Determinants in 9 Subjects

7S	19S	7S	19S	7S	19S
mg/ml	*mg/ml*	*mg/ml*	*mg/ml*	*mg/ml*	*mg/ml*
1.4	0	0	8	1.8	37
2.4	4	3.5	19	1.2	12*
32	10	0	32	2.6	17*

* The same patient, samples 1 year apart.
(From Solomon, 1969.)

γM also contained both forms. By labeling techniques it was definitely determined that the 7S globulin was not a degradation product of 19S but rather arose by synthesis along with 19S. It remained to be determined whether 7S was a precursor and defective product in 19S synthesis by the same cells or an independent globulin synthesized in separate cells.

In addition to the ultrastructural view that suggests a pentameric (Chesebro *et al.*, 1968; Parkhouse *et al.*, 1970) and sometimes hexameric (Parkhouse *et al.*, 1970) structure there is also an indirect picture related to the number of antibody binding sites that are available. The most unambiguous investigation has been that of Ashman and Metzger (1969) who were able to determine that a homogeneous Waldenstrom's macroglobulin with binding affinity for nitrophenyl ligands had 10 binding sites in the intact γM, 2 in the 7S subunit γM$_s$, 2 in the (Fab')$_{2\mu}$ peptic subunit, and 1 in the Fab$_\mu$. The binding affinity was uniform in the intact and fragmented portions. Therefore, it can be concluded for certain that γM *may* exist in pentameric form. Results are not always so clear-cut. Stone and Metzger (1967), for example, contrast the valency of two macroglobulins, the γM *Lay* and the γM *War*. The one after dissociation into Fab fragments in two separate experiments was 84% and 88% active in binding whereas the other in two separate experiments was 47% and 48% active. The one could be taken to mean that all the Fab protrusions in an intact γM may be active, whereas the other could be taken to mean that only half of the Fab protrusion may be capable of binding ligands.

Onoue, Yagi, Grossberg, and Pressman (1965) isolated a rabbit γM with an antiligand activity which had 6 available sites in the intact γM and 1 in the 7S γM$_s$ subunit (after correction for 20% loss in activity due to the reduction-alkylation procedure). Thus, it appeared that here also only half of the Fab portions were capable of binding. It also appeared that the quaternary structure of this particular rabbit γM was hexameric rather than pentameric.

Merler, Karlin, and Matsumoto (1968) tested the binding of a tetrasaccharide ligand from *Salmonella typhi* by a human γM antibody and obtained a valence of 9.8 (i.e., 10) as the best fit of their data—a result certainly commensurate with a pentameric structure with 10 fully active Fab protrusions.

LeFor and Bauer (1970) compared the complexes obtained when rabbit γM and rabbit γG from the same antisera were separated and individually reacted with the antigen, bovine serum albumin (BSA). The test was an unambiguous primary reaction technique which gave excellent reproducibility (Table 3-9). Their conclusion was that "the intact IgM antibody molecule bound a maximum of five to six antigen molecules" which is certainly true. An intriguing question to which they did not address themselves was whether the available Fab protrusions are fully active or only half active. The implications either way are clear: $(Fab)_{2\mu}$ does not have the same tertiary structure as $(Fab)_{2\gamma}$. If all the sites are free to bind, they must react as pairs of Fab_μ with each BSA molecule as opposed to single Fab_γ units per mole. If only half the sites are free to bind, then either the Fab units in the γM molecule are not uniformly the same or there are steric and/or conformational problems associated with binding that are not in evidence in γG. The results of Coligan and Bauer (1969) showed that over 90% activity was contained in 7S subunits as tested on a BSA-cellulose immunoadsorbent; thus, one presumes that in that case there was at least one active binding site in each $(Fab)_{2\mu}$. This question, which will be explored more fully later, particularly as it applies to γA, is raised here to emphasize the relevance not only of primary structure to the antibody problem but also of tertiary and quaternary as well.

11. Conformational aspects of γG

A less than cursory examination of γM tertiary structure may not yet be possible, but the available information on γG is not so superficial. A systematic approach to the problem, based upon sound physical chemistry and thorough knowledge of protein characteristics, was first made in a significant way in Tanford's laboratory. From that application Noelken, Nelson, Buckley, and Tanford (1965) were able to produce a conceptually satisfactory model of a 7S γG molecule that both accounted for the biophysical parameters and preserved the immunochemical features. Discarded was the tradi-

TABLE 3-9

Comparison of Rabbit γM and γG Antibodies in their Primary Binding with BSA

Antigen Concentration*	Mole Ratio BSA/γM	Mole Ratio BSA/γG
1	5.08	—
1:2	5.54	1.95
1:4	6.22	2.01
1:8	5.31	1.92
1:16	4.60	—
Mean	5.35 ± 0.53	1.96 ± 0.04

* 1 = 2.6 mg in γM tests and 3.3 mg in γG tests.
(Modified from LeFor and Bauer, 1970.)

tional inflexible cigar-shaped model with its tips bitten off for binding sites* and offered in its place was the now universally accepted Y-model with its two Fab binding sites firmly anchored in Fc but capable of varying their distance from each other "by virtue of a flexible link."

Ultrastructural support for the new model was suggestive in the electron micrographs of Feinstein and Rowe (1965) (Fig. 3–8) and clearly indicated in those of Valentine and Green (1967) as shown in Figures 3-9–11. Valentine and Green reacted a small haptenic bivalent molecule, bisdinitrophenyloctamethylenediamine, [(DNP)$_2$-OMD, with dinitrophenyl determinants at each end] with highly specific, purified, rabbit antibody γG and obtained many types of complexes; linear polymers, dimers, and cyclic oligomers. The ring structures were most helpful in evaluating ultrastructural data since they could be treated with pepsin to digest away the Fc portions. The structures that remained were still closed polygonic rings made up of alternating regions of (Fab')$_2$ and (DNP)$_2$OMD, e.g., a triangle containing the hinge region at each corner, and with Fc portions projecting from each corner when undigested intact γG was used.

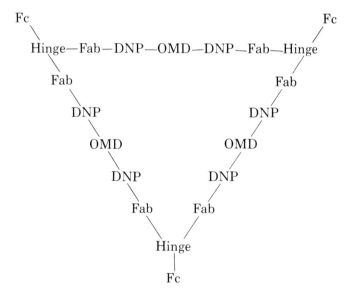

---

* For example, see Figure 2-6 in Boyd (1966) and Figure 2 in Campbell (1968).

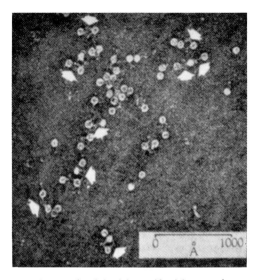

Fɪɢ. 3-8. Electron micrograph of ferritin-antiferritin complexes near equivalence, showing cross-linking strands between ferritin molecules suggestive of Y-shaped anti-bodies. (From Feinstein and Rowe, 1965.)

Perhaps more meaningful than the direct visual electron microscopy confirmation of the Y-structure is the crystallographic evidence. Goldstein, Humphrey, and Poljak (1968), in extending the studies of Poljak, Goldstein, Humphrey, and Dintzis (1967), determined that crystallized human Fc fragment from a homogeneous myeloma protein of γG1 subclass had a 2-fold axis of symmetry rather than a 2-fold screw axis and that it would fit a parallelepiped enclosure of $50 \times 40 \times 7$ Å. These dimensions, which allowed for a 40% H_2O insertion, were very much in keeping with the dimensions given by Valentine and Green and emphasized the intrinsic globular domains of Fc. Edmundson, Wood, Schiffer, Hardman, Ainsworth, Ely, and Deutsch (1970) were fortunate to crystallize from water a human γG1, *Mcg*, in the orthorhombic space group C222 (Fig. 3-12). The unit cell contained 4 γG molecules and had the overall dimensions of $a = 87.8 \pm 0.3$, $b = 111.3 \pm 0.4$, and $c = 186.3 \pm 0.6$ A. From their investigations it was found that the intact γG molecule—not just Fc—also had a 2-fold rotation axis that related two halves and that each half had crystallographic asymmetric units composed of one light and one heavy chain.

Small angle X-ray scattering can be used to deduce the molecular behavior of macromolecules in solution on the basis of radii of gyration and scattering curves. With this technique Pilz, Puchwein,

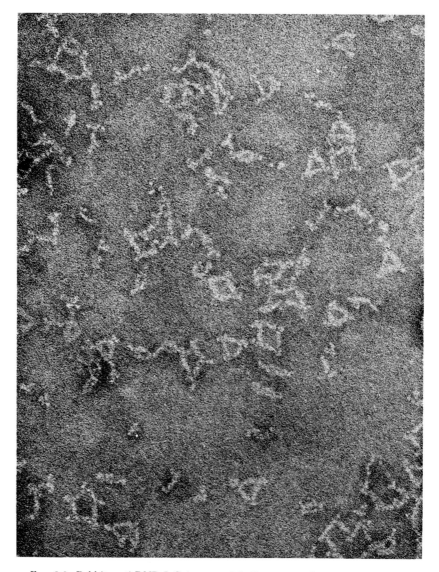

Fɪɢ. 3-9. Rabbit anti-DNP IgG immunoglobulin saturated with a divalent DNP hapten (bis-N-DNP-octamethylenediamine). Many of the antibody molecules are linked together to form closed rings with regular shapes. A projection at each corner of the polygonal shapes can be seen. (From Valentine and Green, 1967.)

Kratky, Herbst, Haager, Gall, and Edelman (1970) were able to determine that in a homogeneous γG1 immunoglobulin the three main regions—two Fab and one Fc—"are relatively compact, but that the whole molecule has an extended structure in solution." The data

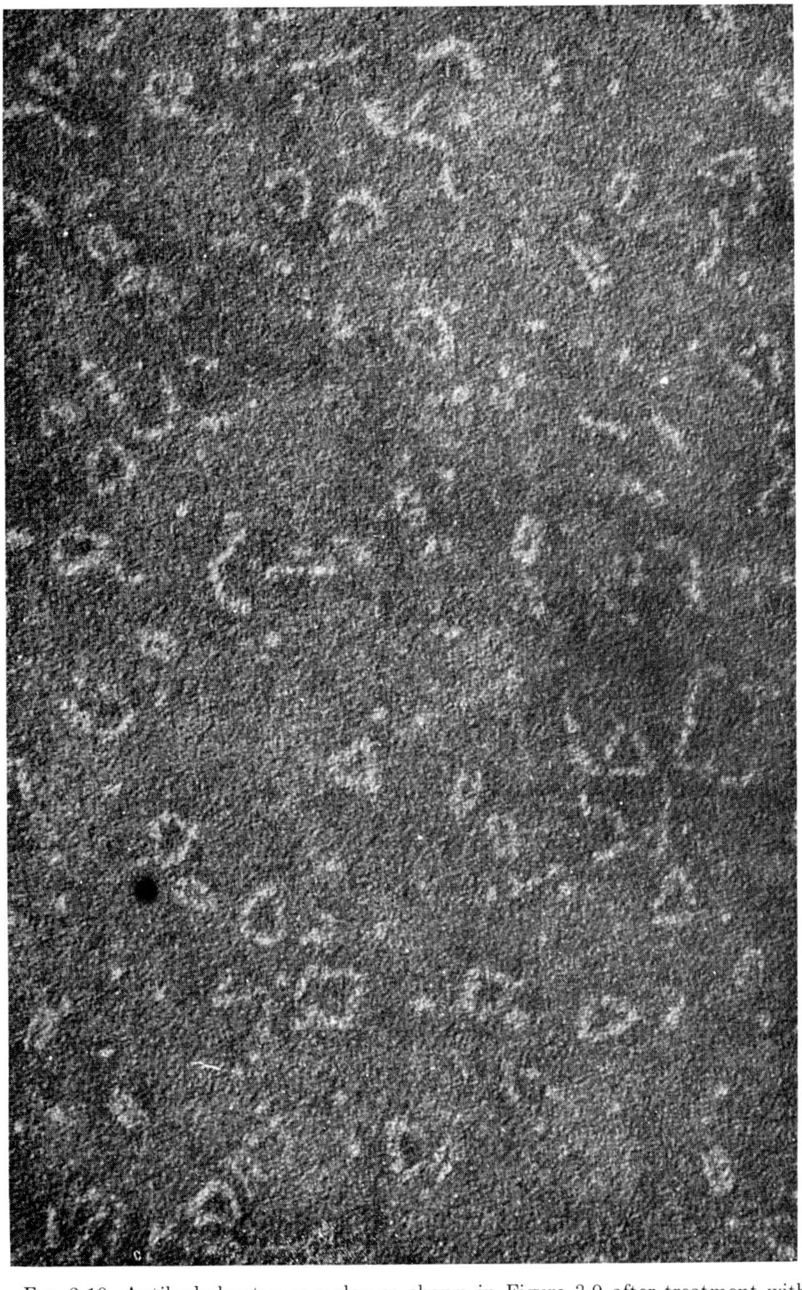

Fig. 3-10. Antibody-hapten complex as shown in Figure 3-9 after treatment with pepsin at pH 4.5 to digest the Fc fragment. The projections at the corners of the regular shapes have been detached and appear as small pieces (×500,000). (From Valentine and Green, 1967.)

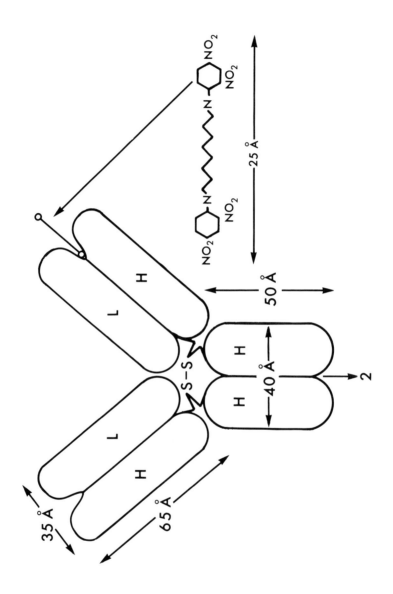

were in agreement with the views of Noelken *et al.* and of Valentine and Green and extended them on the following grounds:

(a) Fab and Fc fragments are relatively compact, since their scattering curves are not anomalous and are approximated by theoretical curves for ellipsoids.

(b) The whole γG molecule is not compact since its scattering curves *are* anomalous and since the radii of gyration of the whole molecule are larger than expected for overall close-packing of regions.

A comparison of calculated cross-section curves for various models with the experimental cross section curve suggested that perhaps the individual ellipsoidal regions might better be visualized as slightly overlapping rather than completely separated as in the Noelken-Tanford model (Figs. 3-13 and 3-14). The flexibility of the Noelken-Tanford model was preserved, so much so, in fact, that the authors were forced to conclude: "If the whole molecule is flexible in solution, however, it is clear that no single structure of γG immunoglobulin in a crystal is likely to be identical with the structures present in solution."

The domain hypothesis of Edelman and Gall (1969) suggested that the homology regions within each domain would contribute to the tertiary structure in that domain (Fig. 3-15). In keeping with crystallographic data, the model made the 2-fold axis of symmetry bisect the interchain H-H disulfide bridges and pass perpendicularly through them giving a unit cell of dimensions $195 \times 93 \times 51$ Å, commensurate with both extended and compact Y-shaped molecules.

Predicted from the Pilz-Edelman concept is an increase in frictional coefficient of γG as the angle between the two Fab portions increases.

FIG. 3-11. Scale diagram of a molecule of rabbit IgG based on measurements of the dimensions of cyclic trimers and on chemical evidence (Cohen and Porter, 1964). The lengths of the Fab and Fc fragments are 10% greater than those published previously (Valentine and Green, 1967) following a more extended set of measurements. The mean distance between the extremes of Fc fragments in 20 cyclic trimers was 245 Å (range 215–270 Å). The variable orientation of the Fc fragment probably accounts for the rather wide range of the measurements. The molecular weight of each fragment would be 52,000, assuming a cylindrical cross section and making no allowance for the rounded corners illustrated. The relative positions of the L and H chains in the Fab fragments and the orientation of the cleavage plane between them are unknown and, therefore, arbitrary. This has been emphasized by reversing the positions of the L and H chains. The *arrow* between the two halves of the Fc fragment indicates the position of the 2-fold symmetry axis observed both in crystals of Fc and of human IgG myeloma protein. The location of the binding site in a cleft between L and H chains is consistent with the available evidence on the roles of the two chains. The smooth contour of the junction between hapten-linked Fab's is consistent with the central location of the binding site. (From Green, 1969.)

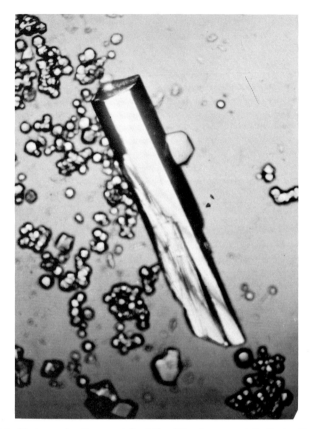

FIG. 3-12. Photograph of a crystal of the Mcg immunoglobulin in the midst of smaller, unidentified crystals. The dimensions of the immunoglobulin crystal are 0.4 × 0.4 × 2.8 mm. (From Edmunson *et al.*, 1970, p. 2763.)

Warner and Schumaker (1970) tested this idea by the application of various chemical treatments that would result in conformational changes. Their data were completely consistent with this prediction and supported further still the flexible Y-model conceived by Noelken *et al.*

Perhaps the most elegant touch of all stems from fluorescence polarization. In retrospect, in fact, and not widely appreciated at the time the fluorescence depolarization experiments of Chowdhury and Johnson (1963) set the stage. Using 5-dimethylamino-1-naphthalene-sulphonyl chloride (also called naphthyl dye, dansyl group, or DNS) that was conjugated to bovine γG to provide a fluorescent focus they observed that the relaxation times needed for fluorescence depolarization in neutral solutions was many times lower than expected

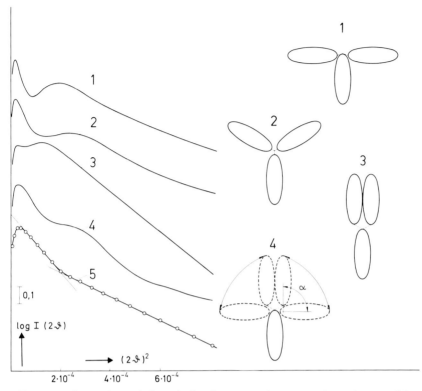

Fɪɢ. 3-13. Comparison of the calculated cross section curves for various models (*1–4*) with the experimental cross section curve (*5*). *Curve 4* represents the best approximation to the experimental curve obtained with these models. The scattering curves of shapes obtained by variation of angle α have been averaged so that the deviation from the experimental curve is smallest. (From Pilz *et al.*, 1970.)

from the rigid translational dynamic properties of the traditional model. They concluded that nonpolar amino acids were important in folding a core but that flexibility must remain outside this core. Metzger, Perlman, and Edelhoch (1966) by fluorescence polarization then determined that human macroglobulin in its conformation must have subunits with internal degrees of rotational freedom. Then, in a very straightforward fashion Zagyansky, Nezlin, and Tumerman (1969) established the flexibility of γG beyond all doubt. They compared dansylated conjugates of rabbit or human γG with those of the naphthyl dye conjugated to bovine serum albumin or ovalbumin. In the albumins the lifetime of the excited state was 12.1 nanoseconds, the quantum yield was high, the wavelength of maximum fluorescence was 523 mμ; in the globulins the excited state was less at 7.3 nano-

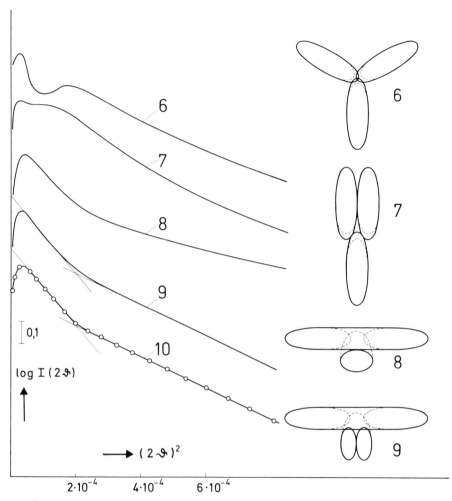

FIG. 3-14. Comparison of the calculated cross section curves for various models (*6–9*) with the experimental cross section curve (*10*). The *dashed lines* correspond to the ellipsoids equivalent to the individual fragments. (From Pilz *et al.*, 1970.)

seconds, the quantum yield was low, the wavelength of maximum fluorescence was higher at 543 mμ. It was calculated from all available data that the rotational relaxation time of dansylated human γG (DNS-HGG) was only 60 nanoseconds. If the molecule had been rigid the value would have been 220 nanoseconds. In a very quantitative way the full meaning of flexibility was encountered in the dynamic state, and the Noelken-Tanford model was fully established.

Having presented the flexible Y-structure in the manner of three

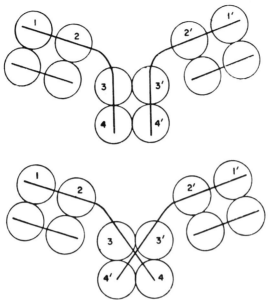

FIG. 3-15. Hypothetical compact domains in γG-immunoglobulin. Numbers indicate domains of the heavy chains and show two different arrangements in the Fc fragment. (From Edelman and Gall, 1969.)

major globular domains, each composed of four regional globular units, one might have given the impression that the three were actually in all physical ways equivalent. Before leaving the subject, however, one would do well to point out that this is not true. Abaturov, Nezlin, Vengerova, and Varshavskii (1969) investigated regional secondary structure by infrared spectroscopy and the change in their shape by hydrogen-deuterium exchange, all as a function of pH. At neutral pH light chains, Fab, and Fc all *did* show similar responses and compactness, but below pH 5.1 Fc fragments lost their conformational properties and native properties. Fab fragments and light chains, on the other hand, resisted significant change even at pH 2. Whole γG below pH 3.9 underwent conformational changes as well that were attributable to Fc deterioration. These results are in keeping with those of Charlwood and Utsumi (1969) on conformational changes in Fc and with Harrington and Fenton (1970) on heavy chains. The results of Azuma, Hirai, Hamaguchi, and Migita (1970) and of Takahashi, Hirai, Azuma, Hamaguchi, and Migita (1970) go one step further and show changes in Bence-Jones proteins as well. Using circular dichroism and ultraviolet spectroscopy they found that these light chains were stable in structure within the pH range 4–10. Above pH 10.2 denaturation occurred with randomly coiled polypeptide chains resulting. Below pH 4.0 an ordered structure was obtained and no random coil; nevertheless, denaturation did occur and an irreversible conformational change to a different ordered structure occurred. It is not known what stabilizing effect the presence of Fd might have in such instances, but the answer is important immuno-chemically. Much of the purification of antibody from antigen-antibody complexes has involved the separation at a pH well below 4 and closer to 2.

REFERENCES

Abaturov, L. V., Nezlin, R. S., Vengerova, T. I., and Varshavskii, Ya.M. (1969). Conformational studies of immunoglobulin G and its subunits by the methods of hydrogen-deuterium exchange and infrared spectroscopy. Biochim. Biophys. Acta 194: 386–96.

Abel, C. A., and Grey, H. M. (1967). Carboxy-terminal amino acids of γA and γM heavy chains. Science 156: 1609–1610.

Abel, C. A., and Grey, H. M. (1968). Studies on the structure of mouse γA myeloma proteins. Biochemistry 7: 2682–2688.

Amiraian, K., and Leikhim, E. J. (1961). Preparation and properties of antibodies to sheep erythrocytes. J. Immunol. 87: 301–309.

Apicella, M. A., and Allen, J. C. (1970). Antigenic specificity of γA polymers. J. Immunol. 104: 455–62.

Ashman, R. F., and Metzger, H. (1969). A Waldenstrom's macroglobulin which binds nitrophenyl ligands. J. Biol. Chem. 244: 3405–3414.

Askonas, B. A., and Williamson, A. R. (1966). Biosynthesis of immunoglobulins on polyribosomes and assembly of the IgG molecule. Proc. Roy. Soc. Lond. 166: 232–243.

Askonas, B. A., and Williamson, A. R. (1967a). Biosynthesis and assembly of immunoglobulin G. Symp. Quant. Biol. 32: 233–231.

Askonas, B. A., and Williamson, A. R. (1967b). Balanced heavy and light chain synthesis in immune tissue and disulphide bond formation in IgG assembly. In Gamma Globulins, 3rd Nobel Symposium, Killander, J., ed. (Interscience, 643 pp.), pp. 369–383.

Azuma, T., Hirai, T., Hamaguchi, K., and Migita, S. (1970). Hydrogen ion equilibria of a Bence-Jones protein. J. Biochem. 67: 801–808.

Baglioni, C. (1969). Initiation and assembly of the immunoglobulin peptide chains. Fed. Eur. Biochem. Soc. Proc. 15: 93–104.

Baglioni, C., Cioli, D., Gorini, G., Ruffili, A., and Alescio-Zonta, L. (1967). Studies on fragments of light chains of human immunoglobulins: genetic and biochemical implications. Symp. Quant. Biol. 32: 147–159.

Beale, D., and Feinstein, A. (1970). Evidence for C-terminal intra-subunit disulfide bridges between immunoglobulin M heavy chains. Fed. Eur. Biochem. Soc. Letters 7: 175–176.

Bienenstock, J., and Strauss, H. (1970). Evidence for synthesis of human colostral γA as 11S dimer. J. Immunol. 105: 274–277.

Bienenstock, J., and Tomasi, T. B., Jr. (1968). Secretory γA in normal urine. J. Clin. Invest. 47: 1162–1171.

Boyd, W. C. (1966). *Fundamentals of Immunology*, Ed. 4, Interscience (New York, 773 pp.), p. 67.

Bradtzaeg, P. (1970). Unfolding of human secretory immunoglobulin A. Immunochemistry 7: 127–130.

Bush, S. T., Swedlund, H. A., and Gleich, G. J. (1967). The occurrence of low molecular weight γA in human serums. Fed. Proc. 26: 529 incl.

Buxbaum, J., Franklin, E. C., and Scharff, M. D. (1970). Immunoglobulin M heavy chain disease: intracellular origin of the mu chain fragment. Science 169: 770–772.

Cammack, K. A. (1962). Molecular weight of rabbit γ-globulin. Nature 194: 745–747.

Campbell, D. H. (1968). Antibody formation: from Ehrlich to Pauling and return. In *Structural Chemistry and Molecular Biology*, Rich, A., and Davidson, N., eds. Freeman (San Francisco, 907 pp.), pp. 166–171.

Cebra, J. J., and Robbins, J. B. (1966). γA-immunoglobulin from rabbit colostrum. J. Immunol. 97: 12–24.

Cebra, J. J., and Small, P. A., Jr. (1967). Polypeptide chain structure of rabbit immunoglobulins. III. Secretory γA-immunoglobulin from colostrum. Biochemistry 6: 503–512.

Charlwood, P. A., and Utsumi, S. (1969). Conformation changes and dissociation of Fc fragments of rabbit immunoglobulin G as a function of pH. Biochem. J. 112: 357–365.

Chen, J. P., Reichlin, M., and Tomasi, T. B., Jr. (1969). Studies on the chymotrypsin C and papain fragments of human immunoglobulin M. Biochemistry 8: 2246–2254.

Chesebro, B., Bloth, B., and Svehag, S.-E. (1968). The ultrastructure of normal and pathological IgM immunoglobulin. J. Exp. Med. 127: 399–410.

Chowdhury, F. H., and Johnson, P. (1963). Physicochemical studies of bovine γ-globulin. Biochem. Biophys. Acta 66: 218–228.

Cohen, S., and Porter, R. R. (1964). Structural and biological activity of immunoglobulins. Adv. Immunol. 4: 287–349.

Coligan, J. E., and Bauer, D. C. (1969). Distribution of antigen-binding sites on rabbit IgM subunits. J. Immunol. 103: 1038–1043.

Connell, G. E., Dorrington, K. J., Lewis, A. F., and Parr, D. M. (1970). The conformation of an atypical IgG myeloma protein and its papain fragments. Can. J. Biochem. 48: 784–789.

Costea, N., Yakulis, V., Schmale, J., and Heller, P. (1968). Light chain determinants of exocrine isoagglutinins. J. Immunol. 101: 1248–1252.

D'Amico, R. P., and Kern, M. (1970). Synthesis and secretion of γ-globulin by lymph node cells. VII. The cell-free incorporation of galactose and sialic acid into the carbohydrate component of endogenous immunoglobulin. Biochem. Biophys. Acta 215: 78–87.

Dammaco, F., Giustino, V., and Bonomo, L. (1970). The occurrence of serum 7S IgM in diseases associated with immunoglobulin abnormalities. Int. Arch. Allergy Appl. Immunol. 38: 618–626.

Dayhoff, M. O. (1969). *The Atlas of Protein Sequence and Structures*, Vol. 4, National Biomedical Research Foundation (Silver Spring, Md., xxvi + 109 text pp. + 252 data pp.).

Deutsch, H. F., and Morton, I. J. (1957). Dissociation of human serum macroglobulins. Science 125: 600–601.

DiGuglielmo, R. (1966). Unusual morphologic and humoral conditions in the field of plasmacytomas and M-dysproteinemia. Acta Med. Scand. 179: Suppl. 445, 206–211.

Doolittle, R. F., Singer, S. J., and Metzger, H. (1966). Evolution of immunoglobulin polypeptide chains: carboxy-terminal of an IgM heavy chain. Science 154: 1561–1562.

Dorrington, K. J., and Rockey, J. H. (1970). Differences in the molecular size of the heavy chains from γA1- and γA2-globulins. Biochim. Biophys. Acta 200: 584–586.

Edelman, G. A. (1959). Dissociation of γ-globulin. J. Am. Chem. Soc. 81: 3155–3156.

Edelman, G. M. (1970). The covalent structure of a human γG-immunoglobulin. XI. Functional implications. Biochemistry 9: 3197–3204.

Edelman, G. M., and Gall, W. E. (1969). The antibody problem. Annu. Rev. Biochem. 38: 415–466.

Edelman, G. M., and Poulik, M. D. (1961). Studies on the structural units of the γ-globulins. J. Exp. Med. 113: 861–884.

Edmundson, A. B., Wood, M. K., Schiffer, M., Hardman, K. D., Ainsworth, C. F., Ely, K. R., and Deutsch, H. L. (1970). A crystallographic investigation of a human IgG immunoglobulin. J. Biol. Chem. 245: 2763–2764.

Ein, D., and Waldmann, T. A. (1969). Metabolic studies of a heavy chain disease protein. J. Immunol. 103: 345–348.

Fahey, J. L., and Finegold, I. (1967). Synthesis of immunoglobulins in human lymphoid cell lines. Symp. Quant. Biol. 32: 283–289.

Feinstein, A., and Rowe, A. J. (1965). Molecular mechanism of formation of an antigen-antibody complex. Nature 205: 147–149.

Filitti-Wurmser, S., Gentou, C., and Hartmann, L. (1966). Poids moléculaires des macroglobulines IgM des sérums humains normaux. Association IgM-IgG. Biochim. Biophys. Acta 121: 175–177.

Filitti-Wurmser, S., Tempete-Gaillourdet, M., and Hartmann, L. (1970). Various molecular weights for the heavy chains of human monoclonal IgM immuno-globulins. Immunochemistry 7: 443–452.

Fleischman, J. B. (1967a). Synthesis of the γG heavy chain in rabbit lymph node cells. Biochemistry 6: 1311–1320.

Fleischman, J. B. (1967b). Synthesis of the rabbit γG heavy chain. Symp. Quant. Biol. 32: 233–234.

Fleischman, J. B., Porter, R. R., and Press, E. M. (1963). The arrangement of the peptide chains in γ-globulin. Biochem. J. 88: 220–228.

Forssman, O., and Nilsson, G. (1967). A case of myeloma with flaming plasma cells but no significant M-compound in serum or urine. Acta Med. Scand. 181: 33–36.

Franek, F. (1961). Dissociation of animal 7S γ-globulins by cleavage of disulfide bonds. Biochem. Biophys. Res. Commun. 4: 28–32.

Franek, F., and Riha, I. (1964). Purification and structural characterization of 5S γ-globulin new-born pigs. Immunochemistry 1: 49–63.

Frangione, B., Milstein, C., and Pink, J. R. L. (1969). Structural studies of immuno-globulin G. Nature 221: 145–148.

Franklin, E. C. (1964). Structural studies of human 7S γ-globulin (G immunoglobulin). Further observation of a naturally occurring protein related to the crystallizable (fast) fragment. J. Exp. Med. 120: 691–709.

Franklin, E. C., Lowenstein, J., Bigelow, B., and Meltzer, M. (1964). Heavy chain disease—a new disorder of serum γ-globulins. Am. J. Med. 37: 332–350.

Gallagher, J. S., and Voss, E. W., Jr. (1969). Molecular weight of a purified chicken antibody. Immunochemistry 6: 199–206.

Gergely, J., Fudenberg, H. H., and van Loghem, E. (1970). The papain susceptibility of the IgG (immunoglobulin) myeloma proteins of different heavy chain sub-classes. Immunochemistry 7: 1–6.

Gergely, J., Stanworth, D. R., Jefferis, R., Normansell, D. E., Henney, C. S., and Pardoe, G. I. (1967). Structural studies of immunoglobulins. I. The role of cysteine in papain hydrolysis. Immunochemistry 4: 101–111.

Goldstein, D. J., Humphrey, R. L., and Poljak, R. J. (1968). Human Fc fragment: crystallographic evidence for two equivalent subunits. J. Mol. Biol. 35: 247–249.

Green, N. M. (1969). Electron microscopy of the immunoglobulins. Adv. Immunol. 11: 1–30.

Grey, H. M. (1969). Presence of L—L interchain disulfide bonds in reconstituted γG molecules. J. Immunol. 102: 848–851.

Grey, H. M., Abel, C. A., Yount, W. J., and Kunkel, H. G. (1968). A subclass of human γA-globulins (γA2) which lacks the disulfide bonds linking heavy and light chains. J. Exp. Med. 128: 1223–1236.

Grey, H. M., Sher, A., and Shalitin, N. (1970). Subunit structure of mouse IgA. J. Immunol. 105: 75–84.

Habeeb, A. F. S. A., Schrohenloher, R. E., and Bennett, J. C. (1970). Studies of maleylated chains of human IgM. J. Immunol. 105: 846–855.

Halpern, M. S., and Koshland, M. E. (1970). Novel subunit in secretory IgA. Nature 228: 1276–1278.

Hansson, U.-B., Laurell, C.-B., and Bachmann, R. (1966). Sedimentation constants of IgG and IgD myeloma proteins compared with those of normal IgG. Acta Med. Scand. 179: Suppl. 445, 89–92.

Harrington, J. C., and Fenton, J. W., II. (1970). Evidence for conformational unfolding of immunoglobulin heavy chains in propionic and acetic acids. J. Immunol. 104: 525–527.

Hashimoto, N., Chandor, S., Mandy, W., and Yokoyama, M. (1970). Atypical IgA with hidden light chain. Clin. Exp. Immunol. 6: 941–950.

Heimer, R., Jones, D. W., and Maurer, P. H. (1969). The immunoglobulins of sheep colostrum. Biochemistry 8: 3937–3944.

Heimer, R., Martinez, J., and Abruzzo, J. (1970). Polyclonal 13S human γG immunoglobulin. J. Immunol. 104: 738–745.

Hersh, R. T., Kubo, R. T., Leslie, G. A., and Benedict, A. A. (1969). Molecular weights of chicken, pheasant, and quail IgG immunoglobulins. Immunochemistry 6: 762–765.

Hong, R., Pollara, B., and Good, R. A. (1966). A model for colostral IgG. Proc. Nat. Acad. Sci. 56: 602–607.

Hurez, D., Preud'Homme, J.-L., and Seligmann, M. (1970). Intracellular "monoclonal" immunoglobulin in non-secretory human myeloma. J. Immunol. 104: 263–264.

Ishizaka, K. (1970). Human reaginic antibodies. Annu. Rev. Med. 21: 187–200.

Jefferis, R., Weston, P. D., Stanworth, D. R., and Clamp, J. R. (1968). Relationship between the papain sensitivity of human γG immunoglobulins and their heavy chain subclass. Nature 219: 646–649.

Jerry, L. M., Kunkel, H. G., and Grey, H. M. (1970). Absence of disulfide bonds linking the heavy and light chains, a property of a genetic variant of γA2 globulins. Proc. Nat. Acad. Sci. 65: 557–563.

Karlsson, F. A., Peterson, P. A., and Berggard, I. (1969). Properties of halves of immunoglobulin light chains. Proc. Nat. Acad. Sci. 64: 1257–1263.

Kern, M., and Swenson, R. M. (1967). Biochemical studies of the intracellular events involved in the secretion of γ-globulin. Symp. Quant. Biol. 32: 265–268.

Klein, F., Mattern, P., Radema, H., and van Zwet, T. L. (1967). Slowly sedimenting serum components reacting with anti-IgM sera. Immunology 13: 641–647.

Kubo, R. T., and Benedict, A. A. (1969). Unusual conditions for crystallization of the

Fc fragment of chicken IgG. J. Immunol. *102:* 1523–1525.

Lamm, M. E., and Small, P. A., Jr. (1966). Polypeptide chain structure of rabbit immunoglobulins. II. γM-immunoglobulin. Biochemistry *5:* 267–276.

Lawton, A. R., Asofsky, R., and Mage, R. G. (1970a). Synthesis of secretory IgA in the rabbit. II. Production of alpha, light, and T chains by in vitro cultures of mammary tissue. J. Immunol. *104:* 388–396.

Lawton, A. R., Asofsky, R., Mage, R. G. (1970b). Synthesis of secretory IgA in the rabbit. III. Interaction of colostral IgA fragments with T chain. J. Immunol. *104:* 397–408.

Lawton, A. R., and Mage, R. G. (1969). The synthesis of secretory IgA in the rabbit. I. Evidence for synthesis as an 11S dimer. J. Immunol. *102:* 693–697.

LeFor, W. M., and Bauer, D. C. (1970). Relative concentrations of IgM and IgG antibodies during the primary response. J. Immunol. *104:* 1276–1286.

Mach, B., Koblet, H., and Gros, D. (1967). Biosynthesis of immunoglobulin in a cell-free system. Symp. Quant. Biol. *32:* 269–275.

Mamet-Bratley, M. D. (1970). Molecular weight of a rabbit antibody. Biochim. Biophys. Acta *207:* 76–91.

Markus, G., Grossberg, A. L., and Pressman, D. (1962). The disulfide bonds of rabbit γ-globulin and its fragments. Arch. Biochem. Biophys. *96:* 63–69.

Marrack, J. R. (1938). *The Chemistry of Antigens and Antibodies.* His Majesty's Printing Office, (London, 194 pp.), pp. 52–53.

Matsuoka, Y., Yagi, Y., Moore, G. E., and Pressman, D. (1969a). Isolation and characterization of free λ-chain of immunoglobulin produced by an established cell line of human myeloma cell origin. I. λ-Chain in culture medium. J. Immunol. *102:* 1136–1143.

Matsuoka, Y., Yagi, Y., Moore, G. E., and Pressman, D. (1969b). Isolation and characterization of free λ- chain of immunoglobulin produced by an established cell line of human myeloma cell origin. II. Identity of λ-chains in cells and in medium. J. Immunol. *103:* 962–969.

McVeigh, T. A., Jr., and Voss, E. W., Jr. (1969). Properties of purified mouse homocytotropic antibody. J. Immunol. *103:* 1349–1355.

Melchers, F. (1969a). The attachment site of carbohydrate in a mouse immunoglobulin light chain. Biochemistry *8:* 938–947.

Melchers, F. (1969b). As reported in Dayhoff, M. O. (1969), p. D-109.

Melchers, F. (1969c). Carbohydrate composition of a myeloma protein from different subcellular fractions of plasma cells. Behringwerk-Mitteil. *49:* 169–183.

Melchers, F., and Knopf, P. M. (1967). Biosynthesis of the carbohydrate portion of immunoglobulin chains: possible relation to secretion. Symp. Quant. Biol. *32:* 255–262.

Merler, E., Karlin, L., and Matsumoto, S. (1968). The valency of human γM immunoglobulin antibody. J. Biol. Chem. *243:* 386–390.

Mestecky, J., Zikán, J., and Butler, W. T. (1971). IgM and secretory IgA: presence of a common polypeptide chain different from light chains. Science *171:* 1163–1165.

Metzger, H. (1970). The antigen receptor problem. Annu. Rev. Biochem. *38:* 889–928.

Metzger, H., Perlman, R. L., and Edelhoch, H. (1966). Characterization of a human macroglobulin. IV. Studies of its conformation by fluorescence polarization. J. Biol. Chem. *241:* 1741–1744.

Mihaesco, C., and Seligmann, M. (1968). Papain digestion fragments of human IgM globulins. J. Exp. Med. *127:* 431–453.

Miller, F., and Metzger, H. (1965a). Characterization of a human macroglobulin. I. The molecular weight of its subunit. J. Biol. Chem. *240:* 3325–3333.

Miller, F., and Metzger, H. (1965b). Characterization of a human macroglobulin. II. Distribution of the disulfide bonds. J. Biol. Chem. *240:* 4740–4745.

Miller, F., and Metzger, H. (1966). Characterization of a human macroglobulin. III. The products of tryptic digestion. J. Biol. Chem. *241:* 1732–1740.

Milstein, C. (1969). The variability of human immunoglobulin G. Fed. Eur. Biochem. Soc. Proc. *15:* 43–56.

Milstein, C., and Frangione, B. (1969). Abnormalities in immunoglobulin synthesis: the heavy chain disease protein Zuc. Behringwerk-Mitteil. *49:* 59–65.

Moav, B., and Harris, T. N. (1970a). Biosynthesis and assembly of immunoglobulin in rabbit lymph node cells. I. Immunoglobulin on the ribosomes. J. Immunol. *104:* 957–964.

Moav, B., and Harris, T. N. (1970b). Biosynthesis and assembly of immunoglobulin in rabbit lymph node cells. II. Assembly in the soluble phase. J. Immunol. *104:* 965–975.

Moroz, C., and Uhr, J. W. (1967). Synthesis of the carbohydrate moiety of γ-globulin. Symp. Quant. Biol. *32:* 263–264.

Newcomb, R. W., Normansell, D., and Stanworth, D. R. (1968). A structural study of human exocrine IgA globulin. J. Immunol. *101:* 905–914.

Nezlin, R. S., and Rokhlin, O. V. (1969). Biosynthesis of γG-globulin and its peptide chains in a cell-free system. Fed. Eur. Biochem. Soc. Proc. *15:* 117–132.

Nisonoff, A., and Thorbecke, G. J. (1964). Immunochemistry. Annu. Rev. Biochem. *33:* 355–402.

Nisonoff, A., Wissler, F. C., and Lipman, L. N. (1960). Properties of the major component of a peptic digest of rabbit antibody. Science *132:* 1770–1771.

Nisonoff, A., Wissler, F. C., Lipman, L. N., and Woernley, D. L. (1960). Separation of univalent fragments from the bivalent rabbit antibody molecule by reduction of disulfide bonds. Arch Biochem. Biophys. *89:* 230–244.

Nisonoff, A., and Woernley, D. L. (1959). Effect of hydrolysis by papain on the combining sites of an antibody. Nature *183:* 1325–1326.

Noelken, M. E., Nelson, C. A., Buckley, C. E. III, and Tanford, C. (1965). Gross conformation of rabbit 7S γ-immunoglobulin and its papain-cleaved fragments. J. Biol. Chem. *240:* 218–224.

Northrop, J. H. (1942). Purification and crystallization of diphtheria antitoxin. J. Gen. Physiol. *25:* 465–485.

O'Daly, J. A., and Cebra, J. J. (1968). Structure and cellular localization of secretory IgA. Protides Biol. Fluids *16:* 205–219.

O'Daly, J. A., and Cebra, J. J. (1971). Rabbit secretory IgA. I. Isolation of secretory component after selective dissociation of the immunoglobulin. II. Free secretory component from colostrum and its specific association with IgA. J. Immunol. *107:* 436–455.

O'Donnell, I. J., Frangione, B., and Porter, R. R. (1970). The disulfide bonds of the heavy chain of rabbit immunoglobulin G. Biochem. J. *116:* 261–268.

Onoue, K., Kishimoto, T., and Yamamura, Y. (1967). Papain fragmentation of the subunits of human macroglobulin. J. Immunol. *98:* 303–313.

Onoue, K., Yagi, Y., Grossberg, A. L., and Pressman, D. (1965). Number of binding sites of rabbit macroglobulin antibody and its subunits. Immunochemistry *2:* 401–415.

Orlans, E., Rose, M. E., and Marrack, J. R. (1961). Fowl antibody. I. Some physical and immunochemical properties. Immunology *4:* 262–277.

Osserman, E. F., and Takatsuki, K. (1964). Clinical and immunochemical studies of four cases of heavy (H-γ2) chain disease. Am. J. Med. *37:* 351–373.

Pahud, J. J., and Mach, J. P. (1970). Identification of secretory IgA, free secretory piece, and serum IgA in the ovine and caprine species. Immunochemistry 7: 679–686.

Palmer, J. L., Mandy, W. J., and Nisonoff, A. (1962). Heterogeneity of rabbit antibody and its subunits. Proc. Natl. Acad. Sci. 48: 49–53.

Palmer, J. L., and Nisonoff, A. (1964). Dissociation of rabbit γ-globulin into half-molecules after reduction of one labile disulfide bond. Biochemistry 3: 863–869.

Palmer, J. L., Nisonoff, A., and Van Holde, K. E. (1963). Dissociation of rabbit γ-globulin into subunits by reduction and acidification. Proc. Natl. Acad. Sci. 50: 314–321.

Parfentjev, I. A. (1936). U. S. patent 2065196.

Parkhouse, R. M. E., Askonas, B. A., and Dourmashkin, R. R. (1970). Electron microscopic studies of mouse immunoglobulin M; structure and reconstitution following reduction. Immunology 18: 575–584.

Phelps, R. A., Neet, K. E., Lynn, L. T., and Putnam, F. W. (1961). The cupric ion catalysis of the cleavage of γ-globulin and other proteins by hydrogen peroxide. J. Biol. Chem. 236: 96–105.

Pilz, I., Puchwein, G., Kratky, O., Herbst, M., Haager, O., Gall, W. E., and Edelman, G. M. (1970). Small angle x-ray scattering of a homogeneous γG1 immunoglobulin. Biochemistry 9: 211–219.

Poljak, R. J., Goldstein, D. J., Humphrey, R. L., and Dintzis, H. M. (1967). Crystallographic studies of rabbit and human Fc fragments. Symp. Quant. Biol. 32: 95–98.

Pope, C. G. (1938). Disaggregation of proteins by enzymes. Brit. J. Exptl. Pathol. 19: 245–251.

Pope, C. G. (1939a). The action of proteolytic enzymes on the antitoxins and proteins in immune sera. I. True digestion of the proteins. Brit. J. Exptl. Pathol. 20: 132–149.

Pope, C. G. (1939b). The action of proteolytic enzymes on the antitoxins and proteins in immune sera. II. Heat denaturation after partial enzyme action. Brit. J. Exp. Pathol. 20: 201–212.

Porter, R. R. (1950). The formation of a specific inhibitor by hydrolysis of rabbit antiovalbumin. Biochem. J. 46: 479–484.

Porter, R. R. (1958). Separation and isolation of fractions of rabbit γ-globulin containing the antibody and antigenic combining sites. Nature 182: 670–671.

Porter, R. R. (1959). The hydrolysis of rabbit γ-globulin and antibodies with crystalline papain. Biochem. J. 73: 119–126.

Putnam, F. W. (1965). Structure and function of the plasma proteins. In The Proteins, 2nd Ed., Vol. III, Neurath, H., ed., Academic Press (New York, pp. 153–267), p. 234.

Putnam, F. W., Tan, M., Lynn, L. T., Easley, C. W. and Migita, S. (1962). The cleavage of rabbit γ-globulin by papain. J. Biol. Chem. 237: 717–726.

Ralph, P., Becker, M., and Rich, A. (1967). Immunoglobulin synthesis in a cell-free system. Symp. Quant. Biol. 32: 277–282, 1967.

Richie, E. R., Woolsey, M. E., and Mandy, W. J. (1970). New serum factor in normal rabbits. VI. Reaction with buried determinants of IgG exposed sequentially with cyanogen bromide, pepsin, and papain. J. Immunol. 104: 984–991.

Rothfield, N. F., Frangione, B., and Franklin, E. C. (1965). Slowly sedimenting mercaptoethanol-resistant antinuclear factors related antigenically to M immunoglobulins ($\gamma_{1\,M}$-globulin) in patient with systemic lupus erythematosus. J. Clin. Invest. 44: 62–72.

Rowe, D. S., Dolder, F., and Welscher, H. G. (1969). Studies on human IgD. I. Molecular weight and sedimentation coefficient. Immunochemistry 6: 437–443.

Saha, A., Chowdhury, P., Sambury, S., Behelak, Y., Heiner, D. C., and Rose, B. (1970). Human IgD. II. Physicochemical characterization of human IgD. J. Immunol. *105:* 238–247.

Schachman, H. K. (1963). The ultracentrifuge: problems and prospects (acceptance address, Sargent Award in Chemical Instrumentation). Biochemistry *2:* 887–905.

Scharff, M. D., Shapiro, A. L., and Ginsberg, B. (1967). The synthesis, assembly, and secretion of gamma globulin polypeptide chains by cells of a mouse plasma-cell tumor. Symp. Quant. Biol. *32:* 235–241.

Schubert, D., and Cohn, M. (1968). Immunoglobulin biosynthesis. III. Blocks in defective synthesis. J. Mol. Biol. *38:* 273–288.

Schubert, D., and Horibata, K. (1968). Immunoglobulin biosynthesis. II. Four independently isolated myeloma variants. J. Mol. Biol. *38:* 263–271.

Schultze, H. E. (1962). Influence of bound sialic acid on electrophoretic mobility of human serum proteins. Arch. Biochem. Biophys. Suppl. *1,* 290–294.

Shapiro, A. L., Scharff, M. D., Maizel, J. V., Jr., and Uhr, J. W. (1966). Polyribosomal synthesis and assembly of the H and L chains of gammaglobulin. Proc. Natl. Acad. Sci. *56:* 216–221.

Small, P. A., Jr., and Lamm, M. E. (1966). Polypeptide chain structure of rabbit immunoglobulins. I. γG-immunoglobulin. Biochemistry *5:* 259–267.

Solomon, A. (1969). Molecular heterogeneity of immunoglobulin. J. Immunol. *102:* 496–506.

Solomon, A., Killander, J., Grey, H. M., and Kunkel, H. G. (1966). Low-molecular weight proteins related to Bence-Jones proteins in multiple myeloma. Science *151:* 1237–1239.

Solomon, A., and Kunkel, H. G. (1967). A "monoclonal" type, low molecular weight protein related to γM-macroglobulins. Amer. J. Med. *42:* 958–967.

Solomon, A., and McLaughlin, C. L. (1970). Biosynthesis of low molecular weight (7S) and high molecular weight (19S) immunoglobulin M. J. Clin. Invest. *49:* 150–160.

Sox, H. C., Jr., and Hood, L. (1970). Attachment of carbohydrate to the variable region of myeloma immunoglobulin light chains. Proc. Natl. Acad. Sci. *66:* 975–982.

Steinberg, I. Z., and Schachman, H. K. (1966). Ultracentrifugation studies with absorption optics. V. Analysis of interacting systems involving macromolecules and small molecules. Biochemistry *5:* 3728–3747.

Stobo, G., and Tomasi, T. B. (1967). A low molecular weight immunoglobulin antigenically related to 19S IgM. J. Clin. Invest. *46:* 1329–1337.

Stone, M. J., and Metzger, H. (1967). The valence of a Waldenstrom macroglobulin antibody and further thoughts on the significance of paraprotein antibodies. Symp. Quant. Biol. *32:* 83–88.

Sutherland, E. W. III, Zimmerman, D. H., and Kern, M. (1970). Synthesis and secretion of γ-globulin by lymph node cells. VIII. Order of synthesis of the interchain disulfide linkages of immunoglobulins. Proc. Natl. Acad. Sci. *66:* 987–994.

Suzuki, T., and Deutsch, H. F. (1967). Dissociation, reaggregation, and subunit structure studies of some human γM-globulins. J. Biol. Chem. *242:* 2725–2738.

Svehag, S. E. (1969). Ultrastructure of human IgM and IgA globulins. Behringwerk-Mitteil. *49:* 74–76.

Svehag, S. E. and Bloth, B. (1970). Ultrastructure of secretory and high-polymer serum immunoglobulin A of human and rabbit origin. Science *168:* 847–849.

Svehag, S.-E., Bloth, B., and Seligmann, M. (1969). Ultrastructure of papain and pepsin digestion fragments of human IgM globulins. J. Exp. Med. *130:* 691–705.

Svehag, S.-E., Chesebro, B., and Bloth, B. (1967). Ultrastructure of γM-immunoglobulin and α-macroglobulin: electron microscopic study. Science 158: 933-936.

Svehag, S.-E, Chesebro, B., and Bloth, B. (1968). Ultrastructure of IgM immuno-globulins. Bull. Soc. Chim. Biol. 50: 1013-1021.

Takahashi, H., Hirai, T., Azuma, T., Hamaguchi, K., and Migita, S. (1970). pH-Dependent conformation change of a Bence-Jones protein. J. Biochem. 67: 795-800.

Terry, W. D., and Ohms, J. (1970). Implications of heavy chain disease protein se-quences for multiple gene theories of immunoglobulin synthesis. Proc. Natl. Acad. Sci. 66: 558-563.

Tomasi, T. B., Jr., and Bienenstock, J. (1968). Secretory immunoglobulins. Adv. Immunol. 9: 1-96.

Tomasi, T. B., Jr., Tan, E. M., Solomon, A., and Prendergast, R. A. (1965). Charac-teristics of an immune system common to certain external secretions. J. Exp. Med. 121: 101-124.

Utsumi, S. (1969). Stepwise cleavage of rabbit immunoglobulin G by papain and isola-tion of four types of biologically active Fc fragments. Biochem. J. 112: 343-355.

Utsumi, S., and Karush, F. (1967). Chemical characterization of the peptic fragment of rabbit γG-immunoglobulin. Biochemistry 6: 2313-2325.

Vaerman, J.-P., and Heremans, J. F. (1969). The immunoglobulins of the dog. II. The immunoglobulins of canine secretions. Immunochemistry 6: 779-786.

Vaerman, J.-P., and Heremans, J. F. (1970). Immunoglobulin A in the pig. I. Pre-liminary characterization of normal pig serum IgA. Int. Arch. Allergy Appl. Immunol. 38: 561-572.

Valentine, R. C., and Green, N. M. (1967). Electron microscopy of an antibody-hapten complex. J. Mol. Biol. 27: 615-617.

Van Eyk, H. G., and Myszkowska, K. (1967). On the localisation of antigenic de-terminants in a Bence Jones protein. Clin. Chim. Acta 18: 101-106.

Warner, C., and Schumaker, V. (1970). Change in conformation of the rabbit γG-immunoglobulin molecule with various chemical treatments. Biochemistry 9: 3040-3046.

Watanabe, S., and Kitagawa, M. (1970). Naturally occurring rabbit antibodies against the tryptic 3.5S and 5S fragments of rabbit IgG. II. Immunochemistry 7: 363-372.

Woods, R., Blumenschein, G. R., and Terry, W. D. (1970). A new type of human γ-heavy chain disease protein: immunochemical and physical characteristics. Immunochemistry 7: 373-381.

Zagyansky, Yu. A., Nezlin, R. S., and Tumerman, L. A. (1969). Flexibility of immuno-globulin G molecules as established by fluorescent polarisation measurements. Immunochemistry 6: 787-800.

Zappacosta, S., Nisonoff, A., and Mandy, W. J. (1968). Mechanism of cleavage of rabbit IgG in two stages by soluble papain and reducing agents. J. Immunol. 100: 1268-1276.

Zolla, S., Buxbaum, J., Franklin, E. C. , and Scharff, M. D. (1970). Synthesis and assembly of immunoglobulins by malignant plasmacytes. I. Myelomas producing γ-chains and light chains. J. Exp. Med. 132: 148-162.

4

THE ANTIBODY BINDING SITE

---

1. Antibody specificity and primary structure

After much exposure to the sequential homologies of protein structures one is made particularly aware of other sequential homologies such as semantic ones. Thus, in the opening sentence of five different papers in the Cold Spring Harbor Symposium on Antibodies (1967) and in Jerne's summary statement of that conference, one may find remarkable homology of opinion:

"There is considerable evidence that the specificity of antibodies is determined by differences in their primary structure (Koshland and Englberger, 1963; Little and Eisen, 1965)."
                                        —Appella and Perham (1967).

"There is evidence that the antibody activity of immunoglobulins is related to their primary sequence (Whitney and Tanford, 1965a, b; Haber, 1964)."
                                        —Press and Piggot (1967).

"The specificity of antibodies appears to result from variations in the amino acid sequence of their constituent polypeptide chains (Koshland and Englberger, 1963; Haber, 1964; Whitney and Tanford, 1965a, b)."
                                        —Waxdal, Konigsberg, and Edelman (1967).

"The activity of an antibody, like that of an enzyme, appears to be determined by its primary structure (Haber, 1964; Whitney and Tanford, 1965a, b)."
                                        —Eisen, Little, Osterland, and Simms (1967).

"It is now generally accepted that the specificity of antibody is consequent to its amino acid sequence and mediated through the effects of sequence on the conformation of the combining site. Evidence for this has been obtained from reversible denaturation experiments on specific antibodies (Haber, 1964; Whitney and Tanford, 1965a, b; Freedman and Sela, 1966)."
                                        —Haber, Richards, Spragg, Austen, Vallotton
                                                and Page (1967).

"Antibody specificity is determined by amino acid sequence (Haber, 1964; Whitney and Tanford, 1965a, b;
Freedman and Sela, 1966)."   —Jerne (1967).

Prior to Haber's experiment of 1964, Buckley, Whitney, and Tanford (1963) had effected the recovery of 75% binding capacity of
rabbit γG Fab fragments—inactivated with the unfolding reagent,
guanidine hydrochloride—by simple dialysis. The rabbit antibodies
had been prepared against bovine serum albumin (BSA) and the Fab-
BSA complexes had been assayed by sedimentation velocity studies
in an analytical ultracentrifuge. What made Haber's experiment so
important was that he not only disrupted noncovalent bonds with
unfolding reagent but also cleaved all of the disulfide bonds with a
reducing agent. Rabbit antibody Fab, specific for ribonuclease,
when treated in this manner and then allowed to refold and reoxi-
dize *in the absence of antigen*, recovered a substantial amount of its
ability to combine specifically with ribonuclease. Whitney and Tanford (1965a, b) completely confirmed those results through use of
rabbit antibody specific for dinitrophenyl (DNP) ligands (Figs. 4-1
and 4-2) as measured by the technique of fluorescence quenching.

Freedman and Sela (1966), by using polyalanylation to keep fragments soluble, went on to demonstrate recovery of binding activity
of *whole* polyalanylated rabbit γG after it had been completely reduced and then reoxidized. Jaton, Klinman, Givol, and Sela (1968)

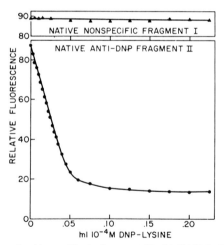

FIG. 4-1. Titration of native antibody fragment II with DNP-lysine. The *upper curve*
is from a control experiment using fragment I from nonspecific γ-globulin. Fluorescence
intensities are reported relative to a standard solution of N-acetyl-L-tryptophanamide.
Differences in the *initial* values of the relative intensity, here and in Figure 4-2, simply
reflect differences in protein concentration. (From Whitney and Tanford, 1965a.)

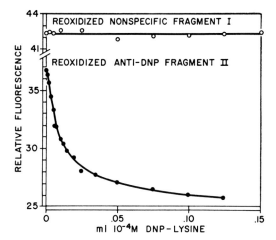

FIG. 4-2. Titration of nonspecific fragment I and antibody fragment II after reoxidation in the presence of a 100-fold excess of DNP-lysine. (The hapten was removed from the reoxidized protein before the titration was carried out.) (From Whitney and Tanford, 1965a.)

later showed that the polyalanylated heavy chain and its Fd fragment from anti-DNP antibody could also be completely unfolded and reduced to destroy antibody activity and then reoxidized to restore binding capacity.

As in a number of enzymes so then in antibodies the classic demonstration of activity dependence upon primary structure was proved. With the proof came the realization that antibody specificity indeed must depend upon sequences of amino acids, not upon the generation of antigen-directed folding of a protein chain and maintenance of stability by noncovalent forces. To appreciate the force of this demonstration, which caused the Cold Spring Harbor conferees to declaim in unison, a review of the previous climate of opinion is needed.

2. Defeat of the Instructionists

Although the active site properties of antibodies and enzymes are closely similar, two other general characteristics distinguish them from each other. The main distinction is that antibodies, unlike enzymes, do not ordinarily participate in synthetic and degradation processes involving the compounds bound to them. The other distinction is concerned with valency. Enzymes are usually regarded as univalent, i.e., molecules with single substrate-binding sites. In fact, chymotrypsin, with serine as an integral member of its binding site, is necessarily univalent since it possesses only one serine residue. Antibodies, on the other hand, are not limited to univalency, but can and most generally do possess at least two binding sites per molecule.

Immunochemists during the 1930s and 1940s and even into the 1950s were in somewhat of a quandary concerning the multivalency of antibodies. On the one hand, they found it difficult to explain precipitation reactions on the basis of univalency, and felt it was therefore most reasonable to accept Marrack's (1938) lattice hypothesis involving multivalency of both antibody and antigen. On the other hand, they found it difficult to believe "that the peptide chain of an antibody molecule during the short period of its formation, which may be only a few seconds, should always react with two identical determinant groups as templates, although other determinant groups were available." Haurowitz (1963), who wrote these words and who had earlier expressed his concern over this point, continued as follows:

"The discovery of the univalence of the Fragments I and II and of their combination by a dithio bond suggests that the formation of I and II precedes their combination by an SS bridge and makes it unnecessary to postulate immunological bivalence of a single peptide chain."

Rothen and Landsteiner (1939) had proposed that the folding of a peptide chain of an antibody in many different ways could account for the large number of antigenic specificities, and Pauling (1940) used this concept in the formulation of his explanation of bivalency formation. He conceived of an antibody globulin as differing from normal globulin only in the two end parts of a coiled polypeptide chain. The two active ends by folding would first assure configurations complementary to an antigen surface and then one end would be freed. The central part of the protein would subsequently fold up into globular form and an antibody molecule with two oppositely placed active sites would result. From this description arose the familiar picture of a structurally rigid antibody molecule—an elongated ellipsoid with two bites symmetrically removed from the longitudinal ends.

It was a remarkable concept for 1940, but its acceptance as a substantially accurate model by others during the subsequent two decades influenced immunochemical thinking to such a degree that it was still rampant when Haber performed his experiments. For example, Pressman, Grossberg, Roholt, Stelos, and Yagi (1963), in their discussions of the chemical nature of antibody molecules were still suggesting that the formation of univalent fragments against the same antigenic moiety, before union as a bivalent entity, might perhaps follow the 1940 mechanism proposed by Pauling.

Jerne's "natural selection theory of antibody formation" had been enunciated in 1955 and Burnet's "clonal selection theory" had been delineated in 1957, but the hard-core "instructionists" still held their ground firmly with the opinion that antibody diversity resulted from antigen diversity, i.e., that the former was instructed by the latter through antigen templates. The selectionists won the battle through the victories of Haber, Whitney and Tanford, and Freedman and Sela.

3. The enzyme analogy

It having been determined that the antibody, like most enzymes, depends upon its primary structure to specify the binding sites in its tertiary structures, logic permits one to pursue the enzyme analogy further to gain additional insight into the nature of an antibody binding site.

A routine procedure for investigating the binding site topology of enzymes involves the identification of specific amino acid residues that participate in the reaction of enzyme with substrate, the determination of amino acid sequences in the various chains that make up the enzyme, and the location of the active amino acids in their proper positions in these chains. From such information patterns of substrate specificity can be constructed, the size of the active region can be determined, and the influence of tertiary protein structure upon the specificity of the primary structures can be inferred. At one time it was widely believed that an active site pattern most certainly should involve a set sequence of amino acids in a given chain of an enzyme. This may still be true in certain cases but certainly not in all. Interaction of substrate with semi-sites at two or more different parts of an enzyme protein molecule, as in the case of α-chymotrypsin, can also occur. Through folding and coiling of a protein molecule these semi-sites are brought adjacent to each other to act as an "active patch" on the protein surface.

The enzymatic properties of α-chymotrypsin, as discussed by D. Koshland (1963), depend upon at least three different amino acids— serine, methionine, and histidine—but these three do not form a sequential pattern in linear array. In fact, the active histidine is present on the B chain of the enzyme while the active methionine and serine are located on the C chain. In three-dimensional orientation, the histidine, methionine, and serine are close to each other, when bound to substrate, with histidine and serine most intimately involved. Methionine can be photooxidized with loss of only two-thirds of enzyme activity, whereas phosphorylation of serine or photooxidation of histidine results in complete loss. Koshland regards the active (surface) methionine, therefore, to reside at the periphery of the active site and, in spite of its nearness to serine (only three residues away), not to be completely involved in substrate binding.

Although photooxidation of histidine had resulted in enzyme activity loss, D. Koshland pointed out that this effect in itself did not establish histidine as a part of the active site. Its position might have been a distant point where its presence might have been necessary to maintain tertiary structure. Modification there might have resulted in protein unfolding and loss of support for the active site. The experiments of Schoellman and Shaw (1962), however, established the direct role of histidine in the enzyme site. By choosing a substrate that was also an alkylating agent they were able to effect specific alkylation of amino acids at the enzyme site where substrate was bound. Alkylated histidine was recovered when the reaction mixture was analyzed. Thus, *affinity labeling* could be used to study enzyme-substrate reactions. Would it, by analogy, prove useful in the study of antibody-antigen reactions as well?

4. Affinity labeling of antibody binding sites

The question was answered affirmatively in the same year, and in the same general way, when Wofsy, Metzger, and Singer (1962) labeled the active site of an antihapten antibody preparation. The antibody was prepared against p-azobenzenearsonate (Rpz) and was reacted with p-(arsonic acid)-benzenediazonium fluoborate (Rpz-FB); the Rpz-FB was preferentially guided to the active site by virtue of its haptenic specificity; side chains in the active site were then made to react with the functional diazonium group; and tyrosine was found to be the principal amino acid at the site that was labeled. The technique was also successfully applied to the 2,4-dinitrophenyl-lysine system (Metzger, Wofsy, and Singer, 1963). The scheme, shown in Figure 4-3, is based upon a conception of Singer and Doolittle (1966).

Tyrosine had previously been implicated in the active sites of various antibodies but not with such convincing evidence as presented by the affinity-labeling experiments. Pressman and Roholt (1961), for example, attempted to label exposed tyrosine in an Fab fragment except those at the active site, which were protected by adsorbed hapten. In essence this would seemingly have provided a mirror image to affinity labeling. Papain-fragmented rabbit anti-p-azobenzoate (anti-Xpz) was purified for Fab fragment, mixed with p-aminobenzoate (Xpa), and iodinated with 6–7 atoms of carrier containing ^{131}I, the iodine reacting mainly with tyrosine residues. Another portion, not protected with Xpa, was iodinated with a similar amount of carrier containing [125]I. The two labeled preparations were then

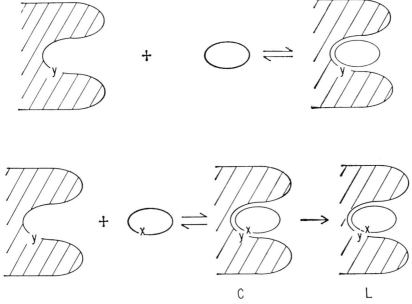

FIG. 4-3. Method of affinity labeling. (*Top*) Typical reversible combination is represented of a hapten with its specific antibody site. (*Bottom*) The hapten, modified by the attachment of the group *x*, first combines reversibly with the specific site to give a complex *C*; while in the site, the group *x* reacts to form a covalent bond with a suitable amino acid residue *y* in the site, yielding the labeled product *L*. (From Singer and Doolittle, 1966.)

freed of unbound iodide and hapten, digested in formic acid with pepsin, and subjected to two-dimensional paper electrophoresis and chromatography to separate the various peptides. Two peptide regions contained relatively more ^{125}I than ^{131}I, compared to the total, while one region contained less. The remaining regions (about 75% of the total) contained equivalent amounts of each. It was suggested at that time that the unbalanced regions represented tyrosine-containing peptides derived from the active site.

But, as D. Koshland (1963), pointed out at the 1962 conference on *Antibody to Enzymes*, the classical interpretation of a "protection" experiment remains in doubt:

"A residue labeled in the absence of hapten and not labeled in the presence of hapten is conventionally presumed to be at the active site. It is possible however that the protection occurs because of a refolding of the molecule and the labeled group is actually a group made less reactive by refolding at some distant position of the tertiary structure."

Indeed, Roholt, Radzimski, and Pressman (1963) found that when they repeated their experiments (except this time also to separate the light and heavy chains prior to final digestion for peptides) the peptides with unbalanced ratios of the two isotopes were contained wholly in the light chains!

The bulk of present evidence points to the heavy chains as the main center for the active site but it does not exclude light chains by any means. Fleischman, Pain, and Porter (1962) obtained the first substantial indication that the heavy chains, when separated by mild reduction from the light chains, carried with them a large share of the binding activity for protein. Metzger and Singer (1963), using a rabbit antibody to dinitrophenyl-lysine, found that when the antibody was mildly reduced in the presence of hapten and separated into heavy and light chains, the hapten-binding capacity was again wholly associated with heavy chains. In this case, however, some of the light chains remained with the heavy chain-hapten fraction, reducing the yield of free light chains by one-third. No hapten was associated with light chains alone.

Utsumi and Karush (1964) prepared from purified antihapten antibody a mildly reduced and alkylated rabbit IgG that retained its antihapten activity, and then separated it carefully into its subunits by molecular-sieve filtration in the presence of a neutral and dilute detergent. Immunological activity was present in the heavy chains as revealed by binding of the homologous hapten during equilibrium dialysis. Negative energy of binding was 8.28 kcal/mole, a loss of only 13% from that of original reduced and alkylated antibody. The authors concluded tentatively:

"... that the antibody-combining region is exclusively associated with the A [heavy] chain and that the stated difference [13% loss] was probably due to aggregation and/or denaturation of the A chain. It is suggested that the B [light] chain serves to prevent these effects and thereby indirectly contributes to the immunologic reactivity. The apparent partial specificity of the B chain in enhancing the activity of the isolated A chain, reported by others, is attributed to a selection among the varieties of B chain of those which are most appropriate for complex formation with that portion of the A chain whose conformation is associated with its specific reactivity."

The partial specificity of the light chains (B chains in the quotation) referred to by Utsumi and Karush is exemplified by the work of Edelman, Benacerraf, and Ovary (1963). Antibodies were prepared in guinea pigs against a number of antigens and were then purified by dissociation from specific precipitates, reduced, alkylated, and separated by zone electrophoresis in 8 M urea at pH 3.5. A distinctive pattern of light chains was obtained for each type of antigen and confirmed their previous view that light chain patterns of guinea pig antibodies of widely different specificities were different. These differences persisted from animal to animal and were therefore not due to variations among the guinea pigs themselves.

To bring the problem around full circle, Metzger, Wofsy, and Singer (1964) applied the technique of affinity labeling to the question of active site participation by heavy vs. light chains. *They found specifically labeled tyrosines, representative of the combining site, in both types of chains.* It would appear that the total active patch of an antibody surface is composed of semi-sites from two different chains, as in the case of chymotrypsin, but with the major binding energy contribution stemming from the heavy chain semi-site pattern.

5. Location of antibody binding site by affinity labeling

Follow-up affinity-labeling studies by Fenton and Singer (1965) with the positively charged p-azophenyltrimethylammonium (Apz) hapten, as compared with negatively charged p-azophenylarsonate (Rpz), gave essentially the same results—label present on both heavy and light chains, tyrosine implicated, and ratio of labeling of heavy and light chains near 2:1. The conclusion was drawn that tyrosine must be in a relatively fixed position and that its orientation must be such that it is placed within the active sites of antibodies of different specificities. Additional work (Good, Traylor, and Singer, 1967; Singer, Slobin, Thorpe, and Fenton, 1967; Good, Ovary, and Singer, 1968), utilizing the radioactive tritiated derivative, [^{3}H]m-nitrobenzenediazonium fluo(ro)borate (Traylor and Singer, 1967), demonstrated that not only in antibodies of rabbits but also in those of sheep, guinea pigs, and mice the same conclusion could be drawn. Even the two-to-one labeling of heavy and light chains was felt to be adequately borne out in spite of the actual range of 1.3 to 4.5. The average at least was 2.4.

By 1968 Singer and Thorpe were ready to conclude:

"Our results (1) demonstrate that the labeled residues are indeed unique; (2) establish that the variable segment of the L chain is directly involved in forming the antibody active site; (3) strongly suggest that the labeled tyrosine is residue 86 from the amino-terminal end of the L chain; and (4) lead to the suggestion that in the Fab fragment (and, in particular,

in the active site) of each half of an IgG molecule, the H
and L chains are structurally related by a dyad axis of
pseudosymmetry." (Fig. 4-4.)

Kennel and Singer (1970), while adding yet another haptenic example,
trinitrophenyl (TNP) groups, to the list of affinity labeled sites, re-
asserted their belief in position 86 as the most likely.

One will recall that the "insertion hypothesis" of Wu and Kabat
(1970) associates the complementarity region with the light chain
segments, 24–34 and 89–97, that are linked by cysteines I_{23} and II_{88}.
The tyrosine in position 86 represents an intermediate invariant
position that occurs in 20/20 sequenced light chains—6 κ_I, 2 κ_{II}, 4
κ_{III}, 2 λ_I, 1 λ_{II}, 2 λ_{IV}, and 1 λ_V from human light chains; 1 κ_I and 1 κ_{II}
from mouse light chains. Although there are also tyrosines in 16/20
of these same light chains at position 87, 13/17 at position 36, and
13/14 at position 49, the likelihood of position 86 involvement is considered to be greatest based upon light-heavy linked peptide analy-

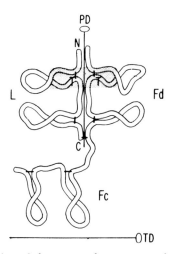

FIG. 4-4. Representation of the proposed symmetry relationships in each half of
an IgG immunoglobulin molecule. (*TD* represents the true dyad axis, which presumably relates the two identical halves of the whole molecule.) The L chain and Fd
fragment of the H chain are related by a dyad axis of pseudosymmetry (*PD*). *N* and *C*
refer to the amino- and carboxyl-terminals, respectively, of the L chain. The *solid bars*
between chains and between chain segments indicate the disulfide bridges within the
half molecule. The *stippled region* very schematically represents the Ab active site
of the half molecule; it is intended to show the general location of the active site and
illustrate the proposal that the *PD* axis relates the portions of the active site contributed by the L and H chains. The *T* symbols denote the tyrosine residues on the
L and H chains, which, it is proposed, are the unique residues that become affinity-
labeled in the active sites. (From Singer and Thorpe, 1968.)

sis and upon the nearest-neighbor analysis of Thorpe and Singer
(1969). A look at heavy chain positions of tyrosine reveals that a
relatively invariant tyrosine at position 94 (Eu numbering), just in
advance of the second segment of the insertion-deletion region of
heavy chain hypervariability, exists in human Eu, Daw, Cor, Ou,
and He human heavy chains as well as in rabbit γG heavy chain and
that an adjacent tyrosine resides at position 95 in all the human
chains as well. There is, however, no direct proof as yet of the actual
residues involved; in fact, Franek (1969) has implicated a different
region in the case of affinity labeled pig anti-DNP, a position somewhere between 22 and 47 on λ-chains. In his experiments a 2:1 ratio
between heavy and light chains was obtained also, once again showing the preferential labeling of the heavy chain moiety.

Singer and Doolittle (1966) likened the antibody binding site to an
enzyme site in which both conservative and variable regions are also
implicated. For example, in the case of trypsin and chymotrypsin
both share a conservative region of binding to peptides but differ in
their variable regions (Fig. 4-5). In the case of anti-Rpz and anti-Apz
both share a conservative region of binding to the phenyl group but
differ in their variable region specificities for the negatively charged
arsonate and positively charged phenyltrimethylammonium regions.
Such an extension of the enzyme analogy implies a function for the
tyrosine residue which is not yet in evidence. It will be interesting in

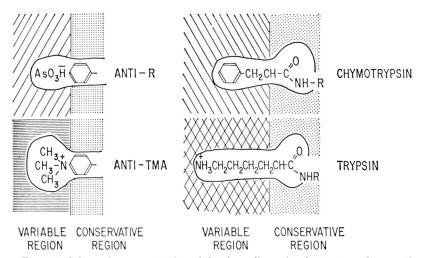

FIG. 4-5. Schematic representation of the three-dimensional structure of two antibody and the two enzyme active sites in which specific function is achieved by the
juxtaposition of a region of variable composition and structure to a conservative region
of essentially constant composition and structure. (From Singer and Doolittle, 1966.)

the years to come, as active site topology becomes unveiled, to find out just how big a role invariant tyrosine-86 actually does play.

That the role is not universal or paramount is seen in the experiments carried out by Wofsy and colleagues (Wofsy, Kimura, Bing, and Parker, 1967; Wofsy, Klinman, and Karush, 1967; Wofsy and Parker, 1967). o-Diazoniumphenyl glycosides were developed as affinity labeling reagents for antibodies against p-azophenyl-β-lactoside (anti-Lac) and p-azophenyl-β-galactoside (anti-Gal). The structure of o-diazoniumphenyl-β-lactoside (OD-Lac), the affinity label for anti-Lac, shows that the reactive group has a diazonium function just as in the case of the labels for the antiphenyl-type antibodies; moreover, the phenylglycosidic link has enough rotational freedom to allow the diazonium group to approach the adjacent sugar residue in a number of ways. Analysis of affinity labeled rabbit anti-Lac and anti-Gal antibodies showed labeled peptide patterns that were

OD-Lac

nearly identical involving both heavy and light chains and involving tyrosine. But for the fact that the labeling patterns were different than for anti-DNP antibodies it would have appeared that the ideas of Singer were completely supported. Going on to equine anti-β-lactoside antibodies Wofsy, Klinman, and Karush (1967) obtained labeling patterns and azospectra different yet from rabbit antibodies, that left tyrosine completely out of the picture, and that implicated histidine instead. The results were the same whether γG or γT immunoglobulins of the horse were involved. The only common feature to all other affinity labeling results was the participation of both heavy and light chains in the active site region. Wofsy and Parker (1967) concluded:

"Until fairly recently, the hope implicit in the study of antibody sites was that, despite the many manifestations of antibody heterogeneity, there would be found a uniformity of amino acid sequence in the peptides comprising the active sites of antibodies of a given specificity. While this appears naive in the light of present knowledge, there do seem to be subsets of H and L chains which may be differentiated on the basis of their suitability for one or another kind of ligand binding."

Koyama, Grossberg, and Pressman (1968) investigated the variability of affinity labeling results among seven different rabbit anti-Rpz antisera, and found that five had extensive labeling on tyrosine only, that one had a mixed pattern involving tyrosine and a different residue, probably histidine, and that one exhibited no evidence of labeling of any sort. From these results one would conclude that although the technique of affinity labeling had most certainly established the neighborhood of complementarity it had not yet been able to prove, on its own, the intimate and diverse nature of binding *per se* and that other affinity labels and other techniques altogether were needed to establish the nature of points of contact. The photolyzable diazoketones of Converse and Richards (1969) may prove useful in this regard, but even more so may be the spectral shifts associated with fluorescent probes and tryptophan fluorescence.

6. Tryptophan in antibody binding sites

Little and Eisen (1967) showed that anti-DNP and anti-TNP antibodies from rabbit, guinea pig, goat, and horse all exhibited spectral shifts associated with tryptophan whenever specific binding was involved. After controlling for possible effects of binding upon distant tryptophan residues, these investigators found ample evidence for tryptophan within or near the binding sites themselves. Little, Border, and Freidin (1969) then obtained essentially the same results for rabbit anti-2,6-DNP as had been obtained earlier for anti-2,4-DNP and anti-2,4,6-TNP. Basing their experimental design upon these preliminary findings Rubinstein and Little (1970) decided to investigate the association between active site tryptophan residues and haptens in a systematic way. Polynitrobenzene compounds had been known to have a high affinity for electrons while tryptophan, among all amino acid residues, had been known to have the greatest ability to serve as an electron donor; moreover, charge-transfer complex formation had been suggested to account for the previously observed red shifts in the absorbance spectra of DNP and TNP as the ligands formed complexes with antibodies. Rubinstein and Little decided, therefore, to find out what kind of spectral data might be associated with folic acid in the specific interaction with antifolate antibodies. Here was a determinant that was very well known as a good electron acceptor and as a ligand in the formation of complexes with a num-

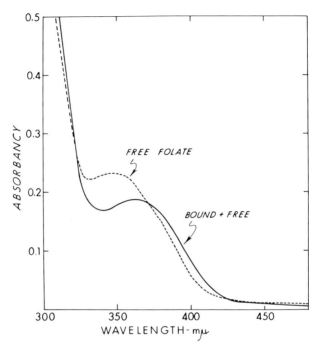

FIG. 4-6. Absorbance spectra of free and antibody-bound folic acid. The *dotted curve* was obtained with 2.72×10^{-5} M folic acid at 4°C, in buffered saline in a Cary Model 14 spectrophotometer equipped with a temperature-controlled cell housing. The solid curve was obtained with the same concentration of folate mixed with 1.38×10^{-5} M antifolate antibodies isolated from the early antiserum pool. The λ_{max} of free folate was 350 mμ and the λ_{max} of the solid curve (bound + free) was 362–363 mμ. (From Rubinstein and Little, 1970).

ber of electron donors. Would specific antibodies formed against it produce the same hypsochromic-bathochromic changes in folate absorbance spectra during binding as had been seen with the polynitrobenzene haptens? As the curves in Figure 4-6 indicate, there

pteridine portion | p-aminobenzoylglutamic acid portion

Folic Acid

was indeed the expected spectral shift due to binding. Another question was raised. Would quenching of antibody (tryptophan) fluorescence result from ligand binding by analogs of folic acid (so-called "antifolates" but not to be confused here with antibodies) in view of the direct relationship often observed between the electron affinity of a ligand molecule and ability to accept excitation energy transfer? The positive results obtained with pteroic acid, pteridine-6-carboxylic acid, and methotrexate are shown in Figure 4-7. Dihydrofolic acid produced a quenching effect superimposable with that of methotrexate. As an additional indication that the pteridine moiety of folic acid was involved, p-aminobenzoylglutamic acid failed to produce any quenching nor would it inhibit the precipitation of antifolate antibodies (Table 4-1).

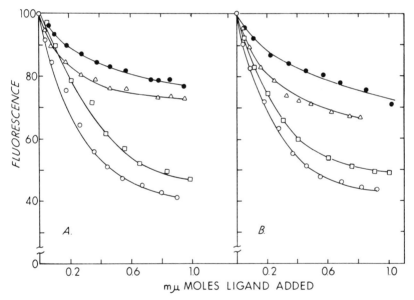

FIG. 4-7. Fluorescence quenching of antibodies isolated from antiserum pools obtained 48 days (A) or 7.5 months (B) after initial immunization of a single group of rabbits. The ligands employed were folic acid (O), pteroic acid (□), pteridine-6-carboxylic acid (△), and methotrexate (●). Each titration was obtained with 1-ml aliquots of antibody at 40–50 μg/ml in buffered saline at 0–2°C. Fluorescence values have been corrected for solvent fluorescence and for volume change due to ligand addition. Each curve is the average obtained from duplicate titrations. When dihydrofolic acid was used as a ligand in similar titrations, the quenching curves obtained were nearly superimposable with those shown above for methotrexate. (From Rubinstein and Little, 1970.)

TABLE 4-1

Hapten Inhibition of Precipitation of Antifolate Antibodies and Folate-HSA

Inhibiting Hapten (0.01 M)	Amount of Antibody Precipitated	Inhibition
	mg	*%*
None	0.473	0
p-Aminobenzoylglutamic acid	0.426	10
Pteridine-6-carboxylic acid	0.270	43
Folic acid	0.000	100

(From Rubinstein and Little, 1970.)

7. Conformational changes in binding site due to ligand binding

In continuation of the enzyme analogy the question remains whether, for each type of enzyme (and, presumably, each type of antibody), the "active patch" is preformed in a somewhat rigid structure or whether the semi-sites are brought into proper orientation at the time of substrate interaction. In the case of phosphoglucomutase, D. Koshland (1963) concluded that protein conformation took place at the time of substrate interaction and that the active site was flexible, i.e., that semi-sites were brought into juxtaposition as a result of binding to substrate. If an "active patch" is composed of semi-sites from different parts of a molecule and yet is more or less rigid and preformed, then tertiary structures (those involved in protein folding and coiling) must play a part in determining specificity. Such structures would determine the preformed orientation of the various parts of the "active patch."

Any substantial conformational rearrangement at the time of interaction, necessitated by flexibility of active site substructures, would require additional activation energy and heat of reaction, and would result in lower specific rate reaction constants than those for preformed active site patterns. In the case of antibodies reactive with DNP haptens, preformed active sites would appear to be indicated, for this particular antibody-hapten reaction exemplifies one of the fastest bimolecular reactions in homogeneous solution known to immunochemistry. With a rate constant approaching 1×10^7 M^{-1} sec^{-1} and yet with a required activation energy of only 4 kcal/mole, any major conformational change during the reaction of anti-DNP with DNP would certainly be contraindicated (L. Day, Sturtevant, and Singer, 1963).

As will be discussed more thoroughly in Chapter 6, the measurement of the velocity of forward reactions between antibodies and their antigenic counterparts is difficult to obtain except in very special cases. Thus, it is not yet possible to generalize that all antigen-antibody reactions have such high rate constants as their limit or that all reactions require such minimal activation energies and, therefore, to further generalize that the active sites of all antibodies are preformed and presumably rigid. One can only say that this is true in all the cases studied—in anti-DNP, for example, and also in anti-benzenearsonate (anti-Rp). In the latter case Froese, Sehon, and Eigen (1962) obtained a value of 2×10^7 M^{-1} sec^{-1} as the limiting rate constant, which again is extremely high. Even in these instances there is a display of heterogeneity in kinetic behavior which appears to be associated with heterogeneity among the active sites of individual molecules. This would open the possibility that some sites are preformed and rigid while others, in the same population, are fully formed only when antigen is present but otherwise flexible and disunited.

Three complications make investigations along these lines difficult. The first is that most antibody-hapten reactions are measured by establishment of equilibrium conditions between the forward bimolecular reactions and a reverse monomolecular dissociation. In the first-order reverse dissociation of DNP-anti-DNP the rate constant is only 1 sec^{-1} while that of Rp-anti-Rp is 50 sec^{-1}. Thus, while the rate of combination in each system is nearly the same, the equilibrium constants of the two differ by two orders of magnitude. Heterogeneity of rate constants for a given system is best revealed by studying equilibrium conditions, but then it is not known whether such heterogeneity expresses a distribution among both forward and reverse rate constants or primarily in just one direction.

The second complication arises from the varied nature of antigens that combine with their respective antibodies. While many haptenic groups are relatively small, the reactive determinant groups of many known antigens are considerably larger with perhaps as many as six linked organic residues participating in the reaction with certain active antibody sites. Under such circumstances one could visualize a range of areas for the active patch of an antibody surface to accommodate a range of sizes of antigenic determinant groups. Preformed semi-sites may perhaps react effectively with small haptenic groups as though they were completed sites, whereas conformation of full-sized active sites may have to take place, subsequent to semi-site reaction, before antibodies can bind effectively with larger complex determinant groups.

The third complication has less to do with antibody than with antigen. It involves the rate of diffusion of antibody and antigen toward each other. If every collision of reactants resulted in immediate union then the rate of diffusion would be the rate-limiting step.

For small uncharged haptens with spherical symmetry, diffusion would limit the rate constant to 10^9 M^{-1} sec^{-1} and would require an energy (apparent activation energy) of 4–5 kcal/mole to overcome solvent viscosity (L. Day et al., 1963). Since the reactions of anti-DNP and of anti-Rp with their respective haptens approached but did not reach this limit, one presumes that diffusion was not rate-limiting in these instances. Talmage and Cann (1961) have suggested that since the Q_{10} for certain antigen-antibody reactions is 1.4 and since the Q_{10} for diffusion processes is also about 1.4, such reactions may be diffusion-controlled. (Q_{10} is the increase in rate of reactant association as temperature is increased in increments of 10°C from 0° to 40°C.)

Tsuji, Davis, and Donald (1966) approached the problem from a different point of view. Since high pressures were known to oppose biochemical processes leading to increases in volume, e.g., protein denaturation, they should also oppose any antigen-antibody interaction that involved large conformational increases in volume. Campbell and Johnson (1946) had already shown that a pressure of 667 atmospheres would inhibit the secondary process of immune precipitation between rabbit anti-Rpz antibodies and Rpz-sheep serum conjugate, but their experiment had not involved a measurement of primary binding between Fab and ligand. Casting about for a functional antigen that could be followed in its primary binding with antibody through functional inhibition, that could be measured visibly *when it was not interacting with antibody*, and that would be unaffected in its function under high pressure, Tsuji et al. chose the enzyme, cypridina luciferase from the marine ostracod crustacean, *Cypridina hilgendorfi*. Harvey and Deitrick (1930) had long ago shown that rabbit antibodies could be made against the enzymes which would inhibit its function of catalyzing the oxidation of luciferin in the presence of O_2 and thus of inhibiting the visible emission of blue light. Tsuji and Davis (1959) and Tsuji, Davis, and Gindler (1962) had, themselves, studied the quantitative aspects of luciferase-antiluciferase interaction. In a specially designed high pressure bomb and reaction cell and with a ball bearing to break the cover glass separating reactants upon inversion of the cell, only a small volume change was obtained, 9–12 ml/mole, as measured by an inhibiting pressure that had to reach 1,000 atmospheres. A volume change of 60–100 ml/mole had previously been observed for extensive conformational changes such as thermal denaturation of proteins or inactivation of enzymes. The small volume change was taken to mean that little conformational change had occurred and that the combining sites were readily accessible.

The small volume changes that do accompany antigen-antibody interaction were looked at more closely by Ohta, Gill, and Leung (1970) through the use of the very sensitive dilatometric technique. The reaction device consisted of an inverted, asymmetrical V-tube with its long arm (62 × 13 mm) containing antibody and its other arm (53 × 13 mm) containing antigen. At the apex, attached through a ground glass joint, was a precision bore capillary (0.2685 μl/cm) that contained water-saturated kerosene. Antigen and antibody were mixed by tilting and the volume change, at 30.00 ± 0.0005°C, was measured by a precision cathetometer. The higher the affinity of antibody for antigen (DNP-lysine) the greater the volume change, an effect that was the same per Fab region whether intact immunoglobulin or Fab fragment was used in the measurement (Fig. 4-8). It was the conclusion of the authors that the most probable reason for the volume change was that of intermolecular hydrophobic interactions, that the least likely was charge neutralization, and that only a small contribution was due to conformational changes in Fab. Nevertheless, the major if not exclusive source of volume changes did lie in each Fab fragment independent of its hinged attachment to Fc.

Inherent in the structural model of γG which Feinstein and Rowe (1965) presented, on the basis of their electron microscope observations, was the assumption that a conformational change would take place when antibody interacted with antigen. The two independent Fab regions were supposed to "click-open," i.e., the legs of the Y-shaped molecule were expected to separate to an open position from a normally closed one. Warner and Schumaker (1970) put the hypothesis to a critical test through the technique of differential sedimentation. Should the "click-open" hypothesis be correct then an increase in frictional coefficient and a decrease in sedimentation coefficient would be expected as an antibody combined with hapten and changed its conformation to the open configuration. Rabbit antilactoside antibody not only did not exhibit a "click-open" response upon exposure to lactoside hapten, but it assumed an even more compact configuration than before as if it had "clicked shut." In the case of monovalent glycine-DNP hapten Warner, Schumaker, and Karush (1970) observed no conformational change in anti-DNP in either direction; with a divalent hapten, α, ϵ-2,4-DNP-lysine or 2,4-DNP-cysteine, no more than a 1% conformational change was obtained.

The conclusion that the antibody binding site is open and freely accessible at least to haptenic moieties seems to be in order, and it appears to hold whether the site is within an intact globulin or Fab fragment. In the presence of chaotropic ions such as chloride,

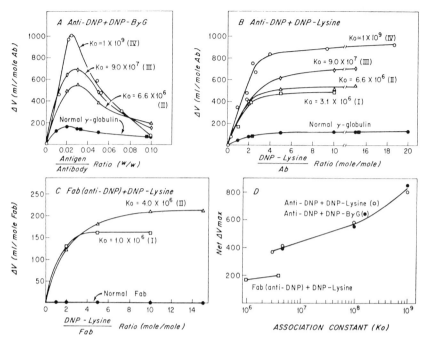

FIG. 4-8. (A) Volume changes accompanying the reactions between purified anti-DNP antibody and DNP-bovine γ-globulin. The amount of antigen added at the maximum of the curve was the same as that added at the maximum of the precipitin curve. (B) The volume change accompanying the reaction between purified anti-DNP antibody and DNP-lysine. The antibody preparation number is given in parentheses after the association constant. Normal γ-globulin (19 mg) was used in the control reaction. (C) The volume changes accompanying the reaction between the Fab fragment of purified anti-DNP antibody and DNP-lysine. The number of the antibody preparation from which the Fab fragment was prepared is given in parentheses after the association constant. The control Fab fragment was prepared from normal γ-globulin (15 mg). The value of ΔV with the normal Fab fragment at a molar rate was also 0. In addition, mixing the normal Fab fragment and DNP-BγG over the Ag/Fab (w/w) range 0–0.15 did not cause any change. (D) the net maximal volume change as a function of the association constant for the reactions between anti-DNP antibody and DNP-lysine or DNP-BγG and for the reaction between the Fab fragment of anti-DNP antibody and DNP-lysine. (From Ohta, Gill, and Leung, 1970.)

perchlorate, and thiocyanate the sites also seem to be relatively open to larger antigens such as egg albumin (Levison, Kierszenbaum, and Dandliker, 1970), and simple second-order rate reaction law prevails whether the antibodies are intact or present as Fab. An interesting phenomenon occurs at the other end of the Hofmeister series, however, in media containing phosphate, sulfate, fluoride, etc. Whereas the interaction of egg albumin with Fab remains simple second order, the bivalent antibody-egg albumin reaction follows a more complicated rate course. The most plausible and fitting reaction mechanism in solutions containing non-chaotropic anions involves an initial rapid second-order reaction between an encounter pair with loose weak binding, few contact points, and many interdispersed solvent molecules, and then a slow unimolecular process with gradual realignment, release of solvent molecules, and higher energy involvement. Levison *et al.*, in accounting for this departure from second-order behavior, explained that a bivalent antibody molecule with its high degree of asymmetric flexibility would be much more sensitive to the intramolecular folding and associative effects of high-charge density anions than the more globular univalent Fab portions.

Cathou and Haber (1967) were more concerned with the intrasite conformation of a single Fab portion in its interaction with a simple hapten as exemplified by the ε-DNP-lysine-anti-DNP complex. They reasoned that if the amino acids responsible for binding were mainly sequential then the effect of unfolding in 4 M guanidine hydrochloride, as measured by ultraviolet optical rotatory dispersion, would not be very different from the unbound state. As a matter of fact, however, they found that the binding of hapten to antibody stabilized the tertiary structure and caused a reduction in the number of possible unfolded conformations. They could conclude only that the amino acid residues involved in a binding site *even to a simple hapten* were located in at least several widely separated areas of Fab and were brought into close spatial relationship by the molecular conformation—ordered by the primary structure, expressed by the tertiary structure, and stabilized by the filled complementation structure.

By measuring circular dichroism and the intrinsic tryptophan fluorescence of Fab, Cathou and Werner (1970) were able to study the effect of hapten stabilization on antibody site conformation in even greater detail. The circular dichroism of native forms would show bands that were very sensitive to the conformational state, and which could be eliminated one by one by guanidine hydrochloride over a period of 5 hr. The presence of hapten stabilized these bands— indicators of intact tertiary structure—and, by strong inference, helped maintain the compactness of the molecule, its rigidity, and the environmental asymmetry. Once again there was a very firm indication that particular amino acids in the binding site that were participating in hapten binding were located in several nonconsecutive portions of the polypeptide chains which were brought into close spatial relationship by the native molecular conformation. A

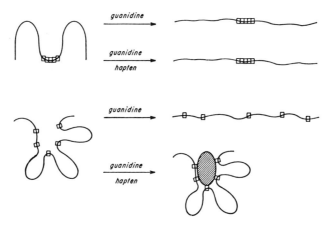

Fɪɢ. 4-9. Schematic models of two possible configurations of the antibody combining site and the effects of Gd·HCl denaturation on each. The *small blocks* represent contact amino acids. The number and size of these are not to be taken literally.
The *large oval* in the lower figure represents hapten. In the *upper set* of figures, the
site is composed of several vicinal amino acids along a single polypeptide chain.
The presence of hapten has no effect on the course of denaturation. In the *lower set*
of figures, the amino acids comprising the binding site are sequentially separated
along the length of the polypeptide chain(s). One or both chains could contribute contact amino acids. The presence of hapten in the site stabilizes this conformation.
(From Cathou and Werner, 1970.)

schematic model was drawn to illustrate the effect (Fig. 4-9) with
heavy chain alone. Of course, light chain participation could also
be implied.

8. Size of antibody sites—lower and upper limits—as estimated by antigen accommodation

One of the classical experiments in immunochemistry that still
enters into lively discussions concerning antibody structure is that of
Landsteiner and van der Scheer (1938). Contained therein are data
related to antigenic specificity, to antibody heterogeneity, and to
the effective lower limit of the size of antibody sites. Landsteiner and
van der Scheer prepared the complex hapten, *sym*-aminoisophthalyl-
glycineleucine (GIL), in which the two amino acids extended outward in opposite directions from the central aminophenyl group:

$$HOOC-CH_2-NH-CO-\underset{NH_2}{\underset{|}{\bigcirc}}-CO-NH-\underset{\underset{CH_2-CH(CH_3)_2}{|}}{\overset{\overset{COOH}{|}}{CH}}$$

By attaching the hapten to the washed stromata of horse red blood cells through a diazo link to the central phenyl group of the hapten, and by immunizing rabbits with azostromata, antisera were obtained that would precipitate the hapten diazotized to otherwise nonreactive chicken serum protein.

Two other azostromata were also prepared, one with *m*-aminobenzoylglycine (G) and the other with *m*-aminobenzoylleucine (L), to be used as insoluble adsorbents for removing antibodies from the test antisera. G and L were also diazotized to chicken serum protein to be used as precipitating antigens in the same way as GIL-serum:

$$HOOC{-}CH_2{-}NH{-}CO{-}\overset{\overset{\displaystyle NH_2}{|}}{\bigcirc}\qquad \overset{\overset{\displaystyle NH_2}{|}}{\bigcirc}{-}CO{-}NH{-}\overset{\overset{\displaystyle COOH}{|}}{CH}$$

$$CH_2{-}CH(CH_3)_2$$

G   L

It can be seen in Table 4-2 that adsorption with G-azostromata removed antibodies that would precipitate with G-azoprotein but left antibodies that would precipitate with L-azoprotein; likewise, that adsorption with L-azostromata removed antibodies that would precipitate with L-azoprotein but left antibodies that would precipitate with G-azoprotein. Adsorption with a mixture of G- and L-azostromata removed both types of precipitating antibodies simultaneously. Adsorptions with either azostromata alone, moreover, did not affect antibody precipitation with GIL-azoprotein. Only when adsorption with combined G- and L-azostromata was carried out did the antiserum show nearly complete loss of precipitating power with GIL-azoprotein.

Landsteiner and van der Scheer concluded that these experiments as well as similar ones with succinic and phenylarsenic acid residues "definitely establish the existence of cases in which discrete antibodies are formed that are individually directed towards separate determinant groups in one substance, even though it be of small molecular size and the determinant groups rather closely adjoining." The authors commented further upon the results and contrasted them with data obtained with "multiple" antibodies (Landsteiner and van der Scheer, 1936):

"The failure of repeated absorption with an antigen which contains only one of the two groupings, to effect a significant diminution of the antibody reacting with the other group, is

TABLE 4-2

Effects of Adsorption of Rabbit Anti-GIL-Azostromata (Horse) with G- and L-Azostromata upon Precipitation with GIL-, G-, and L-Azoproteins

Absorbing Azostromata (Horse)	Test Azoprotein (chicken)	Unabsorbed*	Absorbed Once	Absorbed Twice	Absorbed Three Times
G	GIL	+ + + ±	+ + + ±	+ + + ±	+ + + ±
	G	+	0	0	0
	L	+ + ±	+ + ±	+ + ±	+ + ±
L	GIL	+ + + ±	+ + ±	+ +	+ +
	G	+	+	+	+
	L	+ + ±†	0	0	0
G + L	GIL	+ + + ±	+ ±	±	*tr*
	G	+	0	0	0
	L	+ + ±	tr	0	0

* Intensity of reactions were graded: 0, faint trace, trace (tr), *trace (tr)*, ±, +, + ±, + +, + + ±, + + +, + + + ±, + + + +. Overnight readings only are given above although 1-hour readings were also given in the original paper.

† This value appeared as "0" in the original paper and was also reproduced as such in Landsteiner's (1936) book, Table 36. It obviously was a typographical error in the original article that was carried over uncorrected in the book. A zero reading would mean that no antibody had reacted with L from the unabsorbed serum, which, of course, would have made the whole paper and discussion pointless. The authors state in the text that "the separation of two sorts of antibodies in GIL serum by absorption is demonstrated . . ., there being stronger reactions on the leucine than on the glycine moiety."

(Constructed from Landsteiner and van der Scheer, 1938.)

proof for the serological kinship between the two antibodies demonstrated. It is in contrast to the behavior of multiple but related antibodies developed through the stimulus of a single determinant structure, where continued absorption with a reacting heterologous antigen was often seen to exhaust the immune serum completely."

Campbell and Bulman (1954) calculated the area of an active patch of an anti-GIL antibody surface that would be most complementary to the two classes of GIL determinants and obtained a value of 700 $Å^2$. What made the situation confusing was their suggestion that this might fix the upper limit of the combining site. That it did so for anti-GIL antibodies in the sera that Landsteiner and van der Scheer used is unquestionable. Other discussants, however, tried to generalize that perhaps this was the upper limit of all antibodies and that heterogeneity within a population of antibodies for various adjacent groupings on an antigen would explain seemingly larger combining sites.

Levine (1963), however, demonstrated larger combining sites in rabbit antibody to benzylpenicilloyl (BPO) groups in a Landsteiner-van der Scheer type of experiment. The BPO groups have a phenyl-acetylamine side and a thiazolidine-carboxylic acid side symmetrical to a midway carboxyl group. The carboxyl reacts with the ε-amino groups of lysine in polylysine to produce a haptenic structure quite similar in size and shape to GIL-azostromata.

BPO-lysine

The question was raised whether rabbit antisera would form only to the phenylacetylamine end or to the thiazolidinecarboxylic acid end or perhaps form against intermediate portions thereof. The results quite conclusively showed, even after considerations of heterogeneity had been made, that the pool of six rabbit sera against BPO-rabbit normal serum and tested with BPO-polylysine contained no antibodies against end structures but rather had antibodies encompassing the entire BPO group, lysine side chain, and even adjacent peptides of the carrier protein. It was clear that the active patch of antibody surface in this instance was much greater than 700 $Å^2$. Isliker (1962), on the other hand, calculated on the basis of serologically active fragments that an active surface patch need be only 100–200 $Å^2$. Assuming a total surface area of 26,000 $Å^2$, the active site would in this case represent only 0.4–0.7% of the total protein surface. Since antibody activity can be inhibited by substances that bind with much less than the total active site, the fact that an antibody binds with a small grouping does not delineate the site as being necessarily small. The GIL type of experiment is therefore important in that it presents a potential haptenic grouping slightly larger than can ordinarily accomodate antibody. One has little control over production of antibodies with active sites of a certain size, and one can only take the smallest upper limit described for individual antibody preparations (such as Isliker's 100–200 $Å^2$) as descriptive of the smallest total area that can be attained. Kabat (1961) has emphasized this point—that while available data can establish an upper limit for the complementary area of the antibody combining site, they "provide no insight into how small an antibody cavity can be."

Kreiter and Pressman (1964) reopened the question of heterogeneity among anti-GIL antibodies once more in experiments designed to separate the various antibody species—anti-G, anti-L, and anti-GIL—and to test their cross-reactivity with G, L, and/or GIL. They concluded that although a major part of the binding energy of hapten and antibody was supplied by either leucine or glycine, the opposite amino acid did contribute to the binding energy to a certain extent. Their view, therefore, was that the combining site was directed against a large part of the immunizing hapten. Such conclusions would be valid only for the Kreiter-Pressman sera and not necessarily for the Landsteiner-van der Scheer sera. Because of heterogeneity in reactivity from one serum to the next, it is impossible to prove or disprove a point made with one serum by testing the reaction with another.

In reverse direction Atsumi, Nishada, Kinoshita, Shibata, and Horiuchi (1967) reopened the question of heterogeneity among anti-benzylpenicilloyl antibodies. By preparing columns of immunoadsorbents from benzylpencilloyl groups attached to bisdiazotized benzidine—bovine γ-globulin complexes, by using a series of nine different BPO analogs as eluants (applied in different sequences from one run to the next), and by employing a very definitive and excellent experimental design, these workers were able to establish that the antibodies obtained from a given single rabbit consist of at least five antibody populations adopted to different parts of the BPO molecule. Represented were some antibodies with a preference for 6-acetyl-aminopenicilloic acid, some for phenlyacetic acid, some for phenylacetylglycine, some for benzylpenicilloic acid, and some for benzyl-penicilloyl-ε-aminocaproic acid. These specificities for end-group structures stand in marked contrast to Levine's results. All results together account for another example in the sometimes nightmarish realm of heterogeneity.

Landsteiner and van der Scheer (1932, 1934), in their initial investigations on the serological specificity of peptides, had concluded that terminal amino acids played a major role in the specificity of small peptide chains. When, in a later report (1939), they extended their experimentation to larger synthetic peptide units, they revised their notion, for they noted that strong reactions involved not only end groups but other parts of the molecule as well. The following pentapeptides were prepared:

Tetraglycylglycine	G_5
Tetraglycylleucine	G_4L
d,l-Diglycylleucylglycylglycine	G_2LG_2
Trileucylglycylglycine	L_3G_2

The pentapeptides were coupled to horse azostromata for use in immunizing rabbits and for adsorption, and were coupled to chicken serum protein for use as test antigens in the precipitin reaction. Regardless of whether carboxyl or amino groups were prominent, antibodies appeared to be specific for an entire pentapeptide and not just a portion thereof. Moreover, a disparity in the reaction of antibody with peptides as compared with the corresponding amides revealed a difference between acid and other polar groups in their conferral of specificity. The authors suggested that specific combinations occurring in antigen-antibody reactions were not all of the same kind, i.e., that antibody sites did not always contain the same limited number of elements merely arranged in different ways. And they pointed out that perhaps their pentapeptides were not of sufficient size to reach the uppermost possible limit of antibody site conformation.

Sage, Deutsch, Fasman, and Levine (1964) found that in the polyalanine system the most inhibitory hapten was also the pentamer, and that the six-membered chain of alanine residues was actually less effective. It was noted that beginning with the hexamer there was an increasing tendency toward α-helical formation, but perhaps not enough to account for the 3-fold difference in the inhibiting efficiencies between the pentamer and the hexamer. The size of the penta-L-alanine molecule in extended form was calculated to be 25 Å × 11 Å × 6.5 Å, for which an antibody combining site in the form of Karush's (1956) interhelical cavity, which would encompass the hapten, would present an overall surface somewhere in the neighborhood of 2000 Å². The size was found to be little different from Kabat's isomaltohexaose, which will be discussed subsequently.

To go much beyond the pentapeptide size of chain length may not be too instructive in determining the corresponding size of antibody sites since, as Maurer (1963) points out:

"... when we talk of the amino acid residues constituting an antigenic site, we may not be referring to a sequence of amino acids in a protein chain in a chemical sense, but to the residues which are physically adjacent to each other in the coiled three-dimensional protein structure, that is a patch on the protein surface. In other words, if the same globular proteins were to be extended, the adjacent amino acid residues of the reactive site might in fact be separated by several amino acid residues.''

In essence when an active patch on an antibody protein surface re-acts with an active patch on an antigenic protein surface, each patch may be composed of semi-sites from different parts of each protein molecule which are so oriented as to provide a continuum of activity. Measurements of surface area in such instances would require tech-niques and instrumentation that would stretch even the best immuno-chemist's imagination and know-how.

The experiments of Kabat (1954, 1956, 1960) have approached the problem from a different direction and have provided a little less ambiguity in interpretation. Kabat and Berg (1952, 1953) had shown that dextrans—simple polymers of glucose joined mainly by the α-$(1 \rightarrow 6)$ link—were antigenic in man, and this prompted Kabat to raise two questions: Was the antibody specific for the α-$(1 \rightarrow 6)$ linked anhydroglucopyranose units? How many linked glucose residues were necessary to fill the antibody combining site completely? He first found that the antibodies did not react well with members of the α-$(1 \rightarrow 4)$-linked series such as maltose or with those of the β-$(1 \rightarrow 6)$-linked polymers such as gentiobiose. Only those of the α-$(1 \rightarrow 6)$ series—isomaltose, isomaltotriose, etc.—reacted well.

In his 1954 paper Kabat reported that 3 times more of the amount of 4-α-isomaltotriose-D-glucose were needed to inhibit antidextran activity than of the parent compound, isomaltotriose. Since the derivative was α-$(1 \rightarrow 6)$-linked in the first three residues, in the same manner as the parent, but had an additional glucose unit linked α-$(1 \rightarrow 4)$, Kabat predicted that the antibody site should accomodate more than three α-$(1 \rightarrow 6)$-linked residues, i.e., isomaltotetraose. Two years later when the tetraose, pentaose, and hexaose were made available, the prediction was confirmed. The tetraose fitted better than the triose, the pentaose had even better inhibitory power, and the hexaose, with only slightly better inhibition, appeared to estab-lish the upper limit. Because of heterogeneity there was the possibility that a heptasaccharide might on occasion be superior.

As shown in Figure 4-10 the model of isomaltohexaose would be free to rotate about the α-$(1 \rightarrow 6)$ links and to form a number of shapes in a random coil from a compact molecule to a fully extended one. Heterogeneity would therefore be extensive but with preserva-tion of complementarity to the α-$(1 \rightarrow 6)$ linkages. In the fully extended form, dimensions of the hexasaccharide would be 34 Å $\times$ 12 Å $\times$ 7 Å, and an antibody combining site in the form of Karush's (1956) in-terhelical cavity that would encompass the hapten would present an overall surface somewhere in the neighborhood of 2000 Å^2. Whether

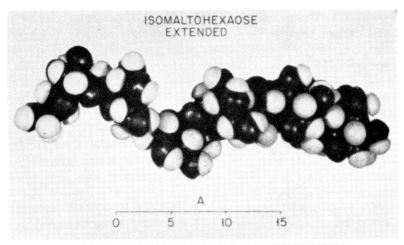

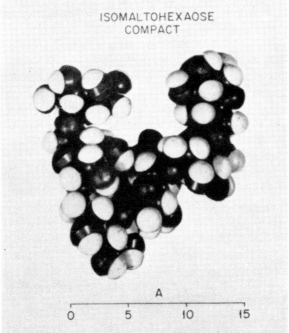

FIG. 4-10. Extended and compact models of isomaltohexaose. (From Kabat, 1957.)

the extended form would actually exist *in vivo* in an antibody-producing host is an open question, but the hypothetical site surface
formed around it would be maximal and still a relatively small part
of the total immunoglobulin surface.

Sage *et al.* (1964) questioned whether such a deep and large-surfaced interhelical cavity at an antibody site actually would exist. They based their reservation upon the fact that binding of the penta-L-alanine depended much more upon the maintenance of an uninterrupted sequence, regardless of position, than upon a terminal status, obviously necessary for deep-cavity binding. A shallow antibody site cavity appeared much more likely with a size, as one can easily calculate, not much more than 700 Å². Mage and Kabat (1963), themselves, considered the ramifications of the shallow-cavity hypothesis of an antibody site. In such a case it would be possible to visualize a site size much smaller than the size of the most effective hapten. The oversized hapten either would have a statistically larger number of ways of fitting the site than a small hapten or would much more easily fold to a specific conformation representative of the specific site surface. The former alternative would best fit the data of Landsteiner and van der Scheer and of Sage et al. (1964), where folded conformation of short polypeptides was unlikely. Either alternative would fit Kabat's dextran data and also those of Stollar, Levine, Lehrer, and Van Vunakis (1962), in which the upper limit of inhibiting power of the polynucleotides of thymine for antideoxyribonucleic acid (DNA) was the pentathymidylic acid. The assumption of a shallow binding site for the pentapeptides, the hexasaccharides, and the pentanucleotides would actually offer substantial agreement with Karush's so-called deep site against a relatively small hapten as well as with Beiser and Tanenbaum's (1963) calculation of a binding site size for antibody against the hapten, β-D-galactoside.

The problem with the shallow-cavity hypothesis of Sage et al. was that it did not apply in cases where it predictably should. Schechter and Sela (1965) had investigated the ability of various members of a series of oligoalanines to inhibit the reaction between rabbit anti-poly-L-alanyl ribonuclease and poly-L-alanyl-rabbit serum albumin. Whenever D-alanine was placed at the N-terminus of an oligoalanine chain the inhibitory effect of the L-alanine peptide sequence was eliminated. The presence of D-alanine at the C-terminus, on the other hand, had no effect and the L-alanine peptide sequence remained fully inhibitory. The N-terminus was highly important in this series. Kabat (1966), in commenting upon these two opposing results and accepting the validity of both, termed them yet another example in the growing list of types of heterogeneity.

Had Landsteiner and van der Scheer constructed their synthetic peptide series with alanine instead of glycine they would most certainly have reached different preliminary conclusions regardless of whether their rabbits responded in the manner of Sage et al. or of Schechter et al. In fact, in the Schechter series (Schechter, Schechter, and Sela, 1966; 1970a, b) the outstanding finding was that the pentapeptide was never a significantly better inhibitor than a tetra-peptide; on some occasions, a tetrapeptide was no better than a tripeptide; the finding held true not only in rabbits but in goats, not only in γG but in γM; and whether the homologous series was poly-L-alanine, poly-D-alanine, or poly-D-alanine-glycine, the response was uniformly the same.

It made a difference what residue appeared in the second and third position from the N-terminus as well as in the first. Replacement of alanine with glycine in those positions drastically reduced inhibitory capacity, but not replacement in the fourth and fifth positions. More-over, if the antisera were made against D-ala-gly-RNase instead of (D-ala)$_3$-gly-RNase, none of the alanine oligomers would satisfy but only an inhibitor such as D-ala-gly-ε-NH$_2$-caproate (Table 4-3).

The concept of Luderitz, Staub, and Westphal (1966), that was developed to account for specificity regions in the side chains of Salmonella group polysaccharides, would appear to embrace the viewpoints both of Sage and of Schechter and their respective col-leagues. Adapting the term "immunodominant" that was suggested to them by M. Heidelberger (to replace their original less applicable one, "immunoterminal") Luderitz et al. were able to construct af-finity regions around the immunodominant sugars for each specificity (e.g., types 3, 15, and 34 in Salmonella group E$_3$) and indicate the participation of adjacent sugar residues (Fig. 4-11).

To probe the problem further Schechter et al. (1970b) prepared an

TABLE 4-3

Concentration of Peptide Causing 50% Inhibition of Precipitates with Antisera Previously Absorbed with RNase

Peptide inhibitor	Anti-(DAla)$_3$-Gly-RNase (Animal 35) with		Anti-DAla-Gly-RNase (Animal 56) with	
	(DAla)$_3$-Gly-RNase	(DAla)$_3$-Gly-RSA	DAla-Gly-RNase	DAla-Gly-RSA
	mM	*mM*	*mM*	*mM*
(DAla)$_2$	>4	>4	>4	>4
(DAla)$_3$	0.22	0.34	>4	>4
(DAla)$_4$	0.062	0.12	>4	>4
(DAla)$_5$	0.065	0.12	>4	>4
DAla–Gly	>4	>4	>4	>4
(DAla)$_2$–Gly	0.65	1.05	>4	>4
(DAla)$_3$–Gly	0.047	0.095	>4	>4
DAla–Gly-ε-AC	0.45	0.76	0.10	0.09
(DAla)$_3$–Gly-ε-AC	0.038	0.075	>4	>4

(From Schechter, Schechter, and Sela, 1970a.)

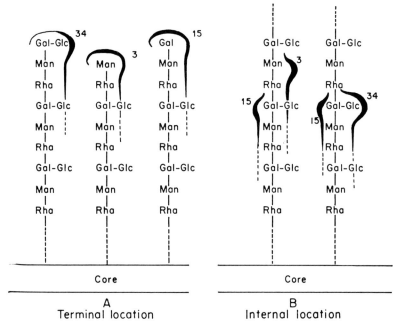

Core   Core

A   B
Terminal location   Internal location

FIG. 4-11. Possible location of factors on the side chains of Salmonella group E_3 (3, 15, 34) polysaccharides. The drawing around the chains symbolizes the intensity of the affinity between the antibody combining sites and the sugars of the determinant groups present on the polysaccharide. The thicker the line, the stronger the affinity. The strongest affinity occurs between the antibody and the "immunodominant" sugar, e.g., the sugar which best inhibits the corresponding antibody. (From Luderitz, Staub, and Westphal, 1966.)

immunoadsorbent by the interaction of poly-D-alanyl-rabbit serum albumin and bromoacetyl cellulose. Rabbit antibodies against poly-D-alanyl RNase and (D-ala)$_3$-gly-RNase were adsorbed by the immunoadsorbent, and then eluted by a three-step procedure: the first fraction was released by suspension of the complex in excess di-D-alanine; the second, in tetra-D-alanine; the third, in 0.1 M acetic acid. Analysis of the fractions revealed that the first one, displaced from the adsorbent by dipeptide, was inhibited by dipeptide 10 times more efficiently than the second fraction, displaced by tetrapeptide; that the first fraction was inhibited 2–3 times more efficiently by tripeptide than was the second; and that both fractions were inhibited by tetrapeptide to the same extent. The authors offer two alternatives to account for the results:

(a) "The first one follows Kabat's interpretation of his studies on anti-dextran antibodies [Schlossman and Kabat, 1962; Gelzer and Kabat, 1964], and suggests that the [first] Ab-2 antibody fraction is a mixture of antibodies with combining sites complementary to peptides of different sizes, with a higher proportion of antibody molecules possessing smaller combining sites, whereas the [second] Ab-4 antibody fraction consists mainly of antibodies complementary to the tetrapeptide."

(b) "A different interpretation is that all the antibodies formed possess combining sites complementary to a tetrapeptide, but that they are heterogeneous in terms of their capacity to bind the dipeptide. The experimental results indeed support such an explanation as antibodies complementary to a tetrapeptide differ in the extent of the interaction with the dipeptide."

A misconception that the binding sites of 19S antibodies are generally smaller than the binding sites of 7S antibodies has threaded its way into the literature. That they sometimes may be smaller is unquestionable; that they generally are smaller is a misreading of the literature. Kaplan and Kabat (1966) had reported finding a fraction of γM in human anti-A antisera that was equally well inhibited by mono-, tri-, and pentasaccharides (homologous to blood group substance A) whereas γG was best inhibited by the pentamer. Moreno and Kabat (1969) had then been able to confirm this finding, emphasizing once more, however, that the portion measured was only a fraction of the total γM antibody. Cowan (1970) has constructed a hypothesis based upon the proposition "that 7S antibody has relatively larger combining sites than 19S antibody, and that antigenic determinants should be described in terms of the antibody class reacting with a given determinant site." The hypothesis suggested that what were viewed as separate determinants by 19S, e.g., a and b, could be viewed as subdeterminants by 7S whose combining site would be sufficiently large to encompass the whole ab.

Completely contrary to this proposition are the results of Haimovich, Schechter, and Sela (1969) in which the upper size limits of γM antibody and γG antibody were determined to be the same, enough to accommodate four alanine residues. Kabat (1970) was moved to correct any misconception that had arisen from the misinterpretation of papers from his laboratory, and made the following remarks at a most appropriate time, the occasion of the Landsteiner Centennial:

"Dr. Kaplan and I found that the γM antibodies eluted by N-acetylgalactosamine, a monosaccharide, had small size sites. We said that there were probably other antibodies on the [fractionation] column that might be extracted with larger oligosaccharides. Dr. Moreno and I have since done this and we find γM antibodies with larger size sites. The distribution, as far as we can tell, is no different between γM antibodies and γG antibodies. It's just harder to elute γM antibodies from the column because they have a higher valence than the γG."

What had stimulated Cowan's hypothesis was his observation that guinea pig sera, obtained 4–8 days following infection with foot-and mouth disease virus, distinguished more determinant variations than sera obtained 20 days or more later. Murphy and Sage (1970) confirmed this type of finding with their demonstration that early antisera in rabbits to poly-L-aspartate hapten were inhibited by an upper limit of triaspartate whereas late antisera required the pentamer for inhibition. In keeping with common knowledge about the immune response, the assumption can safely be made that in both of these studies the early antisera represented γM primarily while the late antisera represented γG, and that, indeed the early γM binding sites were smaller than the late γG binding sites.

Given the modern concept of a variable region that is shared by all classes of immunoglobulins, one cannot exclusively assign a small size Fab categorically to γM and a larger one to γG. One would expect, instead, a complete sharing of all sizes of sites by all immunoglobulin classes *at any given time*. One would predict, therefore, that the γM and γG in the early antisera obtained by Cowan and by Murphy and Sage would have the same binding properties, i.e., small sites, while the antibodies in the late antisera would also share in a larger proportion of larger sites. The difference between early and late would be in the type and number of clones selected during the immune response, not in any particular immunoglobulin isotype. The observed association of γM with small sized sites would be a result of γM prominence as a secreted product early in the immune response, and not to any intrinsic molecular property unique to γM.

The accommodation of antigenic determinants by antibody binding sites is a central issue for discussion in immunochemistry, and the subject will be returned to once again in a later section after the meaning of idiotypy, homogeneous binding, affinity, and related subjects has become clear. As a preview of what lies ahead, however, and as an appropriate close to the present section, the questions Haber *et al.* (1967) asked are most fitting:

"Is this heterogeneous response an intrinsic feature of antibody production? Do many clones necessarily participate in the production of different antibodies directed against the same determinant, or do multideterminant antigens play a major role in determining the heterogeneity of the antibody response?"

9. Idiotypy and the immunogenetics of antibody combining sites

M. Koshland and Englberger as early as 1963 provided a most exacting amino acid analysis of two different purified antiphapten-antibody fractions obtained from the same rabbit. One hapten was the negatively charged phenylarsonate ion (R) and the other was the positively charged phenyltrimethylammonium ion (A), both of which as the p-azo derivatives (Rpz and Apz) were used to immunize the same rabbit. The analyses (Table 4-4) revealed that the anti-Rpz antibody contained two more residues each of arginine and isoleucine than did the anti-Apz antibody whereas the anti-Apz antibody contained two more residues each of leucine and glutamic acid and four more of aspartic acid. The other amino acids, including tyrosine, were remarkably similar in the two antibody preparations.

It was this report to which two of the five different papers referred in their opening sentences at the Cold Spring Harbor Symposium on

TABLE 4-4

Amino Acid Analysis of Two Purified Antibodies Isolated from the Same Rabbit

Amino Acid	Residues/Molecule*	
	Anti-Rpz	Anti-Apz
R	44.7	42.5
I	48.4	46.4
D	106	110
E	125	127
L	89	91
A	81.1	81.4
G	110	110
H	16.4	16.6
K	69.6	69.4
M	13.8	13.5
F	44.3	44.9
P	109	110
S	151	151
T	162	162
Y	56.1	56.2
V	128	128

* Taken as 160,000 molecular weight.
(Reported by Koshland and Englberger, 1963.)

Antibodies, in concert with Haber, Whitney and Tanford, and Freedman and Sela (cf. beginning of this chapter).

The results are made the more convincing when compared with a similar type of assay comparing the amino acid compositions of anti-Rpz and anti-Fpz (anti-p-azophenylphosphonate), two highly cross-reactive antibodies with almost identical binding properties (Koshland, Ochoa, and Fujita, 1970). In this latter case, with anti-bodies derived from separate rabbits of genotype $a^1a^1b^4b^4$, the compositions were identical (Table 4-5) except for a single tyrosine in the heavy chains.

Yet another assay of the same type from Koshland's (1967) work was presented in Chapter 2 in which the allotypic differences in heavy chains were distinguished from antibody differences in the same chains (Table 2-5). The same difference between anti-Rp and anti-Lac was obtained upon two different allotypic backgrounds: an extra proline, two extra serines, and two extra tyrosines; perhaps also an extra threonine and/or valine.

Repeating the original experiment depicted in Table 4-4, but placing it upon a genetically controlled background of three different allotypes a1, a2, and a3, and analyzing only heavy chains, Koshland,

TABLE 4-5

Comparison of Amino Acid Compositions* of Heavy and Light Chains from Cross-Reactive Arsonic and Phosphonic Antibodies

Amino Acid	Heavy Chains		Light Chains	
	Anti-Rpz	Anti-Fpz	Anti-Rpz	Anti-Fpz
K	25.1 ± 0.14†	25.0 ± 0.17	9.3 ± 0.08	9.2 ± 0.06
H	6.3 ± 0.14	6.5 ± 0.08	1.3 ± 0.03	1.2 ± 0.01
R	19.4 ± 0.19	19.6 ± 0.17	3.0 ± 0.13	3.0 ± 0.04
D	33.4 ± 0.18	32.9 ± 0.13	19.8 ± 0.09	19.8 ± 0.10
T	51.7 ± 0.16	51.4 ± 0.16	31.8 ± 0.25	32.1 ± 0.41
S	54.5 ± 0.30	53.7 ± 0.12	22.5 ± 0.11	22.0 ± 0.22
E	39.3 ± 0.23	38.7 ± 0.09	21.7 ± 0.16	21.4 ± 0.17
P	42.8 ± 0.13	43.1 ± 0.38	12.1 ± 0.17	12.2 ± 0.13
G	34.5 ± 0.22	34.4 ± 0.04	20.4 ± 0.11	20.1 ± 0.04
A	22.8 ± 0.19	22.7 ± 0.14	16.9 ± 0.35	16.6 ± 0.13
V	42.4 ± 0.13	42.5 ± 0.22	21.0 ± 0.09	20.8 ± 0.12
I	15.9 ± 0.17	15.7 ± 0.09	7.4 ± 0.04	7.4 ± 0.13
L	33	33	11	11
Y	**17.4** ± 0.13	**16.5** ± 0.14	10.6 ± 0.10	10.8 ± 0.10
F	15.4 ± 0.19	15.5 ± 0.16	6.7 ± 0.04	6.6 ± 0.13
C	13.3 ± 0.34	13.2 ± 0.67	7.2 ± 0.12	7.4 ± 0.22

* After 20-hr hydrolysis.

† Standard error of the mean.

(From Koshland, Ochoa, and Fujita, 1970.)

Reisfeld, and Dray (1968) also established that all anti-Apz antibodies consistently contained one more aspartic acid and one more leucine in their heavy chains than did anti-Rpz.

The data obtained by Spring, Nisonoff, and Dray (1970) beautifully demonstrated the complete independence of allotype and antibody specificity in the ability of rabbit γG to displace ^{125}I-labeled reference Fab fragments in binding with specific anti-allotype antisera. The authors concluded that their data were consistent with Koshland (1967) and with Koshland, Reisfeld and Dray (1968), and that once again differences in amino acid composition associated with allotype specificity in the N-terminal heavy chain occurred independently of compositional changes associated with antibody specificity. They declared:

> "Since many of the amino acid substitutions associated with differences in allotypic specificities a1 and a3 are localized to the 34 residues at the N-terminus, it seems possible that the N-terminus of the [heavy] chain does not contribute significantly to the specificity of the antibody, despite the variability of certain residues in this segment."

By extending their technique of precise total amino acid analyses to μ-chains that were under allotypic a1 and a3 control, Koshland, Davis, and Fujita (1969) were able to show that not only was antibody specificity independent of allotypic specificity but also of immunoglobulin class. From their data they postulated that three categories of genes, at least two of which were germ line, functioned as one in order to account for the three independent regions within a polypeptide heavy chain: one controlling the nonallelic class-specific constant region isotypes, one controlling the allelic products, and one controlling the nonallelic variable region combining sites. Thus, from yet another independent experimental source additional evidence was provided for the ever growing belief in the independence of combining site regions as a genetically controlled phenotypic expression of diversity.

Jacques Oudin (1966) originated the term "idiotypic" and used it in his Royal Society lecture on the genetic control of immunoglobulin synthesis. Pernis (1967) has used the term in a somewhat different way, but here the meaning will be as Oudin declared. Idiotypic specificities are defined as peculiar to antibody against one given antigen and peculiar to one individual or group within which the antibody to the given antigen is different than in another individual or group. The definition of Pernis would include the N-terminal didecapeptide differences among heavy chains and even light chains and is therefore not restrictive enough in the light of current knowledge.

Oudin pointed out that before 1956 the only defined specificities among immunoglobulins were isotypic ones—uniform in all individuals of a given species. Then came the disclosure of allotypic specificities, already discussed, that are different in different groups of individuals within the same species. By 1963, in the same year that Koshland and Englberger published their definitive amino acid tabulation of antibody composition, Rieder and Oudin were able to demonstrate by immunochemical technique what we already know from Koshland's subsequent work: that the allotypic specificities are shared by all antibodies of all specificities, e.g., anti-ovalbumin, anti-DNP, and anti-pneumococcal Type II. But could one show by the same technique anything but heterogeneous individuality, i.e., could one develop a pattern among idiotypes? Beginning to explore the problem in 1963 Oudin and Michel found that the system of antibody production in genetically controlled rabbits to the antigen, *Salmonella typhi*, gave them the necessary foundation upon which to build. Six years later a detailed story could be told (Oudin and Michel, 1969a–c; Oudin, 1969).

The simple basic immunodiffusion pattern is illustrated in Figure 4-12. At the time that a rabbit was actively engaged in synthesizing anti-typhoid antibody, its serum contained an idiotypic globulin—antibody—that was not in detectable evidence either before immuni-

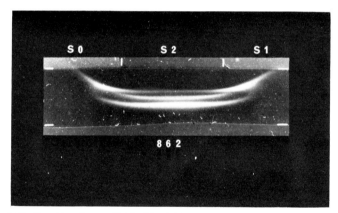

Fig. 4-12. Reaction in a cell (double diffusion in agar) of three serum samples of rabbit 8-03 with the anti-idiotypic serum of rabbit 8-62. *S0* is the serum of a bleeding of rabbit 8-03, made before any immunization. *S2* and *S1* are serum samples, both strongly precipitating against the somatic antigen of *Salmonella typhi*, taken 34–38 days and 13–17 days after the beginning of the immunization of rabbit 8-03 against *S. typhi*. Rabbit 8-62 had been injected with *S. typhi* bacteria agglutinated by S2. The *white dashes* indicate the interface between the various gel layers. (From Oudin and Michel, 1969c.)

zation or after anti-typhoid antibody biosynthesis had, for the most part, ceased a year after immunization. That the reaction was very specific was indicated in two ways: antibody in the same rabbit against a different antigen did not react with the anti-idiotype serum; and anti-typhoid antibody from another rabbit did not cross-react with the anti-idiotype serum. The system was then put to a severe test by comparing the possible cross-reactivities among 21 different anti-idiotypic sera and the 21 different anti-typhoid antibody globulins. Each anti-idiotypic serum precipitated only the corresponding immune serum except for an occasional and extremely faint cross-reaction.

To test whether or not the idiotypic specificities followed simple Mendelian laws of heredity—separate and unlinked from but in the same general way as allotypic specificities—a given rabbit and both parents were immunized against S. typhi. In no case did an anti-idiotypic serum against the progeny anti-typhoid serum ever cross-react with either parent's anti-typhoid serum, and in no case, therefore, was there ever any evidence of hereditary transmission comparable to allotypic specificities. Such a test does not rule out hereditary transmission, but what it does rule out is the restriction of a given antibody to a few clones of determined amino acid sequence. It says that either the complementary binding site region is outside hereditary control or that a very large number of different possible sequences within a complementary binding site region can select for a given antigenic determinant.

That the latter possibility is by no means ruled out is observed by the development of multiple idiotypes within an individual rabbit against S. typhi. For example, it was not unusual to find that a rabbit, after immunization, would produce three idiotypes, that is, three distinct lines in immunodiffusion (Fig. 4-12). After a rest of 28 months (except for an injection of antigenically unrelated Salmonella typhimurium at 11 months) the same three idiotypes could be obtained after boosting. In addition as many as four additional idiotypes could be obtained.

Other variations in pattern within a given individual were also encountered. Three in particular are worth mentioning here.

  (a) Sometimes the same idiotypic specificity is carried by antibodies of two classes, γG and γM (Fig. 4-13).

  (b) Sometimes the same idiotypic specificity is carried by antibodies of two classes, one precipitable and the other not (Fig. 4-14). Such a phenomenon is manifested by comparing an anti-typhoid serum both before and after precipitation with S. typhi polysaccharide.

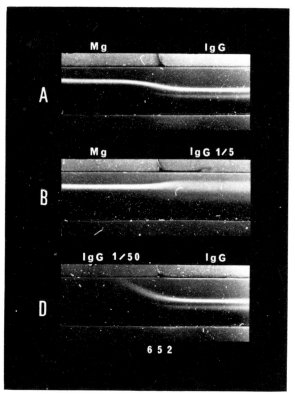

Fig. 4-13. Reaction in three cells (double diffusion in agar) with the anti-idiotypic serum of rabbit 6-52: (A) of a preparation of macroglobulin (Mg) and of IgG of S37 of rabbit 3-24; (B) of the same macroglobulin preparation and a 1:5 dilution of the same IgG preparation as in A; (D) of a 1:50 dilution of the same IgG preparation as in A and this IgG preparation, undiluted. It may be noticed: (a) that the γ precipitation zone is perfectly continuous in front of the macroglobulin (containing IgM) and IgG layers in A; (b) that, when the IgG preparation is diluted 1:5, the position of the γ precipitation zone in front of it is the same as in front of the macroglobulin layer, but that its appearance is definitely different; (c) that, when the IgG layer is diluted 1:50, there is definitely no γ precipitation zone in front of it, although the IgG content is still definitely larger in this dilution than in the macroglobulin layer.

(c) Sometimes a bifuraction in idiotypic specificity occurs between bleeding intervals in a given individual. Thus, in bleeding $n + 1$ (S2 in Fig. 4-15) there are antibodies which carry only a part of the idiotypic determinants that are contained in a single molecular class in bleeding n (S1 in Fig. 4-15).

Whereas Oudin and Michel concentrated mainly on qualitative analysis of idiotypy, Daugharty, Hopper, MacDonald, and Nisonoff

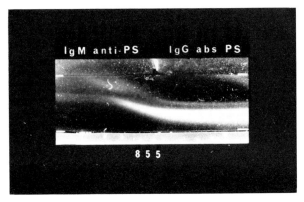

FIG. 4-14. Compared reaction in a cell (double diffusion in agar) of the anti-idiotypic serum of the fifth bleeding of rabbit 8-55 with two fractions of the anti-*Salmonella typhi* serum of the second bleeding of rabbit 8-03: a solution of IgM antibodies recovered from the specific precipitate of a macroglobulin preparation with the polysaccharide of *S. typhi* (IgM anti-PS), and a solution of IgG absorbed with the polysaccharide (IgG abs PS). It may be seen that a precipitation zone is continuous in front of these two antigen layers; this shows that the anti-idiotypic antibodies which react in this precipitation zone with a given idiotypic pattern do not distinguish between the IgM antibodies precipitated by the polysaccharide and the IgG not precipitable by the polysaccharide both of which carry the idiotypic pattern with which we are concerned.

(1969), Hopper, MacDonald, and Nisonoff (1970), and Nisonoff, MacDonald, Hopper, and Daugharty (1970) introduced techniques that would make quantitative analysis of the idiotype response in genetically controlled rabbits possible. Anti-*p*-azobenzoate antibodies (anti-Xp) raised in individual rabbits of known allotype were used as their source of idiotypic immunogen; the antibodies were specifically purified and polymerized with gluteraldehyde for use as immunogen; the same antibodies were specifically purified and radioiodinated with ^{125}I for use as test antigen in direct precipitation tests with anti-idiotype sera; and the same antibodies were converted to their ^{125}I-(Fab')$_2$ fragments to use in indirect inhibition and coprecipitation tests. Of greatest interest was the quantitative tracing of the rise and fall of individual idiotypes in a given rabbit during the immune responses over a period of months. Two examples are shown in Figures 4-16 and 4-17, one from rabbit AZ1 and the other from rabbit AZ5.

As Oudin and Michel had shown in a qualitative way these examples showed in a quantitative manner. The first response profile demonstrated the shift in the 4th month from one idiotype to another, completely non-cross-reacting, idiotype: The second response profile demonstrated the gradual shift from one idiotype to another and the

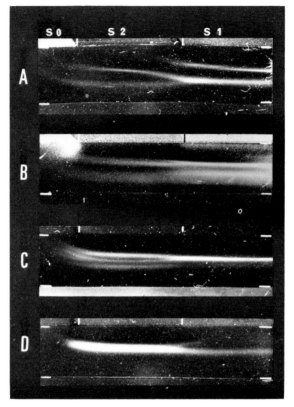

Fɪɢ. 4-15. In each of the four cells, reaction (double diffusion in agar) of an anti-idiotypic serum with three samples of serum of the corresponding immunizing rabbit: *S0*, serum taken before any immunization; *S2* and *S1*, samples taken 34–38 days and 13–17 days after the beginning of the immunization against *Salmonella typhi*. The immunizing serum sample was S2. (*A*) S0, S2, and S1 of rabbit 8-03 reacting with the anti-idiotypic serum of the third bleeding of rabbit 8-55. (*B*) S0, S2, and S1 of rabbit 7-99 reacting with the anti-idiotypic serum of rabbit 8-54. (*C*) S0, S2, and S1 of rabbit 2-63 reacting with the anti-idiotypic serum of rabbit 2-88. (*D*) S0, S2, and S1 of rabbit 2-63 reacting with the anti-idiotypic serum of rabbit 2-89. In *A*, *B*, and *C*, two precipitation zones, distinct in front of S2, are continuous with a single zone in front of S1. An appearance of a bifurcated zone, turned the other way round but, even otherwise, different from the above pictures, is visible in *D* and is likely to be due to the superposition of the precipitation zones of two idiotypes, one of which would be present in S2 and S1, and the other only in S2.

partial sharing of idiotypic determinants by the early and late types. Since a rabbit antibody molecule has a half-life of only about 6 days (Taliaferro and Talmage, 1956; Weigle, 1958) and since an antibody-producing cell likewise does not have a much greater life expectancy (Schooley, 1961; Nossal and Mäkelä, 1962; Makinodan and Albright,

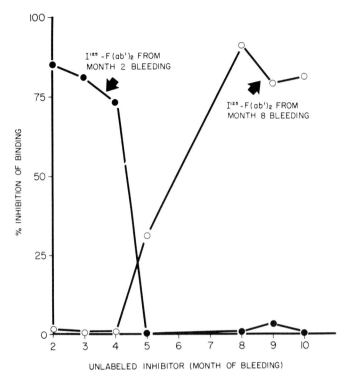

FIG. 4-16. Inhibition of reactions of ^{125}I-F(ab')$_2$ from rabbit AZ1 with its homologous anti-D serum. Inhibitors are anti-p-azobenzoate antibodies specifically purified from sera of the same rabbit, taken at different times during its course of immunization, as specified on the *abscissa*. (●) Anti-D serum prepared against polymerized anti-p-azobenzoate antibodies from bleedings taken approximately 2 months after the start of immunization, the serum was allowed to react with ^{125}I-F(ab')$_2$ prepared from the same (unpolymerized) antibodies by peptic digestion. (○) Anti-D serum prepared against polymerized purified antibody derived from bleedings taken during month 8; the anti-serum was allowed to react with ^{125}I-F(ab')$_2$ prepared from the same antibodies. Each reaction mixture contained 0.5 μg ^{125}I-F(ab')$_2$, 30 μg of unlabeled inhibitor, and 10 μl of anti-D serum. After incubating for 1 hr at 37°C, 0.6 ml of goat anti-Fc serum was added and the percentage of radioactivity precipitated was determined. A different recipient rabbit was used for each of the two purified D preparations. (From Nisonoff, MacDonald, Hopper, and Daugharty, 1970.)

1967), it was the opinion of Nisonoff and his colleagues—one unlikely to be challenged by current thought—that indeed a selected precursor cell for each idiotype had differentiated into an antibody-forming cell, that it was accompanied in this event by the production of memory cells or Y-cells (Sercarz and Coons, 1962), and that subsequent antigenic stimulation had given rise to a clone of cells producing antibody of the same idiotype as that synthesized initially.

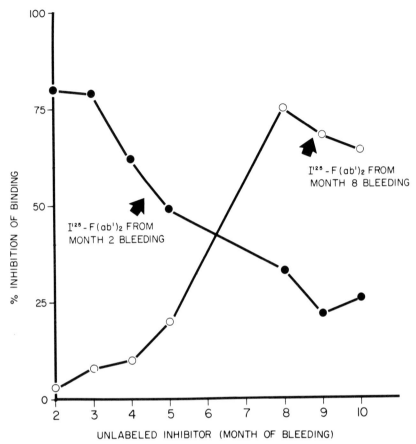

FIG. 4-17. These experiments were carried out as described in Figure 4-16 except that the ^{125}I-F(ab')$_2$ as well as the unlabeled inhibiting antibodies were from rabbit AZ5. Anti-D sera were prepared against purified antibodies of rabbit AZ5 derived from bleedings of months 2 and 8. (From Nisonoff, MacDonald, Hopper, and Daugharty, 1970.)

In the human as well as in the rabbit the idiotypic response has been differentiated from the allotypic. In the year 1963, independent of Oudin's or Koshland's experiments with individual rabbits, Kunkel, Mannik, and Williams observed the same type of individual antigenic specificity of isolated antibodies in human sera. An almost heroic achievement was announced soon thereafter by Bassett, Tanenbaum, Pryzwansky, Beiser, and Kabat (1965)—the amino acid composition of antibodies and "normal" γG from 22 different fractions or pools from a single individual. A summary of significant differences in nine particular amino acid residues among six specificities—anti-levans, anti-dextrans, anti-teichoic acids, anti-blood group A, "normal" γG, and pooled γM—is given in Table 4-6.

Hydroxylysine was found exclusively in only three of the groups (anti-dextran, anti-teichoic acid, and γM); anti-teichoic acids had 12–20 more glycines than any other group; anti-levan, anti-dextrans, and normal γG were rich in valine; anti-levans and γM were poorer in tyrosines than the others; and so on for the other five listings. The authors also noted that the sum of lysine and arginine residues was nearly constant except in γM. Of course, one cannot attribute all of these differences or any particular one to idiotypy of the restricted kind as defined by Oudin (1966) although they would fit the looser definition of Pernis (1967). In their studies on human antibodies, in fact, Yount, Dorner, Kunkel, and Kabat (1968) did find that there was apparent selective association of subgroups with antibody specificity: γG1 was prominent in anti-tetanus antitoxins and anti-A isoagglutinins; γG2, in anti-dextrans, anti-levans, and anti-teichoic acids. One anti-levan immunoglobulin was exclusively composed of γG2 heavy chains and κ-light chains very much in the manner of an individual homogeneous myeloma protein. The idiotypic profile would be expected to prevail over and above any such isotypic subclass that happened to have selection advantage.

Another gross selective process within an individual, not related in any major way with the idiotypy of the combining site region, but still capable of refining the antibody population to a particular anti-

TABLE 4-6

Significant Differences in Average Amino Acid Composition Among 6.5S Antibodies from One Individual*

Specificity→	Anti-Levans	Anti-Dextrans	Anti-Teichoic Acid	Anti-"A"	Normal γG	Pooled γM
Gm group→	a – b –	a – b –	a – b –	a + b –	a + b +	
Glycine	101	99.5	120	108	107	105
Valine	132	134	102	115	139	105
Leucine	116	109	110	115	116	98.0
Tyrosine	45.5	56.0	53.3	53.2	55.9	41.0
Arginine	46.4	48.2	58.6	56.1	47.8	55.5
Lysine	93.5	87.5	81.9	79.1	93.2	64.0
Hydroxylysine	0	3.2	3.7	0	0	4.0
Threonine	113	109	110	127	111	116
Proline	101	101	108	108	107	97.1
[Arginine + lysine]	140	136	141	135	141	120

* All values taken at 22 hr hydrolysis. Residues per mol. wt, 160,000.
(From Bassett, Tanenbaum, Pryzwansky, Beiser, and Kabat, 1965.)

gen, is the net electrical charge. Although unappreciated at the time, Porter's (1959) original separation of rabbit Fab into two separate fractions, I and II, by carboxymethyl (CM)-cellulose ion-exchange chromatography was based upon this charge difference. Sela, Givol, and Mozes (1963) discovered this fact when they prepared antibodies against two antigens of different charge, one against an acidic synthetic polypeptide and the other against lysozyme. After chromatography on diethylaminoethyl (DEAE)-Sephadex the first fraction contained antibodies against the synthetic acidic antigen while the second fraction exclusively contained anti-lysozyme antibodies. Sela and Mozes (1966) went on to show that there was an unambiguous direct correlation between the net electrical charge on a variety of natural and synthetic antigens and the type of antibody they elicit whether in rabbit, goat, or horse. The correlation went further—it was important what net electrical charge was carried by the macromolecular carrier to which antigenic determinants were attached. Thus, antibodies of a given specificity could be made to appear in either fraction I or II depending upon the choice (in this case) of a synthetic carrier with a particular charge. Rüde, Mozes, and Sela (1968) pursued the matter further, showing that the net electrical charge of the complete antigen played a rôle in determining the chemical nature of anti-Rp antibodies. (Rp *per se*, it will be remembered, is negatively charged.) Anti-Rp-azo-poly-L-lysyl-ribonuclease appeared in fraction I; anti-Rp-azo-BSA, in fraction II. The phenomenon persisted not only in γG but also in γM (Robbins, Mozes, Rimon, and Sela, 1967). Confirmation of these effects and their relegation to Fab have since been adequately reported from a number of laboratories (e.g., Strosberg and Kanarek, 1970), but meanwhile Segal, Givol, and Sela (1969) went on to show that when Fd fragments themselves were compared by disc electrophoresis patterns of reduced and alkylated chains, *there was no significant difference whatsoever in mobility between acid and basic fragments. The light chains carried all of the charge differences and within them there remained a correlation between antigen charge and final electrophoretic mobility of the directed antibody light chain.* Within the restricted electrophoretic mobilities of the Fd fragments, as might be expected, greater heterogeneity of pattern was obtained than with light chains and therein still resided the undifferentiated idiotypes of the heavy chains from one individual to another.

The charge difference in antibody heterogeneity brought about by light chain selection does in no way decrease the importance of the unique features of the insertion-deletion portions of the light chains. Kabat (1968) and Wu and Kabat (1970) have made this very clear by a discussion of variety of amino acid residues encountered in every position of the combining-site region. The recombinant studies in Nisonoff's laboratory also give one an assurance that idiotypy does seem to exist among light chains. Hong and Nisonoff (1966) showed that light chains from high affinity antibodies were more effective than light chains from low affinity antibodies in restoring high affinity complementation of heavy chains from high affinity antibodies. It was apparent that different clones of cells utilized different pairs of light and heavy polypeptide chains to achieve the same specificity. Zappacosta and Nisonoff (1968) noted that heavy chains and light chains obtained from anti-DNP antibodies of different animals in general yielded recombinant products of greater activity than did heavy chains of anti-DNP antibodies that were recombined with non-specific light chains of the same individual. Finally and perhaps most like idiotypic phenomena MacDonald, Alescio, and Nisonoff (1969) found that recombinants of heavy and light chains of anti-Xp anti-bodies obtained from the same rabbit over a long period of time yielded much greater complementation units than did other re-combinant pairs.

It is sometimes difficult to keep in mind all the various factors that impinge upon the final makeup of an immunoglobulin molecule, but it is well to keep the words of Sela and Mozes (1966) constantly in mind even in this latter day:

> "*The biosynthesis of the antibody is controlled both by the specificity determinants* (in the formation of specific com-bining sites) *and by other parts of the antigenic molecules* (in defining areas of the antibody which do not include the anti-body combining sites)." (Italics are theirs.)

And since the conclusion to this section on idiotypy is also the con-clusion to the chapter on the antibody binding site, and the con-clusion to Part One on antibody structure, the remarks that Wu and Kabat (1970) have made concerning idiotypy are most apropos:

> "The data on idiotypic specificity of myeloma globulins (Slater, Ward, and Kunkel, 1955) and antibodies (Kunkel, Mannik, and Williams, 1963; Oudin and Michel, 1963; 1969a, b; Daugharty, Hopper, MacDonald, and Nisonoff, 1969; Hurez, Meshaka, Mihaesco, and Seligmann, 1968) are compatible with the insertion model and with the overall concept of the antibody structure proposed. Thus idiotypic determinants which are found in the variable regions would represent antigenic determinants formed by patterns of amino acid sequences involving some of the side chains of residues from the inserted regions—namely those forming

the exterior portions of the site but also including some of the residues involved in three-dimensional folding and belonging to various subgroups, etc. This could give rise to a large number of determinants generally not related to specificity but influenced by or indeed partly created by the sequence of site-determining residues. In many instances in which immunodominant groups of the idiotypic determinants were from those of the inserted regions, one might expect the same idiotypic specificity to be manifested in several classes of immunoglobulins; this has been shown to the case for γM and γG antibodies from the same rabbit (Oudin and Michel, 1969a, b). Thus the findings on idiotypic specificity provide further support for the uniqueness and universality of the antibody-forming mechanism."

REFERENCES

Appella, E., and Perham, R. N. (1967). The structure of immunoglobulin light chains. Symp. Quant. Biol. *32:* 37–44.

Atsumi, T., Nishida, K., Kinoshita, Y., Shibata, K., and Horiuchi, Y. (1967). The heterogeneity of combining sites of anti-benzylpenicilloyl antibodies obtained from individual rabbits: fractionation of antibodies with a specific immunoadsorbent. J. Immunol. *99:* 1286–1293.

Bassett, E. W., Tanenbaum, S. W., Pryzwansky, K., Beiser, S. M., and Kabat, E. A. (1965). Studies on human antibodies. III. Amino acid composition of four antibodies from one individual. J. Exp. Med. *122:* 251–261.

Beiser, S. M., and Tanenbaum, S. W. (1963). Binding site topology of enzymes and antibodies induced by the same determinants. Ann. N. Y. Acad. Sci., *103:* 595–609.

Buckley, C. E., III, Whitney, P. L., and Tanford, C. (1963). The unfolding and renaturation of a specific univalent antibody fragment. Proc. Nat. Acad. Sci. *54:* 827–834.

Campbell, D. H., and Bulman, N. (1954). Some current concepts of the chemical nature of antigens and antibodies. Fortschr. Chem. Org. Naturst. *9:* 443–484.

Campbell, D. H., and Johnson, F. H. (1946). Pressure and specific precipitation. J. Am. Chem. Soc. *68:* 725–incl.

Cathou, R. E., and Haber, E. (1967). Structure of the antibody combining site. I. Hapten stabilization of antibody conformation. Biochemistry *6:* 513–517.

Cathou, R. E., and Werner, T. C. (1970). Hapten stabilization of antibody conformation. Biochemistry *9:* 3149–3154.

Cold Spring Harbor Symposia on Quantitative Biology. (1967). Antibodies. *32:* 1–619.

Converse, C. A., and Richards, F. F. (1969). Two-stage photosensitive label for antibody combining sites. Biochemistry *8:* 4431–4436.

Cowan, K. M. (1970). Immunochemical studies of foot-and-mouth disease. VI. Differences in antigenic determinant site recognition by guinea pig 19S and 7S antibodies. J. Immunol. *104:* 423–431.

Daugharty, H., Hopper, J. E. MacDonald, A. B., and Nisonoff, A. (1969). Quantitative investigations of idiotypic antibodies. I. Analysis of precipitating antibody population. J. Exp. Med. *130:* 1047–1062.

Day, L. A., Sturtevant, J. M., and Singer, S. J. (1963). The kinetics of the reactions between antibodies to the 2,4-dinitrophenyl group and specific haptens. Ann. N. Y. Acad. Sci. *103:* 611–625.

Edelman, G. M., Benacerraf, B., and Ovary, Z. (1963). Structure and specificity of guinea pig 7S antibodies. J. Exp. Med. *118:* 229–244.

Eisen, H. N., Little, J. R., Osterland, C. K., and Simms, E. S. (1967). A myeloma protein with antibody activity. Symp. Quant. Biol. *32:* 75–81.

Feinstein, A., and Rowe, A. J. (1965). Molecular mechanism of formation of an antigen-antibody complex. Nature *205:* 147–149.

Fenton, J. W. II, and Singer, S. J. (1965). Affinity labeling of antibodies to the p-azophenyltrimethylammonium hapten and a structural relationship among antibody active sites of different specificities. Biochem. Biophys. Res. Commun. *20:* 315–320.

Fleischman, J. B., Pain, R., and Porter, R. R. (1962). Reduction of γ-globulins. Arch. Biochem. Biophys. Suppl. *1:* 174–180.

Franek, F. (1969). Affinity labeling of pig anti-DNP (dinitrophenol) antibodies. Behringtwerk-Mitteil. *49:* 69–71.

Freedman, M. H., and Sela, M. (1966a). Recovery of antigenic activity upon reoxidation of completely reduced polyalanyl rabbit immunoglobulin G. J. Biol. Chem. *241:* 2382-2396.

Freedman, M. H., and Sela, M. (1966b). Recovery of specific activity upon reoxidation of completely reduced polyalanyl rabbit antibody. J. Biol. Chem. *241:* 5225–5232.

Froese, A., Sehon, A. H., and Eigen, M. (1962). Kinetic studies of protein-dye and antibody-hapten interactions with the temperature-jump method. Can. J. Chem. *40:* 1786–1797.

Gelzer, J., and Kabat, E. A. (1964). Specific fractionation of human antidextran antibodies. II. Assay of human antidextran sera and specifically fractionated purified antibodies by microcomplement fixation and complement fixation inhibition techniques. J. Exp. Med. *119:* 983–995.

Good, A. H., Ovary, Z., and Singer, S. J. (1968). Affinity labeling of the active sites of anti-2,4-dinitrophenyl antibodies from different species. Biochemistry *7:* 1304–1310.

Good, A. H., Traylor, P. S., and Singer, S. J. (1967). Affinity labeling of the active sites of rabbit anti-2,4-dinitrophenyl antibodies with *m*-nitrobenzenediazonium fluoroborate. Biochemistry *6:* 873–881.

Haber, E. (1964). Recovery of antigenic specificity after denaturation and complete reduction of disulfides in a papain fragment of antibody. Proc. Natl. Acad. Sci. *52:* 1099–1106.

Haber, E., Richards, F. F., Spragg, J., Austen, K. F., Vallotton, M., and Page, L. B. (1967). Modifications in the heterogeneity of the antibody response. Symp. Quant. Biol. *32:* 299–310.

Haimovich, J., Schechter, I., and Sela, M. (1969). Combining sites of IgG and IgM antibodies of poly-D-alanyl specificity. Eur. J. Biochem. *7:* 537–543.

Harvey, E. N., and Deitrick, J. E. (1930). The production of antibodies for *Cypridina luciferase* and luciferin in the body of a rabbit. J. Immunol. *18:* 65–71.

Haurowitz, F. (1963). *The Chemistry and Function of Proteins*, Ed. 2, Academic Press (New York, 455 pp.) p. 377.

Hong, R., and Nisonoff, A. (1966). Heterogeneity in the complementation of polypeptide subunits of a purified antibody isolated from an individual rabbit. J. Immunol. *96:* 622–628.

Hopper, J. E., MacDonald, A. B., and Nisonoff, A. (1970). Quantitative investigations of idiotypic antibodies. II. Nonprecipitating antibodies. J. Exp. Med. *131:* 41–56.

Hurez, D., Meshaka, G., Mihaesco, C., and Seligmann, M. (1968). The inhibition by normal γG-globulins of antibodies specific for individual γG-myeloma proteins. J. Immunol. *100:* 69–79.

Isliker, H. (1962). Chemical structure of antibodies. Gazz. Chim. Ital. *92:* 850–858.

Jaton, J.-C., Klinman, N. R., Givol. D., and Sela, M. (1968). Recovery of antibody activity upon reoxidation of completely reduced polyalanyl heavy chain and its Fd fragment derived from anti-2,4-dinitrophenyl antibody. Biochemistry *7:* 4185–4195.

Jerne, N. K. (1967). Summary: waiting for the end. Symp. Quant. Biol. *32:* 591–603.

Kabat, E. A. (1954). Some configurational requirements and dimensions of the combining site on an antibody to naturally occurring antigen. J. Am. Chem. Soc. *76:* 3709–3713.

Kabat, E. A. (1956). Heterogeneity in extent of the combining regions of human antidextran. J. Immunol. *77:* 377–385.

Kabat, E. A. (1957). Size and heterogeneity of the combining sites on an antibody molecule. J. Cell. Comp. Physiol. *50:* Suppl. 1, 97–102.

Kabat, E. A. (1960). The upper limit for the site of the human antidextran combining site. J. Immunol. *84:* 82–85.

Kabat, E. A. (1961). *Kabat and Mayer's Experimental Immunochemistry*, Ed. 2, Charles C Thomas (Springfield, Ill., 905 pp.) p. 250.

Kabat, E. A. (1966). The nature of an antigenic determinant. (Presidential Address before the American Association of Immunologists, April 13, 1966). J. Immunol. *97:* 1–11.

Kabat, E. A. (1968). Unique features of the variable regions of Bence-Jones proteins and their possible relation to antibody complementarity. Proc. Natl. Acad. Sci. *59:* 613–619.

Kabat, E. A. (1970). Discussion. Heidelberg, M., moderator. Ann. N. Y. Acad. Sci. *169:* 36–37.

Kabat, E. A. and Berg, D. (1952). Production of precipitins and cutaneous sensitivity in man by injection of small amounts of dextran. Ann. N. Y. Acad. Sci. *55:* 471–476.

Kabat, E. A., and Berg, D. (1953). Dextran—an antigen in man. J. Immunol. *70:* 514–532.

Karush, F. (1956). The interaction of purified antibody with optically isomeric haptens. J. Am. Chem. Soc. *78:* 5519–5526.

Kaplan, M. E., and Kabat, E. A. (1966). Studies on human antibodies. IV. Purification and properties of anti-A and anti-B obtained by absorption and elution from insoluble blood-group substances. J. Exp. Med. *123:* 1061–1081.

Kennel, S. J., and Singer, S. J. (1970). Affinity labeling of rabbit antibodies to the 2,4,6-trinitrophenyl determinant. Immunochemistry *7:* 235–238.

Koshland, D. E., Jr. (1963). Properties of the active site of enzymes. Ann. N. Y. Acad. Sci. *103:* 630–642.

Koshland, M. E. (1967). Location of specificity and allotypic amino acid residues in antibody Fd fragments. Symp. Quant. Biol. *32:* 119–127.

Koshland, M. E., Davis, J. J., and Fujita, N. J. (1969). Evidence for multiple gene control of a single polypeptide chain: the heavy chain of a rabbit immunoglobulin. Proc. Natl. Acad. Sci. *63:* 1274–1281.

Koshland, M. E., and Englberger, F. (1963). Differences in the amino acid composition of two purified antibodies from the same rabbit. Proc. Natl. Acad. Sci. *50:* 61–68.

Koshland, M. E., Ochoa, P., and Fujita, N. J. (1970). Amino acid differences between highly cross-reactive antibodies. Biochemistry *9:* 1880–1886.

Koshland, M. E., Reisfeld, R. A., and Dray, S. (1968). Differences in amino acid composition related to allotypic and antibody specificity of rabbit IgG heavy chains. Immunochemistry 5: 471–483.

Koyama, J., Grossberg, A. L., and Pressman, D. (1968). Variability among anti-*p*-azobenzenearsonate antibody preparations as revealed by affinity labeling. Biochemistry 7: 1935–1940.

Kreiter, V. P., and Pressman, D. (1964). Antibodies to a hapten with two determinant groups. Immunochemistry 1: 151–163.

Kunkel, H. G., Mannik, M., and Williams, R. C. (1963). Individual antigenic specificity of isolated antibodies. Science 140: 1218–1219.

Landsteiner, K. (1936). *Specificity of Serological Reactions.* Charles C Thomas. (Springfield, Ill., 178 pp.).

Landsteiner, K., and van der Scheer, J., (1932). On the serological specificity of peptides. J. Exp. Med. 55: 781–796.

Landsteiner, K., and van der Scheer, J. (1934). On the serological specificity of peptides. J. Exp. Med. 59: 769–780.

Landsteiner, K. and van der Scheer, J. (1936). On cross reactions of immune sera to azoproteins. J. Exp. Med. 63: 325–339.

Landsteiner, K., and van der Scheer, J. (1938). On cross reactions of immune sera to azoproteins. II. Antigens with azocomponents containing two determinant groups. J. Exptl. Med. 67: 709–723.

Landsteiner, K., and van der Scheer, J. (1939). On the serological specificity of peptides. J. Exp. Med. 69: 705–719.

Levine, B. B. (1963). Studies on the dimensions of the rabbit anti-benzylpenicilloyl antibody-combining sites. J. Exp. Med. 117: 161–183.

Levison, S. A., Kierszenbaum, F., and Dandliker, W. B. (1970). Salt effects on antigen-antibody kinetics. Biochemistry 9: 322–331.

Little, J. R., Border, W., and Freidin, R. (1969). The binding reactions of antibodies specific for the 2,6-dinitrophenyl group. J. Immunol. 103: 809–817.

Little, J. R., and Eisen, H. N. (1965). Physical and chemical differences between antibodies to the dinitrophenyl and trinitrophenyl groups. Fed. Proc. 24: 333 incl.

Little, J. R., and Eisen, H. N. (1967). Evidence for tryptophan in the active sites of antibodies to polnitrobenzenes. Biochemistry 6: 3119–3125.

Luderitz, O., Staub, A. M., and Westphal, O. (1966). Immunochemistry of O and R antigens of *Salmonella* and related Enterobacteriaceae. Bacteriol Rev. 30: 192–255.

MacDonald, A. B., Alescio, L., and Nisonoff, A. (1969). Biosynthesis of antibody molecules with similar properties during prolonged immunization. Biochemistry 8: 3109–3113.

Mage, R., and Kabat, E. A. (1963). Immunochemical studies on dextrans. III. The specificities of rabbit antidextrans. Further findings on antidextrans with 1,2 and 1,6 specificities. J. Immunol. 91: 633–640.

Makinodan, T., and Albright, J. F. (1967). Proliferative and differentiative manifestations of cellular immune potential. Progr. Allergy 10: 1–36.

Marrack, J. R. (1938). *The Chemistry of Antigens and Antibodies,* His Majesty's Stationery Office (London, 194 pp.).

Maurer, P. H. (1963). Nature of antigenic determinants in proteins and synthetic polypeptides. Ann. N. Y. Acad. Sci. 103: 549–580.

Metzger, H., and Singer, S. J. (1963). Binding capacity of reductively fragmented antibodies to the 2,4-dinitrophenyl group. Science 142: 674–676.

Metzger, H. L., Wofsy, L., and Singer, S. J. (1963). Affinity labeling of the active sites of antibodies to the 2,4-dinitrophenyl hapten. Biochemistry 2: 979–988.

Metzger, H., Wofsy, L., and Singer, S. J. (1964). The participation of A and B polypeptide chains in the active sites of antibody molecules. Proc. Natl. Acad. Sci. *51:* 612–618.

Moreno, C., and Kabat, E. A. (1969). Studies on human antibodies. VIII. Properties and association constants of human antibodies to blood group A substance purified with insoluble specific adsorbents and fractionally eluted with mono- and oligosaccharides. J. Exp. Med. *129:* 871–896.

Murphy, P. D., and Sage, H. J. (1970). Variation in the size of antibody sites for the poly-L-aspartate hapten during the immune response. J. Immunol. *105:* 460–470.

Nisonoff, A., MacDonald, A. B., Hopper, J. E., and Daugharty, H. (1970). Quantitative studies of idiotypic antibodies. Fed. Proc. *29:* 72–77.

Nossal, G. J. V., and Mäkelä, O. (1962). Autoradiographic studies on the immune response. I. The kinetics of plasma cell proliferation. J. Exp. Med. *115:* 209–244.

Ohta, Y., Gill, T. J., III, and Leung, C. S. (1970). Volume changes accompanying the antibody-antigen reaction. Biochemistry *9:* 2708–2712.

Oudin, J. (1966). The genetic control of immunoglobulin synthesis. Proc. Roy. Soc. Lond. *166:* 207–219.

Oudin, J. (1969). Recent data on idiotypy of rabbit antibodies. Behringwerk-Mitteil. *49:* 77–84.

Oudin, J., and Michel, M. (1963). Une nouvelle forme de l'allotypie des globulines γ du sérum de lapin, apparement lié à la fonction et à la spécificité anticorps. C. R. Acad. Sci. *257:* 805–808.

Oudin, J., and Michel, M. (1969a). Sur les spécificités idiotypiques des anticorps de lapin anti-S-typhi. C. R. Acad. Sci. *268:* 230–233.

Oudin, J., and Michel, M. (1969b). Idiotypy of rabbit antibodies. I. Comparison of idiotypy of antibodies against *Salmonella typhi* with that of antibodies against other bacteria in the same rabbits, or of antibodies against *Salmonella typhi* in various rabbits. J. Exp. Med. *130:* 595–617.

Oudin, J., and Michel, M. (1969c). Idiotypy of rabbit antibodies. II. Comparison of idiotypy of various kinds of antibodies formed in the same rabbits against *Salmonella typhi*. J. Exp. Med. *130:* 619–642.

Pauling, L. (1940). A theory of the structure and process of formation of antibodies. J. Am. Chem. Soc. *62:* 2643–2657.

Pernis, B. (1967). Relationships between the heterogeneity of immunoglobulins and the differentiation of plasma cells. Symp. Quant. Biol. *32:* 333–341.

Porter, R. R. (1959). The hydrolysis of rabbit γ-globulin and antibodies with crystalline papain. Biochem. J. *73:* 119–126

Press, E. M., and Piggot, P. J. (1967). The chemical structure of the heavy chains of human immunoglobulin G. Symp. Quant. Biol. *32:* 45–51.

Pressman, D., Grossberg, A. L., Roholt, O., Stelos, P., and Yagi, Y. (1963). The chemical nature of antibody molecules and their combining sites. Ann. N. Y. Acad. Sci. *103:* 582–594.

Pressman, D., and Roholt, O. (1961). Isolation of peptides from an antibody site. Proc. Natl. Acad. Sci. *47:* 1606–1610.

Rieder, R. F., and Oudin, J. (1963). Studies on the relationship of allotypic specificities to antibody specificities in the rabbit. J. Exp. Med. *118:* 627–633.

Robbins, J. B., Mozes, E., Rimon, A., and Sela, M. (1967). Correlation between net charge of antigens and electrophoretic mobility of immunoglobulin M antibodies. Nature *213:* 1013–1014.

Roholt, O., Radzimski, G., and Pressman, D. (1963). Antibody combining site—the B polypeptide chain. Science *141:* 726–727.

Rothen, A., and Landsteiner, K. (1939). Absorption of antibodies by egg albumin films. Science 90: 65–66.

Rubinstein, W. A., and Little, J. R. (1970). Properties of the active sites of antibodies specific for folic acid. Biochemistry 9: 2106–2114.

Rüde, E., Mozes, E., and Sela, M. (1968). Role of the net electrical charge of the complete antigen in determining the chemical nature of anti-p-azobenzenearsonate antibodies. Biochemistry 7: 2971–2975.

Sage, H. J., Deutsch, G. F., Fasman, G. D., and Levine, L. (1964). The serological specificity of the poly-alanine immune system. Immunochemistry 1: 133–144.

Schechter, B., Schechter, I., and Sela, M. (1970a). Antibody combining sites to a series of peptide determinants of increasing size and defined structure. J. Biol. Chem. 245: 1438–1457.

Schechter, B., Schechter, I., and Sela, M. (1970b). Specific fractionation of antibodies to peptide determinants. Immunochemistry 7: 587–597.

Schechter, I., Schechter, B., and Sela, M. (1966). Combining sites of antibodies with L-alanine and D-alanine peptide specificity and the effect of serum proteolytic activity on their estimation. Biochim. Biophys. Acta 127: 438–456.

Schechter, I., and Sela, M. (1965). Combining sites of antibodies to L-alanine and D-alanine peptide determinants. Biochim. Biophys. Acta 104: 298–300.

Schlossman, S. F., and Kabat, E. A. (1962). Specific fractionation of a population of antidextran molecules with combining sites of various sizes. J. Exp. Med. 116: 535–552.

Schoellman, G., and Shaw, E. (1962). A new method for labelling the active center of chymotrypsin. Biochem. Biophys. Res. Commun. 7: 36–40.

Schooley, J. C. (1961). Autoradiographic observations of plasma cell formation. J. Immunol. 86: 331–337.

Segal, S., Givol, D., and Sela, M. (1969). Disc electrophoresis patterns of the Fd fragment of rabbit immunoglobulin fractions and of purified antibodies. Immunochemistry 6: 229–234.

Sela, M., Givol, D., and Mozes, E. (1963). Resolution of rabbit γ-globulin into two fractions by chromatography on diethylaminoethyl sephadex. Biochim. Biophys. Acta 78: 649–657.

Sela, M., and Mozes, E. (1966). Dependence of the chemical nature of antibodies on the net electrical charge of antigens. Proc. Natl. Acad. Sci. 55: 445–452.

Sercarz, E., and Coons, A. H. (1962). The exhaustion of specific antibody producing capacity during a secondary response. In Mechanisms of Immunological Tolerance, Hasek, M., Lengerova, A., and Vojtiskova, M., eds. Academic Press (New York, 544 pp.) p. 73–83.

Singer, S. J., and Doolittle, R. F. (1966). Antibody active sites and immunoglobulin molecules. Science 153: 13–25.

Singer, S. J., Slobin, L. I., Thorpe, N. O., and Fenton, J. W. II. (1967). On the structure of antibody active sites. Symp. Quant. Biol. 32: 99–110.

Singer, S. J., and Thorpe, N. O. (1968). On the location and structure of the active sites of antibody molecules. Proc. Natl. Acad. Sci. 60: 1371–1378.

Slater, R. J., Ward, S. M., and Kunkel, H. G. (1955). Immunological relationships among the myeloma proteins. J. Exp. Med. 101: 85–108.

Spring, S. B., Nisonoff, A., and Dray, S. (1970). Independence of allotypic determinants and antibody specificity. J. Immunol. 105: 653–660.

Stollar, D., Levine, L., Lehrer, H. I., and Van Vunakis, H. (1962). The antigenic determinants of denatured deoxyribonucleic acid (DNA) reactive with lupus erythematosus serum. Proc. Natl. Acad. Sci. 48: 874–880.

Strosberg, A. D., and Kanarek, L. (1970). Ratio of the Fab fragments I and II from goat antibodies and normal γ-globulins. Fed. Eur. Biochem. Soc. Letters 6: 28–30.

Taliaferro, W. H., and Talmage, D. W. (1956). Antibodies in the rabbit with different rates of metabolic decay. J. Infect. Dis. 99: 21–33.

Talmage, D. W., and Cann, J. R. (1961). The Chemistry of Immunity in Health and Disease, Charles C Thomas (Springfield, Ill., 178 pp.) pp. 129–132.

Thorpe, N. O., and Singer, S. J. (1969). The affinity-labeled residues in antibody active sites. II. Nearest-neighbor analyses. Biochemistry 8: 4523–4534.

Traylor, P. S., and Singer, S. J. (1967). The preparation and properties of some tritiated diazonium salts and related compounds. Biochemistry 6: 881–887.

Tsuji, F. I., and Davis, D. L. (1959). A quantitative photometric method for studying the reaction between Cypridina luciferase and specific antibody. J. Immunol. 82: 153–160.

Tsuji, F. I., Davis, D. L., and Donald, D. H. (1966). The effect of hydrostatic pressure on the rate of inactivation of Cypridina luciferase by specific antibody. J. Immunol. 96: 614–621.

Tsuji, F. I., Davis, D. L., and Gindler, E. M. (1962). Effect of sodium chloride and pH on the rate of neutralization of Cypridina luciferase by specific antibody. J. Immunol. 88: 83–92.

Utsumi, S., and Karush, F. (1964). The subunits of purified rabbit antibody. Biochemistry 3: 1329–1338.

Warner, C., and Schumaker, V. (1970). The detection of a conformational change in an antihapten antibody system upon interaction with divalent haptens. Biochemistry 9: 451–459.

Warner, C., Schumaker, V., and Karush, F. (1970). The detection of a conformational change in the antibody molecule upon interaction with hapten. Biochem. Biophys. Res. Commun. 38: 125–128.

Waxdal, M. J., Konigsberg, W. H., and Edelman, G. M. (1967). The structure of a human gamma G immunoglobulin. Symp. Quant. Biol. 32: 53–63.

Weigle, W. O. (1958). Estimation of antigen-antibody complexes from sera of rabbits. J. Immunol. 81: 204–213.

Whitney, P. L., and Tanford, C. (1965a). Recovery of specific activity after complete unfolding and reduction of an antibody fragment. Proc. Natl. Acad. Sci. 53: 524–532.

Whitney, P. L., and Tanford, C. (1965b). Properties of the soluble product obtained from reoxidation of reduced fragment I from rabbit 7S γ-immunoglobulin. J. Biol. Chem. 240: 4271–4276.

Wofsy, L., Kimura, J., Bing, D. H., and Parker, D. C. (1967). Affinity labeling of rabbit antisaccharide antibodies. Biochemistry 6: 1981–1988.

Wofsy, L., Klinman, N. R., and Karush, F. (1967). Affinity labeling of equine anti-β-lactoside antibodies. Biochemistry 6: 1988–1991.

Wofsy, L., Metzger, H., and Singer, S. J. (1962). Affinity labeling—a general method for labeling the active sites of antibody and enzyme molecules. Biochemistry 1: 1031–1039.

Wofsy, L., and Parker, D. C. (1967). Comparative studies of antibody active sites. Symp. Quant. Biol. 32: 111–116.

Wu, T. T., and Kabat, E. A. (1970). An analysis of the sequences of the variable regions of Bence-Jones proteins and myeloma light chains and their implications for antibody complementarity. J. Exp. Med. 132: 211–250.

Yount, W. J., Dorner, M. M., Kunkel, H. G., and Kabat, E. A. (1968). Studies on human antibodies. VI. Selective variations in subgroup composition of genetic markers. J. Exp. Med. *127:* 633–646.

Zappacosta, S., and Nisonoff, A. (1968). Complementarity of heavy and light chains from antibodies of the same specificity derived from different rabbits. J. Immunol. *100:* 781–787.

PART TWO

Reactions of
Antibodies

5

AFFINITY AND THE LAW OF MASS ACTION

Derivations of the Affinity Equations for an Ideal Reaction

1. Introduction

To understand the function of antibodies one must understand affinity, and to understand affinity one must understand the "law of mass action." Karush (1970) has called this intrinsic reversible reaction, that leads to complex formation between antigen and antibody and that establishes affinity, "the pivotal element in the biological activity of the antibody molecule." Burnet (1967) has presented two diagrams that "contain the essentials of a modern selection theory of antibody production" and that "have a good chance of remaining valid indefinitely" in their generalized form. One well acquainted with the necessary ingredients of the law of mass action will recognize in Burnet's diagrams, which will be presented in Chapter 10, yet another variant of the Law. Obviously, if one wishes to understand basic biological immunology in terms of this modern selection theory one has an additional reason for coming to grips with the physical scientist's meaning of affinity. In this chapter the various forms of the affinity equations are derived in simple algebraic form. In the subsequent chapters applications of some of the equations will be presented.

2. Rigorous derivation of ideal affinity equations

Ideal affinity assumes that each reactant, antigen and antibody, is homogeneous with respect to determinants and binding sites; further, that the number of determinants on each antigen molecule (antigenic valence) is uniform and that the number of binding sites on each antibody molecule (antibody valence) is also uniform. After we examine the ideal affinity equation it will then be easier to understand the implications of deviations from the ideal.

181

We have two concerns: (i) to measure the concentrations of antigen and antibody molecules that are joined to each other and of those that are free, and (ii) to measure the fractions of the determinants and of the binding sites that are filled and empty in the antigen and antibody molecules that are bound to each other. Obviously all the determinants of a free and unbound antigen are empty and all the binding sites of a free and unbound antibody are empty.

Let the fraction of free and bound antibody molecules be designated as a and b; and the fraction of free and bound antigen molecules, as p and q. Thus, $a + b = 1$; $p + q = 1$.

Let the fraction of binding sites of *bound* antibody molecules that are empty and filled be designated as i and j; and the fraction of determinants of *bound* antigen molecules that are empty and filled, k and l. Thus, $i + j = 1$; $k + l = 1$.

Let A be the total number of antibody molecules in the system; P, the total number of antigen molecules in the system.

Let n be the antibody valence and s, the antigen valence. The valence is that number of sites on a molecule that participates at any one time in mass action; essentially, it is the maximum number of sites that can be occupied by the opposite complementary member at any one time.

The axiom of all immunochemistry is expressed at all times by the relationship between filled antibody and antigen sites:

$$jbnA = lqsP \tag{5.1}$$

Thus, the concentration of antibody binding sites that are occupied is equal to the concentration of antigenic determinants that are covered.

The concentration of unfilled antibody binding sites is given by the sum of two quantities: the number of free sites in the bound antibody molecules and the total number of sites in the free antibody molecules. The same holds true for unoccupied antigenic determinants. Thus, the total number of antibody binding sites in the system is given by:

$$nA = jbnA + ibnA + anA \tag{5.2}$$

And the total number of antigenic determinants is given by

$$sP = lqsP + kqsP + psP \tag{5.3}$$

Consider the interaction between an individual antibody site F and an individual antigen site H to form a joined complementation unit, FH. With forward and reverse rate reaction constants of k_1 and k_2, respectively, the reaction can be written in simple bimolecular form as

$$F + H \underset{k_2}{\overset{k_1}{\rightleftharpoons}} FH \tag{5.4}$$

Letting $[F]$ be the concentration of free and unbound univalent antibody fragments; $[H]$, the concentration of free and unbound univalent antigenic determinants or haptenic groups or ligands; $[FH)$, the concentration of joined complementation units; and K_{12}, the association constant at equilibrium, equal to k_1/k_2, it follows from the law of mass action that

$$\frac{[FH]}{[F][H]} = \frac{k_1}{k_2} = K_{12} \tag{5.5}$$

In an intact antibody molecule A assume that the n active sites will act independently of each other in mass action; likewise, in an antigen molecule or particle P assume that the s individual sites will act independently of each other in mass action.

In an intact antibody and an intact antigen system one can derive equations either in terms of bound antibody sites (a) or bound antigenic determinants (b).

$$[F] = nA - jbnA \tag{5.6a}$$

$$[H] = sP - jbnA \tag{5.7a}$$

$$[FH] = jbnA \tag{5.8a}$$

$$\therefore K_{12} = \frac{jbnA}{(nA - jbnA)(sp - jbnA)} \tag{5.9a}$$

and

$$K_{12} = \left(\frac{jb}{1 - jb}\right)\left(\frac{1}{sP - jbnA}\right) \tag{5.10a}$$

$$\therefore \frac{jb}{1 - jb} = sPK_{12} - jbnAK_{12} \tag{5.11a}$$

and

$$\frac{jbA}{(1 - jb)A} = sPK_{12} - jbnAK_{12} \tag{5.12a}$$

$$\frac{\frac{jbA}{P}}{(1 - jb)A} = sK_{12} - \frac{jbA}{P}nK_{12} \tag{5.13a}$$

Letting

$$f = jbA/P \text{ and } d = (1 - jb)A$$

$$\frac{f}{d} = sK_{12} - nfK_{12} \tag{5.14a}$$

$$[F] = nA - lqsP \tag{5.6b}$$

$$[H] = sP - lqsP \tag{5.7b}$$

$$[FH] = lqsP \tag{5.8b}$$

$$\therefore K_{12} = \frac{lqsP}{(nA - lqsP)(sP - lqsP)} \tag{5.9b}$$

and

$$K_{12} = \left(\frac{lq}{1 - lq}\right)\left(\frac{1}{nA - lqsP}\right) \tag{5.10b}$$

$$\therefore \frac{lq}{1 - lq} = nAK_{12} - lqsPK_{12} \tag{5.11b}$$

and

$$\frac{lqP}{(1 - lq)P} = nAK_{12} - lqsPK_{12} \tag{5.12b}$$

$$\frac{\dfrac{lqP}{A}}{(1 - lq)P} = nK_{12} - \frac{lqP}{A}sK_{12} \tag{5.13b}$$

Letting

$$r = lqP/A \text{ and } c = (1 - lq)P$$

$$\frac{r}{c} = nK_{12} - srK_{12} \tag{5.14b}$$

3. Various special cases of $[r/c = nK_{12} - srK_{12}]$

The value sr represents the total number of filled antigen sites per total antibody in the system ($sr = lsqP/A$) and the value sc represents the total number of empty antigen sites in the system $[sc = (1 - lq)sP]$.

(A) *Special case of univalent antigen or hapten.* In equilibrium dialysis with dialyzable monovalent antigen or hapten in antigen excess:

$s = 1$, since hapten is monovalent
$l = 1$, since by necessity it can't be less

$$c = (1 - q)P = pP \qquad (5.15)$$

and

$$r = qP/A \qquad (5.16)$$

The value c thus represents in this special case free unbound, dialyzable, antigen molecules and the value r represents antibody-bound antigen molecules per total antibody in the system. Therefore,

$$\frac{r}{c} = nK_{12} - rK_{12} \qquad (5.17)$$

This is the familiar Scatchard (1949) form of the law of mass action and the one most widely used in immunochemistry. It has also been misused from time to time as we shall see later on.

If the data are plotted in terms of r/c vs. r, a straight-line relationship is obtained (Fig. 5-1). Extrapolation of r/c to the abscissa (infinite antigen excess with c infinitely high) gives an intercept value equal to antibody valence since, as $r/c \rightarrow 0$,

$$nK_{12} = rK_{12} \qquad (5.18)$$

$$n = r \qquad (5.19)$$

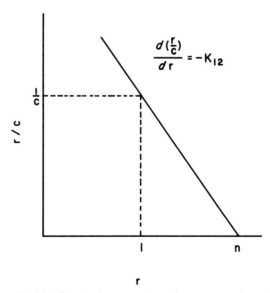

FIG. 5-1. Ideal binding in the case of univalent antigen; Scatchard plot.

The slope of the line gives the value for the association constant since

$$\frac{d\left(\dfrac{r}{c}\right)}{dr} = -K_{12} \tag{5.20}$$

A special case is obtained when the antibody valence n is two and when the antibody-bound univalent hapten molecules equal the total number of antibody molecules, i.e., when r is one and therefore when half the bivalent antibody binding sites are filled. Equation 5.17 then becomes

$$\frac{1}{c} = 2K_{12} - K_{12} = K_{12} = K_0 \tag{5.21}$$

and

$$cK_0 = 1 \tag{5.22}$$

This relation is frequently used to obtain values for association constants since it depends only upon obtaining a value for the reciprocal of the free hapten concentration. The intrinsic association constant obtained in this manner is dependent only upon the conditions that antibody be bivalent and antigen be univalent. Unfortunately, the relation is sometimes misused in an attempt to obtain association constants where these conditions are not met.

In the special case of certain γM molecules when the antibody valence n is 5 and when the antibody-bound univalent hapten molecules equal the total number of antibody molecules, i.e., when r is 1, equation 5.17 then becomes

$$\frac{1}{c} = 5K_{12} - K_{12} = 4K_{12} = 4K_0 \tag{5.23}$$

This relation says that under the conditions necessary to obtain a value for an intrinsic association constant of a pentavalent antibody based solely upon free hapten concentration, i.e., when $r = 1$, the reciprocal of the free hapten concentration must be divided by 4 to give the true value. For antibodies with a valence of 10

$$\frac{1}{c} = 9K_0 \tag{5.24}$$

and for antibodies with a valence of 1 the relation disappears.

$$\frac{1}{c} = 0 \tag{5.25}$$

For antibodies with a valence of n, the general relation becomes

$$\frac{1}{c} = (n - 1)K_0 \qquad (5.26)$$

(B) *Special case in far antigen excess when antigen is not univalent.* When n-valent antibody molecules are overwhelmingly outnumbered by s-valent antigen molecules in a concentration region of far antigen excess, three possible situations may prevail:

(i) Each antibody site on an antibody molecule may be occupied by single antigenic determinants from separate antigen molecules,

(ii) Each antibody site on an antibody molecule may be occupied by antigenic determinants that are all from the same antigen molecule, or

(iii) Antibody sites may be occupied in a mixed manner.

When conditions are such that (i) is obtained, one determinant on each antigen molecule is occupied and $l = 1/s$. Since $j = 1$ and $b = 1$, the antibody valence n is given by the number of bound antigen sites, i.e., since $jbnA = lqsP$,

$$nA = qP \qquad (5.27)$$

$$n = qP/A \qquad (5.28)$$

It holds in this case, therefore, that the valence of antibody is given by the number of bound antigen molecules per antibody molecule regardless of their valence.

Since $r = lqP/A$ and $c = (1 - lq)P$ and, under these conditions, $l = 1/s$, equation 5.14b becomes

$$\frac{\dfrac{qP}{sA}}{\left(1 - \dfrac{q}{s}\right)P} = nK_{12} - \frac{sqP}{sA}K_{12} \qquad (5.29)$$

which, upon rearrangement and elimination of terms, becomes

$$K_{12} = \frac{q}{(s - q)(nA - qP)} \qquad (5.30)$$

Under conditions where q is very small compared to s, the equation may be written in simpler form as

$$K_{12} = \frac{q}{s(nA - qP)} \qquad (5.31)$$

When conditions are such that (ii) is obtained, n determinants on each antigen molecule are occupied and n is indeterminate since

$l = n/s$. From equation 5.27 we then obtained $qP = A$. Equation 5.14b becomes

$$\frac{\dfrac{nqP}{sA}}{\left(1 - \dfrac{n}{s}\, q\right)P} = nK_{12} - \frac{nqP}{sA}\, sK_{12} \tag{5.32}$$

which, upon rearrangement, elimination of terms, and simplification, becomes

$$K_{12} = \frac{q}{(s - nq)(A - qP)} \sim \frac{q}{s(A - qP)} \tag{5.33}$$

(C) *Special case of equivalence.* The definition of ideal equivalence for multivalent antigen and multivalent antibody molecules is that point where the concentrations of reactants are such that all antigen and antibody molecules are bound to each other. There are no free antigen or antibody molecules (except, cf. equation 5.58). The fraction b of bound antibody molecules is 1 and the fraction q of bound antigen molecules is 1. There are, however, many empty sites. The fraction j of filled antibody sites of bound antibody range from $1/n$ at far antibody excess to 1 at far antigen excess with some intermediate value at equivalence; likewise, the fraction l of covered antigenic determinants may range from $1/s$ at far antigen excess to 1 at far antibody excess, again with some intermediate value at equivalence. The relation 5.1 still holds, however, and becomes

$$jnA = lsP \tag{5.34}$$

Equation 5.14b becomes

$$\frac{\dfrac{lP}{A}}{(1 - l)P} = nK_{12} - s\, \frac{lP}{A}\, K_{12} \tag{5.35}$$

which reduces to

$$\frac{l}{1 - l} = nAK_{12} - slPK_{12} = (nA - slP)K_{12} \tag{5.36}$$

Since $slP = jnA$, $1 - l = k$, and $1 - j = i$, we obtain

$$\frac{l}{k} = (nA - jnA)K_{12} = inAK_{12} \tag{5.37}$$

and

$$K_{12} = \frac{l}{kinA} \tag{5.38}$$

For a bivalent antibody at equivalence in the presence of an oligo-valent antigen, it is safe to assume that nearly all the antibody bind-ing sites are filled, i.e., that $n = 2$ and $i = 1$. Equation 5.38 then simplifies to

$$K_{12} = \frac{l}{2kA} \tag{5.39}$$

Thus, to obtain a value for the equilibrium constant from equivalence data, one need only have a knowledge of the ratio of the covered and empty antigenic determinants and the total antibody concentration.

4. Various special cases of $[f/d = sK_{12} - nfK_{12}]$

The value nf represents the total number of filled antibody sites per total antigen in the system and the value nd represents the total number of empty antibody sites in the system; i.e., $(nf = jbnA/P)$ and $[nd = (1 - jb)nA]$.

(A) *Special case of equilibrium filtration near equivalence with bivalent antibody.*

$$n = 2$$
$$j = 1$$
$$\frac{f}{d} = sK_{12} - 2fK_{12} \tag{5.40}$$

The value f now represents the number of bound antibody molecules per total number of antigen molecules; the value d becomes the num-ber of free antibody molecules that filter through the system leaving bound antibodies behind upon unfilterable antigen molecules or particles.

When f/d is plotted against f, a straight-line relationship is obtained for ideal systems (Fig. 5-2). The intercept on the abscissa gives the half-valence of antigen and the slope in absolute terms gives a double value for the association constant. As $f/d \rightarrow 0$,

$$sK_{12} = 2fK_{12} \tag{5.41}$$

$$s = 2f = 2bA/P \tag{5.42}$$

(B) *Special case of equilibrium filtration in far bivalent antibody excess.* When s-valent antigen molecules or particles are over-whelmingly outnumbered by bivalent antibody molecules in a con-centration region of far antibody excess, three possible situations may prevail that would result in complete determinant coverage:

(i) Each antigenic determinant of an antigen molecule may be occupied by an antibody site from an antibody molecule not shared by any other determinant,

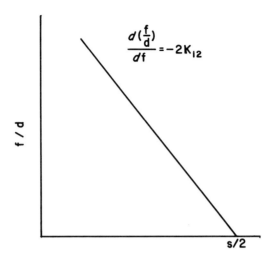

$$\frac{d\left(\frac{f}{d}\right)}{df} = -2K_{12}$$

FIG. 5-2. Ideal binding in the case of equilibrium filtration near equivalence with bivalent antibody; Scatchard plot.

(ii) a pair of antigenic determinants on an antigen molecule may share the bivalent binding sites from a single antibody molecule, or
(iii) antigenic determinants may be covered in a mixed manner.
When conditions are such that (i) is obtained,

$$j = \frac{1}{n} = \frac{1}{2},$$
$$f = bA/2P,$$
$$\begin{aligned}
d &= [1 - (b/2)]A \\
&= [1 - b + (b/2)]A \\
&= (1 - b)A + (bA/2) \\
&= aA + (bA/2)
\end{aligned} \qquad (5.43)$$

and

$$f/d = b/(2aP + bP) \qquad (5.44)$$

Equation 5.40 then becomes

$$\frac{b}{2aP + bP} = sK_{12} - 2\frac{bA}{2P}K_{12} \qquad (5.45)$$

which, upon rearrangement and elimination of terms, reduces to

$$K_{12} = \frac{b}{(2a + b)(sP - bA)} \qquad (5.46)$$

When f/d is plotted against f, as $f/d \to 0$,

$$sK_{12} = 2fK_{12}$$

$$s = 2f = bA/P \qquad (5.47)$$

The slope of the line still remains

$$\frac{d\left(\dfrac{f}{d}\right)}{df} = -2K_{12}$$

Thus it can be seen that regardless of whether (A) or (B, i) pertains, the same equilibrium constant is obtained. The only difference is that the antigenic valence in (A) is double the number of bound antibody molecules per total antigen whereas in (B, i) it is equal to the number bound. When conditions are such that (ii) is obtained, $j = 1$, $n = 2$, and the equations written for (A) pertain. Thus, (B, ii) and (A) are equivalent. It should be noted that, if one were to trace the whole course of *homogeneous binding* by equilibrium filtration from equivalence to far antibody excess, the shape of the curve would be that of curve I in Figure 5-3 for (A) and (B, i), and would be that of curve II for (A) and (B, ii).

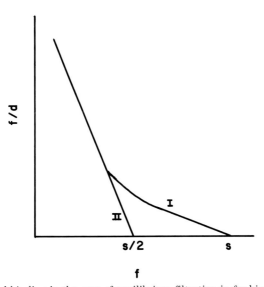

Fig. 5-3. Ideal binding in the case of equilibrium filtration in far bivalent antibody excess. *Curve I*, homogeneous binding when antibody acts in an increasingly univalent fashion with increasing antibody/antigen ratios. *Curve II*, homogeneous binding when antibody acts as a monogamous bivalent entity.

5. Extent of the reaction—the Karush equation

Equations 5.9a and 5.9b can be used to derive two values, α and β, which are named the extent of reaction in accordance with the concept presented by Karush (1970).

$$K_{12} = \frac{jbnA}{(nA - jbnA)(sP - jbnA)} \tag{5.9a}$$

Using the value F for the concentration of free sites, one obains

$$K_{12} = \frac{jbnA}{(F)(sP - jbnA)} \tag{5.48a}$$

$$jbnA = (F)(sP - jbnA)K_{12} \tag{5.49a}$$

$$\frac{jbnA}{sP} = (F)\left(1 - \frac{jbnA}{sP}\right)K_{12} \tag{5.50a}$$

$$\frac{jbnA}{sP} + \frac{jbnA}{sP}(F)K_{12} = (F)K_{12} \tag{5.51a}$$

$$\frac{jbnA}{sP}[1 + (F)K_{12}] = (F)K_{12} \tag{5.52a}$$

$$\frac{jbnA}{sP} = \frac{(F)K_{12}}{1 + (F)K_{12}} \tag{5.53a}$$

Since $jbnA = lqsP$

$$lq = \frac{(F)K_{12}}{1 + (F)K_{12}} \tag{5.54a}$$

When $l = 1$ and $(F) = d$

$$q = \beta = \frac{dK_{12}}{1 + dK_{12}} \tag{5.55a}$$

$$K_{12} = \frac{lqsP}{(nA - lqsP)(sP - lqsP)} \tag{5.9b}$$

Using the value H for the concentration of free determinants, one obtains

$$K_{12} = \frac{lqsP}{(nA - lqsP)(H)} \tag{5.48b}$$

$$lqsP = (H)(nA - lqsP)K_{12} \tag{5.49b}$$

$$\frac{lqsP}{nA} = (H)\left(1 - \frac{lqsP}{nA}\right)K_{12} \tag{5.50b}$$

$$\frac{lqsP}{nA} + \frac{lqsP}{nA}(H)K_{12} = (H)K_{12} \tag{5.51b}$$

$$\frac{lqsP}{nA}[1 + (H)K_{12}] = (H)K_{12} \tag{5.52b}$$

$$\frac{lqsP}{nA} = \frac{(H)K_{12}}{1 + (H)K_{12}} \tag{5.53b}$$

Since $lqsP = jbnA$

$$jb = \frac{(H)K_{12}}{1 + (H)K_{12}} \tag{5.54b}$$

When $j = 1$ and $(H) = c$

$$b = \alpha = \frac{cK_{12}}{1 + cK_{12}} \tag{5.55b}$$

Karush used the same equation to express both states as follows: "We may describe the extent of the reaction in simplified form by the expression

$$\alpha = (Kc)/(1 + Kc)$$

where α is the fraction of antigen reacted when c is the free equilibrium concentration of antibody and K is the association constant. When c is taken as the free equilibrium of antigen, then α measures the fraction of the antibody population in complex with antigen."

In our derivations the notation of c and α are preserved for the latter case only while the notation d and β are used for the former. It can be seen that β is synonymous with q, the fraction of bound antigen molecules, while α is synonymous with b, the fraction of bound antibody molecules, when l and j are both equal to 1. Otherwise, $\beta = lq$ and $\alpha = jb$. Also it can be seen that d is the concentration of unfilled Fab and is equal to unbound antibody molecules only where antibodies are univalent. Likewise, c is the concentration of uncovered antigenic determinants and is equal to unbound antigen molecules only where antigen is univalent. At equivalence the extent of reaction β is equal to l while α is equal to j. The values d and c would then be the concentration of unfilled antibody sites and uncovered antigenic determinants, i.e.,

$$l = \frac{dK_{12}}{1 + dK_{12}} \tag{5.56}$$

and

$$j = \frac{cK_{12}}{1 + cK_{12}} \tag{5.57}$$

Solving these two equations for K_{12}, equating them, and rearranging terms, one obtains the conditions for ideal equivalence:

$$\frac{c}{d} = \frac{jk}{il} \tag{5.58}$$

Regardless of whether one is considering the extent of reaction in terms of equation 5.55a, 5.55b, 5.56, or 5.57, the feature that remains unchanged is the one that Karush wishes to emphasize, namely: "The extent of reaction depends on the product of a concentration and an association constant."

6. Langmuir form of affinity equation

Rearrangement of terms of equations 5.14a and 5.14b into the familiar style of the Langmuir adsorption isotherm gives the following derivations:

$$\frac{f}{d} = sK_{12} - nfK_{12} \tag{5.14a}$$

$$\frac{r}{c} = nK_{12} - srK_{12} \tag{5.14b}$$

$$\frac{1}{d} = \frac{s}{f}K_{12} - nK_{12} \tag{5.59a}$$

$$\frac{1}{c} = \frac{n}{r}K_{12} - sK_{12} \tag{5.59b}$$

$$\frac{s}{f}K_{12} = \frac{1}{d} + nK_{12} \tag{5.60a}$$

$$\frac{n}{r}K_{12} = \frac{1}{c} + sK_{12} \tag{5.60b}$$

$$\frac{1}{f} = \frac{1}{sdK_{12}} + \frac{n}{s} \tag{5.61a}$$

$$\frac{1}{r} = \frac{1}{ncK_{12}} + \frac{s}{n} \tag{5.61b}$$

In the case of univalent hapten and homogeneous n-valent antibody in far antigen excess, equation 5.61b becomes another familiar form in immunochemistry:

$$\frac{1}{r} = \frac{1}{ncK_{12}} + \frac{1}{n} \tag{5.62}$$

The straight-line relationship is graphically shown by plotting $1/r$ vs. $1/c$ (Fig. 5-4). In this case as the concentration of free hapten c becomes infinite the intercept on the ordinate becomes the reciprocal of the antibody valence. When multivalent antigen is used instead, the intercept becomes s/n; and, if the conditions of equation 5.29 pertain, $l = 1/s$, $r = lqP/A$, and

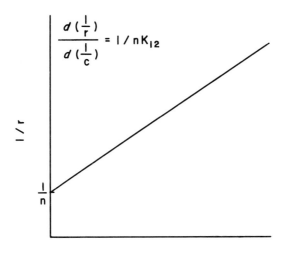

FIG. 5-4. Ideal binding in the case of univalent antigen; Langmuir plot.

$$\frac{1}{r} = \frac{sA}{qP} = \frac{s}{n} \qquad (5.63)$$

$$n = qP/A$$

7. Heterogeneity constants

Another rearrangement of the affinity equations follows:

$$\frac{f}{d} = sK_{12} - nfK_{12} \quad (5.14a) \qquad \frac{r}{c} = nK_{12} - srK_{12} \quad (5.14b)$$

$$\frac{f}{s - nf} = dK_{12} \qquad (5.64a) \qquad \frac{r}{n - sr} = cK_{12} \qquad (5.64b)$$

If the Scatchard or Langmuir forms of the affinity equations do not give rise to linearity, commensurate with homogeneous binding, the reciprocal relationship between association constant and free equilibrium concentration of binding sites or haptenic determinants may be at fault, particularly at the extremes of their relationship. The intrinsic association constant may only be an average of high and low binding antibodies which require, respectively, low and high free component concentrations to satisfy the equilibrium. One method to modify the relationship is to consider the product cK_0 as subject to exponential treatment according to Gaussian distribution (Karush and Sonenberg, 1949), by application of the Sips distribution function (Nisonoff and Pressman, 1958), or by the empirical probability density function of Bowman and Aladjem (1963). The more usual current method is to calculate Sipsian heterogeneity constants in the manner of Karush (1962) by assuming the product cK_0 as an exponential function $(cK_0)^a$ in which a is the heterogeneity constant (equivalent to that of Nisonoff and Pressman, 1958). Equations 5.64a and 5.64b then become

$$\frac{f}{s - nf} = (dK_0)^b \qquad (5.65a)$$

$$\log\left(\frac{f}{s - nf}\right) = b \log d + b \log K_0 \qquad (5.66a)$$

$$\frac{r}{n - sr} = (cK_0)^a \qquad (5.65b)$$

$$\log\left(\frac{r}{n - sr}\right) = a \log c + a \log K_0 \qquad (5.66b)$$

One knows the value of n and s when carrying out equilibrium dialysis experiments with monovalent hapten and bivalent antibody, so that equation 5.66b becomes

$$\log\left(\frac{r}{2 - r}\right) = a \log c + a \log K_0 \qquad (5.67)$$

By plotting the $\log [r/(2 - r)]$ against $\log c$, one obtains the best linear fit and calculates from its slope the heterogeneity constant a. For a homogeneous equation it follows that $a = 1$.

8. Interrelationships

From equations 5.9a and 5.9b, it can also be derived that

$$\frac{jb}{sP} = (1 - lq)(1 - jb)K_{12} \qquad (5.68)$$

and that

$$\frac{lq}{nA} = (1 - jb)(1 - lq)K_{12} \qquad (5.69)$$

In other words

$$\frac{jb}{sP} = \frac{lq}{nA} = (1 - jb)(1 - lq)K_{12} \qquad (5.70)$$

This form of the affinity equation can be used should it happen that one heterogeneity distribution does not hold for antigen, antibody, and association constant alike. For example, one might find that

$$\frac{jb}{sP} = \frac{lq}{nA} = (1 - jb)^u (1 - lq)^v (K_{12})^w \qquad (5.71)$$

would satisfy certain conditions. One might also wish to transform the system into a probability density function in the manner of Bowman and Aladjem (1963), but treat antigenic heterogeneity, antibody heterogeneity, and affinity heterogeneity as separate independent functions. Note that jb and lq are extents of antibody and antigen reaction as described above in paragraph 5.

REFERENCES

Bowman, J. D., and Aladjem, F. (1963). A method for the determination of heterogeneity of antibodies. J. Theor. Biol. 4: 242–253.

Burnet, F. M. (1967). The impact on ideas of immunology. Symp. Quant. Biol. 32: 1–8.

Karush, F. (1962). Immunologic specificity and molecular structure. Adv. Immunol. 2: 1–40.

Karush, F. (1970). Affinity and the immune process. Ann. N.Y. Acad. Sci. 169: 56–71.

Karush, F., and Sonenberg, M. (1949). Interaction of homologous alkyl sulfates with bovine serum albumin. J. Am. Chem. Soc. 71: 1369–1376.

Nisonoff, A., and Pressman, D. (1958a). Heterogeneity and average combining constants of antibodies from individual rabbits. J. Immunol. 80: 417–428.

Nisonoff, A., and Pressman, D. (1958b). Heterogeneity of antibody sites in their relative combining affinities for structurally related haptens. J. Immunol. 81: 126–135.

Scatchard, G. (1949). The attractions of proteins for small molecules and ions. Ann. N.Y. Acad. Sci. 51: 660–672.

6

ANTIBODY REACTIONS WITH HAPTENS

1. Definition of a hapten

The word *hapten*, in its original Greek verb form means *to touch*, *to grasp*, and *to fasten*. No other single word can describe in such an exquisitely simple manner the whole process of binding of an antigenic determinant with an antibody binding site. Many variations in the definition of a hapten have arisen since the word was first used by Landsteiner in 1921 (to refer to simple organic residues that react specifically with antibodies), but none describe so well what is really meant as the original Greek meaning. In modern usage *hapten*, *determinant group*, and *ligand* are synonymous. To stretch the usage of hapten to the full extent of its analytical meaning, the following simple definition contains the necessary essence:

> A hapten is that specific chemical grouping to which a single antibody site conforms and with which it reacts.

A corollary to this definition is a postulate which is basic to the processes of hapten inhibition, antigen neutralization, and antibody purification:

> As long as a hapten occupies an antibody site no other hapten can occupy the same site.

A second corollary that is obvious but nevertheless needs to be stated refers to the physical state of a hapten:

> A hapten, whether free and soluble or attached to a carrier in an exposed position, will react with an antibody site.

A third corollary is implicit in the "law of mass action" and, perhaps, is the most important of all. Epstein, Doty, and Boyd (1956) and Karush (1956) gave it form in their pioneering thermodynamic studies:

> The hapten-antibody bond is completely reversible and never fixed except through the avenue of affinity labeling.

2. Heterogeneous binding

A. Early studies by equilibrium dialysis. Although much of the early work on haptenic cross-reactivity and specificity involved techniques of hapten inhibition, as developed by Landsteiner, much more meaningful data were obtained through direct studies of hapten binding. Inhibition methods involved a second step such as precipitation: the more hapten inhibition, the less antigen reactivity, and the less precipitation, etc. Knowledge of antigenic specificities could be obtained in this way. However, direct methods, such as equilibrium dialysis, were required to probe the nature of the binding reaction itself.

The first attempt to determine an equilibrium constant for the binding of hapten to antibody was made by Marrack and Smith (1932) for the reaction between the azo dye, p-phenylazobenzenearsonic acid, and antibody prepared in rabbits against arsanilic acid coupled to horse serum protein. This occasion was also the first application of the method of equilibrium dialysis to immunochemical problems. An association constant of $K_a = 1 \times 10^4$ M^{-1} was obtained, using arsenic analysis as the measure of free hapten concentration. The value should be considered only as a historical marker since the haptenic product could not be obtained in sufficient purity and since the extent of nonspecific binding was not established. Haurowitz and Breinl (1933) controlled for nonspecific binding by including normal serum in the outer dialysis phase when antiserum was in the inner. They also studied the binding of the weaker hapten, arsanilic acid. It was not until Eisen and Karush (1949) made a number of improvements in procedure that the process of equilibrium dialysis became fully applicable to obtaining thermodynamically acceptable data (Fig. 6-1). Purity of hapten was emphasized as was the use of purified antibody globulin to reduce nonspecific effects. An equilibrium constant for the reaction between p-(p-hydroxyphenylazo)benzenearsonic acid and antibody to p-azobenzenearsonic acid (anti-Rpz) was obtained:

$$K_a = 3.5 \times 10^5 \text{ } M^{-1}$$

With this directly obtained value it was then possible to estimate the free energy change ΔF associated with the equilibrium.

$$\Delta F = -RT \text{ } ln(K_a)$$
$$= -7.7 \text{ kcal/mole}$$

The valence n for the antibody was also obtained within 10%, corresponding to a value of 2.

B. *Heterogeneity constant.* It became immediately apparent that linearity was not to be expected when data were plotted in the Scatchard or Langmuir forms even though extrapolations to obtain intercepts invariably indicated a valence of two. From this nonlinearity

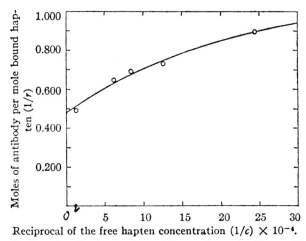

FIG. 6-1. Binding of an Rpz hapten by anti-Rpz as determined by equilibrium dialysis. The Langmuir form of the affinity equation (Equation 5.62 of Chapter 5) was used. (From Eisen and Karush, 1949.)

arose the concept of binding site heterogeneity since the linear form would hold only for homogeneous solutions with independently acting binding sites. To correct for heterogeneity it was assumed that a continuous distribution of association constants existed, and that at each point in the distribution there was a homogeneous equilibrium between antibody and hapten (Karush, 1962) for which a given free energy state held. If the distribution was Gaussian (normal), then a standard deviation σ of the distribution could be expressed. If the distribution followed a function such as that of Sips, then a different index of heterogeneity a would be obtained (Nisonoff and Pressman, 1958a). The choice of distribution generally was made on the basis of ease of integration rather than upon actual knowledge of the distribution shape, but improvement in fitting theoretical curves to actual data was obtained regardless. The Gaussian form was more sensitive, the Sips was easier to integrate, and neither were any more expressive of the actual distribution than as an approximation. A better relation was that of Bowman and Aladjem (1963), in which no assumption concerning the distribution form is made, but a computer was needed to program and calculate binding data from such functions.

In practice a standard value for an association constant (K_0) is obtained from that point where antibody sites are half-saturated with hapten, i.e., where there is an average of one bound hapten per bivalent antibody molecule, and, thus, where $r = 1$ and $n = 2$. From the Scatchard equation (5.17) one can thus obtain equation 5.21.

$$r/c = nK_a - rK_a \qquad (5.17)$$

$$1/c = 2K_a - K_a = K_0 \qquad (5.21)$$

The association constant becomes the reciprocal of concentration at that point. (The standard association constant, of course, must be obtained at 25°C in keeping with accepted thermodynamic conditions.) Regardless of the degree of heterogeneity there is only a single value for K_0 where $cK_a = 1$ since all distributions are expressed in terms of the product cK_a. Each single homogeneous reaction within the distribution, whatever its nature, can be expressed by the fraction of the total combining sites (S) filled with hapten, r/n or dS/S. From the law of mass action one can easily obtain

$$\frac{r}{n} = \frac{dS}{S} = \frac{cK_a}{1 + cK_a}$$

$$\frac{dS}{S} = \frac{1}{\dfrac{1}{cK_a} + 1}$$

$$\frac{dS}{S} = \frac{1}{(cK_a)^{-1} + 1}$$

which shows that the distribution of the fraction of filled combining sites at any point in the distribution is a function of the product of concentration and an association constant. For the total distribution, whatever its nature, the function must express what happens to the product, but at $cK_a = 1$ the function becomes 1/2. The concentration c obtained by analysis at this point represents the average concentration of the many discrete homogeneous c values; therefore, K_a at this point is the average equilibrium constant regardless of the type of distribution.

The easiest linear form of the homogeneous mass action law from which to demonstrate heterogeneity stems from the reciprocal relation n/r since

$$\frac{n}{r} = \frac{1 + cK_a}{cK_a}$$

$$\frac{n}{r} = \frac{1}{cK_a} + 1$$

This was the plot form used by Karush and Sonenberg (1949) to evaluate σ by curve fitting and was used by Nisonoff and Pressman

(1958b) to develop the Sips distribution function:

$$\frac{n}{r} = \frac{S}{dS} = \frac{1}{(cK_o)^a}$$

$$\frac{1}{dS} = \frac{1}{b} = \frac{1}{(cK_o)^a S} + \frac{1}{S}$$

where b was the fraction of bound hapten, c the fraction of free hapten, a the heterogeneity index, K_o the average standard association constant, and S the total available number of binding sites. To obtain the best value of the heterogeneity index, $1/b$ was plotted against $1/(c)^a$ until an a value was obtained which would give the best linear plot. In the cases of p-iodobenzoate and p-(p-hydroxyphenyl-azo)benzoate, a values of 0.7 and 0.75 were obtained, respectively, in their reactions with a single antibody preparation against p-azobenzoate (anti-Xpz). The curved and linear plots are shown in Figures 6-2 and 6-3 (Nisonoff and Pressman, 1958b).

   C. *Anti-lac antibodies.* In a now classic study which has appeared in a number of texts Karush (1957, 1958) prepared rabbit antibodies against the uncharged disaccharide, p-azophenyl-β-lactoside (Lac) that had been combined with dimethyl aniline to form Lac-azo dye. Relatively strong binding was obtained as indicated by the association constants and free energy values (Table 6-1), and hydrogen bonding between the disaccharide and the conforming antibody site was inferred from the relatively large value for $-\Delta H^o$.

   A Gaussian heterogenity index of 1.5 was calculated, and heterogeneity was also demonstrated by the marked curvature of the Scatchard plots (Fig. 6-4). A similarly shaped curve was obtained between Lac-dye hapten and horse γT antibody against the Lac hapten (Rockey, Klinman, and Karush, 1965) showing that heterogeneity was not just a peculiar property of the rabbit system or of γG. An extrapolated valence of 2 was obtained for this nonprecipitating antibody and, as judged from the value of $1/c$ when $r = 1$, the average intrinsic association constant, K_o, was very high [greater than 10^6 M^{-1} according to Klinman, Rockey, and Karush (1964) and later actually reported to be 1.8×10^7 M^{-1} by Klinman and Karush (1967)].

   D. *Anti-DNP antibodies.* Within the genetically controlled system of Hartley strain female guinea pigs one could also demonstrate rampant heterogeneity (Mancino, Paul, Benacerraf, Siskind, and Ovary, 1970). Whether the immunizing antigen was a relatively complex immunogen, dinitrophenylated bovine serum albumin (DNP-BSA), or a simple complete antigen—the dinitrophenylated dodecapeptide,

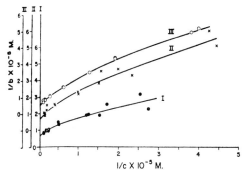

FIG. 6-2. Binding of haptens by specifically purified anti-Xpz at 5° ± 0.1°C in saline-borate buffer, pH 8, μ = 0.16. *Curve I, p-(p'*-hydroxyphenylazo)benzoate; *curve II,* labeled *p*-iodobenzoate; *curve III,* labeled *p*-iodobenzoate with a second antibody. (From Nisonoff and Pressman, 1958b.)

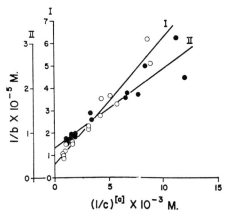

FIG. 6-3. Binding of haptens by specifically purified antibody corrected for heterogeneity. *Curve I,* labeled *p*-iodobenzoate, [a] = 0.7; *curve II, p-(p'*-hydroxyphenylazo)-benzoate, [a] = 0.75. (From Nisonoff and Pressman, 1958b.)

TABLE 6-1

Binding Data for Two Different Anti-Lac Antibodies and Lac-Dye

n	σ	25°C		7.1°C		$-\Delta H°$	$\Delta S°$
		$10^5 K_0$	$-\Delta F°$	$10^5 K_0$	$-\Delta F°$		
		M^{-1}	kcal/mole	M^{-1}	kcal/mole	kcal/mole	eu/mole
2.0	1.5	1.57	7.09	4.48	7.25	9.7	−8.8
2.0	1.5	1.04	6.85	2.90	7.01	9.7	−9.5

(From Karush, 1957, 1958.)

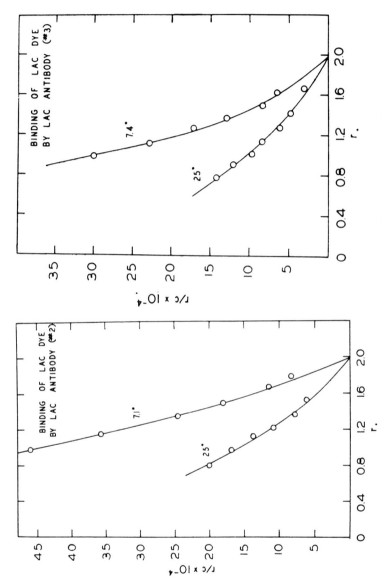

Fig. 6-4. Reaction between Lac-dye and rabbit γG antibody against Lac hapten at two different temperatures. The Scatchard form of the affinity equation (Equation 5.17 of Chapter 5) was used. (From Karush, 1957.)

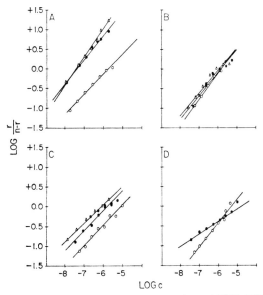

Lac-dye

tri-DNP-bacitracin A—the antibody interaction with tritiated DNP haptenic moieties in equilibrium dialysis was the same. Responses between individual animals varied greatly and each individual antiserum was characterized in particular by a low heterogeneity constant. (Fig. 6-5). One can calculate the constants directly from the curves through use of equation 5.67: [log $(r/2-r)$ = $a \log c + a \log K_0$]. A value of 0.52 for a is obtained, for example, in the case of α-^{3}H-DNP-L-isoleucine in its interaction with anti-DNP-BSA serum 15, and a value of 0.57 is obtained for ^{3}H-DNP-ϵ-aminocaproate in its interaction with anti-tri-DNP-bacitracin A, serum 9.

E. *Antibodies to blood group A substance.* Among the natural human antibodies to blood group A substance can be found yet another example of the ubiquitous phenomenon of affinity heterogeneity.

FIG. 6-5. Equilibrium binding characteristics of: *A*, anti-DNP-BSA, serum 15; *B*, anti-tri-DNP-bacitracin A, serum 9; *C*, anti-tri-DNP-bac, serum 2; *D*, anti-tri-DNP-bac, serum 3, for the following haptens: [^{3}H]-DNP-ϵ-aminocaproate, Δ; [^{3}H]-DNP-α-aminovalerate ($\bullet$); α-[^{3}H]-DNP-L-isoleucine (O). (From Mancino, Paul, Benacerraf, Siskind, and Ovary, 1970.)

Moreno and Kabat (1969) fractionated the antibodies from individual sera according to a scheme in which columns of insoluble polyleucyl hog blood group A + H substance were used. After adsorption of antibodies on the columns, N-acetylgalactosamine (Gal NAc) was passed through in large excess to displace antibodies of that specificity or cross-reactivity; then the reduced but A active pentasaccharide AR_L 0.52 was added to elute additional antibodies.* The purified γG antibodies were found to retain their original characteristics of extreme heterogeneity.

F. Quantum-sensitive probes and the discovery of high-affinity antibodies. Equilibrium dialysis techniques, although powerful in measuring hapten binding and perhaps more widely used today than any other in determining extent of binding, yet are not exclusive. Actually the subatomic techniques, that utilize disturbances in quantum levels of atoms to indicate energy changes brought about by binding, are much more sensitive to the process of binding *per se*. An example is the spin-labeled hapten study of Stryer and Griffith (1965). Another is the nuclear magnetic resonance study of Hauglund, Stryer, Stengle, and Baldeschwieler (1967) in which a mercury-labeled hapten, 2,4-dinitro-4'-(chloromercuri)diphenylamine, is reacted with anti-DNP antibodies in chloride. As binding of Cl^- from the environment to Hg within the hapten-antibody complex takes place, a rapid exchange of previously bound Cl with solvent Cl^- results, and causes a broadening of ^{35}Cl nuclear magnetic resonance spectra. The quantitative equilibrium binding of hapten by various amounts of antibody at the micromole level can therefore be measured by the line-width of the nuclear magnetic resonance band per radioactive unit of ^{35}Cl. Among the quantum-related phenomena, however, the fluorescent properties of certain hapten and of binding site regions have proved to be the most useful.

When Berson and Yalow (1959) reported that the association constant for human anti-insulin with multivalent insulin could apparently be as high as $K_0 = 1 \times 10^9$ M^{-1}, there was considerable doubt in many circles that this high binding should be attributed to an antigen-antibody reaction alone. Perhaps some other factor in the human serum had contributed to the binding and brought it to equilibrium far to the right of the ordinary reaction. The reason for such skepti-

---

* It was from this same series of experiments that Moreno and Kabat obtained eluted γM antibodies with smaller sized binding sites than those of eluted γG. Antibodies eluted by Gal Nac were inhibited as well by Gal NAc as by A active tri- and pentasaccharides in low concentration; pentasaccharide eluted antibodies that came off the column later were not inhibited by Gal NAc but only by the oligossacharides, indicating larger sized sites.

cism was partially contained in the Pauling instructional theory of 1940, in which a rather narrow range of values, 10^4–10^6 M^{-1}, was predicted. The upper limit would be necessary to permit dissociation of the formed antibody from its cell-bound antigen and allow it to enter the circulation. The lower limit, if any lower, would indicate binding so poor as to be ineffective in specificity discrimination except in cases of high antigenic valency. In the same year that Talmage (1960) reported another high association constant, 5×10^8, for multivalent serum albumin and its antibody (which also could conceivably have been attributed to an impurity), Velick, Parker, and Eisen (1960) measured high binding in an elegant and unambiguous way and, by so doing, proved that another of the conditions of the Pauling theory need not be met. They utilized the method of tryptophan fluorescence quenching as the basis of their technique, and showed that tryptophan residues of intact antibody molecules and of univalent fragments gave a fluorescence quantum yield diminished by 70% when reacted with their conforming hapten, ϵ-N-DNP-lysine (formed from 2,4-dinitrophenol and the ϵ-amino groups of lysine). An equilibrium constant of 2×10^8 M^{-1} at 26°C was obtained along with a standard free energy change of -11.3 kcal/mole. Incidental to the study was the finding that the fluorescence-quenching properties of the individual antibody sites of intact antibody molecules were additive, thus showing that the binding properties of one were not affected by the other. Separate nonoverlapping domains of eight to nine tryptophan residues were implicated.

   G. Comparison of fluorescence quenching with equilibrium dialysis. DNP and TNP. Little and Eisen (1966) continued the study by exploring the comparative fluorescence quenching curves for the DNP-anti-DNP and TNP-anti-TNP systems (where DNP and TNP were 2,4-dinitro- and 2,4,6-trinitrophenyl ligands, respectively) (Fig. 6-6). Very high affinity antibody in excellent yield was obtained by elution from precipitates formed between homologous hapten-protein conjugates and rabbit antibody. Quenchability was shown to be a property of the antibodies and not the ligands. Proteolytic cleavage with papain showed that there was no detectable influence of whole γG on binding strength or heterogeneity as compared to Fab. And the Scatchard plots obtained by the fluorescence quenching method were shown to be equivalent to equilibrium dialysis data, each technique in a sense validating the other. Once again extreme heterogeneity was obtained (Fig. 6-7).

   Little, Border, and Freidin (1969) established later that rabbit antibodies against 2,6-DNP hapten reacted with ϵ-2,6-DNP-aminocaproate very strongly with a K_0 greater than 1×10^8 M^{-1} in both early and late antisera. The same antibodies had binding affinities for ϵ-2,4,6-TNP-aminocaproate, early and late, of 6.0×10^6 and 4.8×10^7 M^{-1}; for ϵ-2,4-DNP caproate, early and late, 9.9×10^4 M^{-1} and 2.7×10^5 M^{-1}.

Little and Counts (1969) substituted 2,4-DNP groups exclusively on the sole lysine residue of bovine insulin hoping to prepare a relatively homogeneous antibody in guinea pigs as compared with heavily dinitrophenylated bovine γ-globulin.

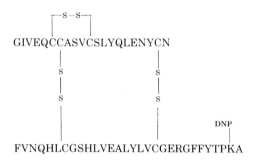

ϵ-2,4-DNP-insulin

Using fluorescence quenching titrations they found that a high average association constant could be obtained, but that extreme heterogeneity once again was the rule. With ϵ-DNP-insulin $K_0 = 2.5 \times 10^7$ and $a = 0.30$ for antibodies from a single guinea pig; with α-[^{3}H]Ac-ϵ-DNP-L-lysine in equilibrium dialysis $K_0 = 2.9 \times 10^6$ and $a = 0.59$. The results were no less heterogeneous than those of Eisen, Simms, Little, and Steiner (1964) with ϵ-41-mono-DNP-ribonuclease.

H. DNS and ANS haptens. Fluorescent probes with a different ligand did not seem to improve the heterogeneity problem. Parker, Yoo, Johnson, and Godt (1967) and Parker, Godt, and Johnson (1967) raised antibodies to the dansyl hapten (5-dimethylaminonaphthalene-1-sulfonyl group or DNS group) and fractioned the antibody population into two separate γG lots according to charge upon elution from diethylaminoethyl (DEAE) cellulose. The emission spectrum of ϵ-DNS-lysine in its reaction with the first fraction was in the 496–501 mμ range; that of the second population, in the 502–505 mμ range (Fig. 6-8). This was taken as confirmation of two different conservative regions in the two types of binding sites, but in spite of the conservative nature of the binding site amino acids involved (Fig. 6-9), a low heterogeneity index and high association constant once again were obtained, e.g., $K_0 = 2.4 \times 10^7$ M^{-1} at 30°C and $a = 0.45$ for the ϵ-DNS-lysine ligand.

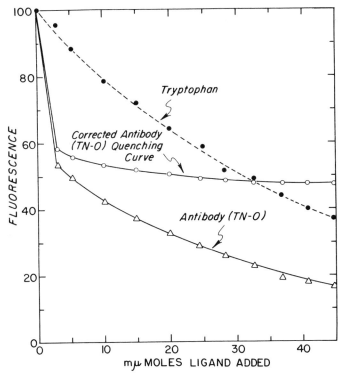

FIG. 6-6. Quenching curves of tryptophan fluorescence in antibody with addition of ligand. (From Little and Eisen, 1966.)

A related hapten to DNS is 1-anilino-8-naphthalene sulfonate (ANS). With antibodies raised to 1-azo-8-naphthalene sulfonate and its 1-4 isomer and tested with ANS, Yoo and Parker (1968) found that the quantum yield of ANS fluorescence was increased over 100-fold in the presence of specific antibody and that a blue shift of 45 mμ accompanied the reaction. Here was a *hydrophobic* molecular probe at a specific antibody site, in confirmation of Winkler's (1962) concept of fluorescence enhancement. With this technique one could explore a greater variety of globulin fractions since normal globulin chains and fragments had no effect. In this assay also, however, with a value of K_o of 5.6 $\times$ 10^6 M^{-1} as average association constant the heterogeneity index was only 0.5.

I. Arsonate hapten with single and double charges. In antisera against a mixture of the single and double charged forms of *p*-azobenzenearsonate (Rpz), Kitagawa, Grossberg, Yagi, and Pressman (1967) found abundant evidence of heterogeneity in both the single charge fraction (eluted at pH 5 with *p*-aminobenzenearsonate) and

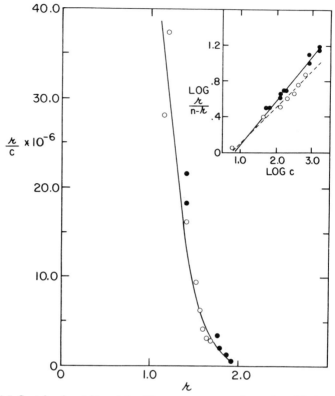

FIG. 6-7. Scatchard and Sips plots of fluorescence quenching and equilibrium dialysis data. $K_0 = 1.59 \times 10^8$ M^{-1} by equilibrium dialysis; $K_0 = 1.42 \times 10^8$ M^{-1} by fluorescence quenching; $a = 0.5$ by equilibrium dialysis, 0.6 by fluorescence. (From Little and Eisen, 1966.)

the double charge fraction (eluted at pH 9.5 with benzenephosphonate). Using p-^{131}I-iodobenzenearsonate as test ligand in equilibrium dialysis they obtained equilibrium and heterogeneity constants of 5×10^5 M^{-1} and 0.42 for the pH 5 fraction at pH 9; 6×10^5M^{-1} and 0.70 for the pH 9.5 fraction at pH 9; 1.1×10^5 M^{-1} and 0.52 for the pH 5 fraction fraction at pH 5; and 0.11×10^5 M^{-1} and 0.75 for the pH 9.5 fraction at pH 5. It was concluded that the antibodies that were largely directed against the single charged hapten could still accommodate the doubly charged hapten. Yet not much improvement in the restriction of heterogeneity was obtained in this way.

J. Heterogeneity in inbred mice. Even in inbred strains of mice in which greatest genetic uniformity can be expected heterogeneity was much in evidence—the index ranging from 0.55 to 0.83 in anti-p-azobenzoate (anti-Xpz) antibodies raised in C57BL/6Ja strain mice

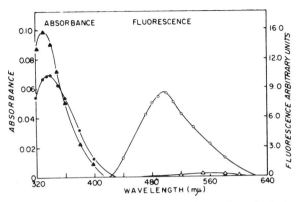

FIG. 6-8. Absorption and emission spectra for free and antibody bound ϵ-DNS-lysine. ($\blacktriangle$) Absorbance of free ϵ-DNS-lysine. ($\triangle$) Emission of free ϵ-DNS lysine. ($\bullet$) Emission of bound ϵ-DNS-lysine. Free and bound hapten were at a concentration of 2.1×10^{-5} M. The absorption and emission spectra of bound ϵ-DNS-lysine were corrected for protein and free dye. The amount of dissociated dye was calculated from parallel equilibrium dialysis experiments at the same antibody concentration. Temperature, 25°C; solvent, phosphate-saline. (From Parker, Yoo, Johnson, and Godt, 1967.)

and from 0.55 to 0.79 in A/Ha strain mice (Mattioli, Yagi, and Pressman, 1968).

K. Effect of carrier residues on heterogeneity. Lysine vs. guanosine. The carrier residues adjacent to 2,4,6-trinitrophenyl groups were investigated as to their effect upon heterogeneity (Winkelhake and Voss, 1970). Lysine residues of a protein carrier were compared with guanosine residues in a DNA carrier as an anchor for TNP. Scatchard and Sips plots were presented showing extensive heterogeneity in both instances: [^{3}H]-ϵ-TNP-L-lysine with rabbit anti-TNP-lysyl antibodies gave a value of 1.3×10^7 M^{-1} for K_0 and 0.57 for a; with anti-TNP-guanosyl antibodies the same ligand gave values of 0.9×10^7 and 0.57, respectively. A 5'-monophosphate-guanosine was tested also with the anti-TNP-guanosyl antibodies giving a much lower binding constant of 2.3×10^4 M^{-1} and a correspondingly higher heterogeneity constant of 0.81.

L. Heterogeneity and heavy chains. Haber and Richards (1966) asked whether the heavy chains themselves might have a more restricted heterogeneity, and used fluorescence quenching to investigate the question. They found that the heavy chains differentiated among haptens in much the same manner as the parent antibody molecules while homologous light chains increased the affinity somewhat without changing selectivity. Nevertheless, while the K_0 for ϵ-DNP-L-lysine hapten binding with solubilized alanylated

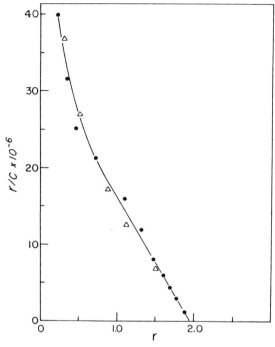

F<small>IG.</small> 6-9. Curves for the binding of ε-DNS-lysine by anti-DNS antibody as measured by fluorescence enhancement (●) and equilibrium dialysis (△). The rabbit anti-DNS purified antibody was at a concentration of 40 μg/ml; c is free hapten concentration (millimicromoles/milliliter) and r is moles of hapten bound per mole of antibody (assuming an antibody molecular weight of 145,000. Temperature, 30°C. Calculation of the fluorometric data was based on changes in ε-DNS-lysine fluorescence (excitation 340 mμ, fluorescence 480 mμ). (From Parker, Yoo, Johnson, and Godt, 1967.)

anti-DNP heavy chains began at 6.2×10^6, increased to 1.2×10^7 with the addition of light chains, and reached 3.0×10^8 M^{-1} in the intact molecule, the heterogeneity constant remained at about 0.6.

M. *Affinity, heterogeneity, and the immune responses.* Eisen and Siskind (1964) studied the relationship between affinity and the timing of the primary and secondary responses in rabbits, and used association and heterogeneity constants as guides as to what was occurring. The earlier revelations of equilibrium constants that were two or more orders of magnitude higher than the Pauling (1940) theory limit of 10^6 had meant that the initial formation of antibody *in vivo* was *not* made around a haptenic template according to antigen-directed instruction. The selection theories of Jerne and of Burnet (1967) fitted the new immunochemistry much better. Now that it was a very common occurrence to obtain heterogeneity constants of 0.5, the upper limit of actual association constants was realized to be even higher than the average K_0 values themselves. Translated into actual distribution terms, a value of 0.5 meant, for example, that an average equilibrium constant of 2.5×10^7 M^{-1} had a range for 80% of the antibodies from 6.2×10^5 to 1×10^9 M^{-1}, i.e., a range over three orders of magnitude, while the remaining 20% would range even more widely. Eisen and Pearce (1962) raised the additional possibility that the very highest binding antibody might be eliminated in hyperimmunized animals if excessive amounts of antigen were used and that *in vitro* measurements might therefore have missed those antibodies of highest affinity that an animal was capable of synthesizing.

What Eisen and Pearce suspected to be true for some antibodies *in vivo*, Stevenson, Eisen, and Jones (1970) found to be true *in vitro*. In the liberation of anti-DNP antibodies from the bound radioactive ligand, ϵ-2,4-DNP-lysine-[^{3}H] and in the liberation of anti-azobenzene-4-sulfonate from the bound nonradioactive ligand, methyl orange, there was a residue of persistent tightly bound hapten-antibody complex that failed to break up in the presence of unlabeled hapten in the first case or with radioactive ^{35}S-labeled hapten in the second case. This effect illustrates one of the hazards of carrying out binding studies with purified antibodies that have been prepared by the technique of free-hapten displacement of antibodies after solid-phase-hapten adsorption. Not all of the liberated antibodies are, in fact, free to participate in subsequent binding experiments, and present instead an aura of nonspecificity. They also subtract from the full expression of heterogeneity in the antibody sample by neutralizing the high side of the affinity distribution.

Eisen and Siskind explored the question raised by Eisen and Pearce in a very systematic way. They found that in rabbits receiving only 5 mg of DNP-bovine γG (DNP-BGG), the average K_0 rose from 0.8×10^6 M^{-1} at 2 weeks to as high as 2.5×10^8 M^{-1} at 8 weeks whereas in rabbits receiving 250 mg the average K_0 remained at 0.2×10^6 M^{-1} during the whole period. It was certainly clear that even within a single animal uniformity in equilibrium constants could not be expected, not even in average ones. Moveover, no marked improvement in heterogeneity constants could be anticipated as a general rule.

What Eisen and Siskind found to be true for the rabbit Klinman, Rockey, Frauenberger, and Karush (1966) found for the horse. The K_0 for γG at 6 weeks was 10^5 M^{-1}; at 6 months, 10^7 M^{-1}. Accompanying the theme were the usual overtones of gross heterogeneity.

Saha, Karush, and Marks (1966) had synthesized a large haptenic moiety called SUp from the interaction of lysyl residues with Sacetylmercaptosuccinnic anhydride, subsequent treatment with an iodoacetamide reagent, and final reaction of thiol groups with *p*-(*p*-iodoacetylaminobenzenezo) hippurate. The result was a 540-formula-weight derivative of lysine.

$$-(CH_2)_4-NH-CO-CH-(CH_2COO-)-S-CH_2-$$
$$CO-NH-\phi-N=N-\phi-CO-NH-CH_2-COO-$$
$$SUp$$

Fujio and Karush (1966) followed the Eisen-Siskind immunization schedule, raised antibodies to SUp-hemocyanin and looked for the appearance of antibodies that would react with the tritiated amino dye, [^{3}H]-*p*-(*p*-aminobenzeneazo) hippurate. Scatchard plots showed the increase in binding constants (Fig. 6-10), and the maintenance of a Sipsian heterogeneity constant of about 0.5 and a Gaussian heterogeneity constant of 3.5 (Table 6-2). Antibody against hippurate itself reached a limiting value of 1×10^4 M^{-1} within 4 weeks and remained there, but anti-SUp antibodies in their reaction with amino dye climbed to 1.23×10^6 M^{-1} in 2 weeks, reached 1.3×10^7 M^{-1} in 13 weeks. The analysis of fragments of antibody revealed that cleavage resulted in only slight decreases in binding and no change in

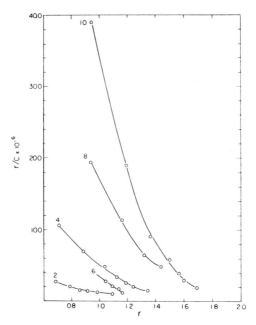

FIG. 6-10. The effect of immunization interval on the binding at 25°C of amino dye by purified anti-SUp antibody. The interval in weeks between the primary and secondary injections is indicated for each binding curve. (From Fujio and Karush, 1966.)

heterogeneity. Measurements of the 10-week antisera at 25 and 37.5° C (Fig. 6-11) gave K_0 values of 3.4×10^7 M^{-1} and 0.84×10^7 M^{-1}, respectively; a $\Delta F\mu$ ° of -12.65 kcal/mole; a $\Delta H°$ of -21.6 kcal/mol; and a unitary entropy change $\Delta S\mu$ of -30.1 eu/mole. The large decrease in enthalpy and the large and unfavorable change in entropy spoke against hydrophobic interactions as the main source of binding stability (on the average), but the actual meaning was not readily interpretable. One of the problems in interpretation would appear to

TABLE 6-2

Binding Constants of Amino Dye-Anti-SUp Equilibrium Reactions

Immunization Interval	Equilibrium Constants		Heterogeneity Constants	
	$10^6 K_0$	$-\Delta F°$	a (Sipsian)	σ^* (Gaussian)
weeks	M^{-1}	*kcal/mole*		
2	1.23	10.7	0.60	2.6
4	5.15	11.5	0.50	3.5
6	3.40	11.3		
8	17.3	12.2		
10	34.3	12.7	0.50	3.5
13†	13.0	12.1		

$* \ \sigma = 2\sqrt{\pi} \, (\cot \pi a/2).$

† No booster.

(From Fujio and Karush, 1966.)

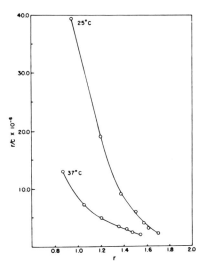

FIG. 6-11. Temperature dependence of the binding of amino dye by anti-SUp antibody purified from 10-week antiserum. (From Fujio and Karush, 1966.)

be the actual broad range of negative free energy changes that were operative among the heterogeneous molecules, some even less than 8.0 kcal/mole and others even greater than 12.4 kcal/mol around a mean value of 10.2 kcal/mol.

3. Kinetics of hapten-antibody interaction

After the breakthrough experiments of Velick, Parker and Eisen (1960) that transformed immunochemistry from instructional to selectional mechanics the time was ripe for kinetic studies as well, and the ingenuity of a few graduate students under Sehon at McGill and Singer at Yale gave rise to some exceedingly important and fundamental results. The requirements for a successful kinetic study were set down by L. Day, Sturtevant, and Singer (1963): (a) The antigen-antibody system must be well defined, the concentration of reactions must be accurately determined, and the reversible biomolecular reactions must be distinguishable from reversible aggregation reactions. (b) The combination of antigen with antibody must result in a kinetically correlated and accurately measurable change in some property of the system. (c) The means of measurement of the change in property must be capable of following the change over extremely short time intervals.

The cathode ray polarographic technique of Schneider and Sehon (1961) for following the reaction of rabbit antibodies with p-(p-aminophenylazo)phenylarsonic acid fulfilled the first two criteria but not the last. The hapten as a free molecule was detectable as a reducible azo group at the mercury cathode of a polarograph but, when bound to antibody, was not available. Thus, free hapten could be measured in terms of peak heights on an oscilloscope at intervals of 1 sec in the micromolar range. The time intervals were still not short enough and, although an equilibrium constant was easily obtained (6.15×10^5 M^{-1}), the forward reaction could not be evaluated.

Sehon's group then turned to a temperature-jump relaxation method (Froese, Sehon, and Eigen, 1962) in which rapid reactions involving changes in heat of reaction (enthalpic changes) could be followed in microsecond intervals. A condenser was discharged through a conducting solution containing the reaction mixture and in 0.1–1 μsec created a temperature jump of about 10°C. The reaction mixture was then measured as it adjusted to the new conditions brought on by the perturbation, and the time taken to reach the new equilibrium was obtained from oscillographic recordings. This time, called relaxation time τ, was found by derivation (Eigen and De Maeyer, 1962) to be related to the forward and reverse reaction rate constants of the new equilibrium by

$$1/\tau = k_r + k_f ([Ab] + [H])$$

where $[Ab]$ and $[H]$ were antibody and hapten concentrations at the new equilibrium. The third criterion for a good kinetic study would thereby be met but now a suitable hapten was required to meet the first two criteria. One such hapten was the dye molecule, 1-naphthol-4-[4-(4'-azobenzeneazo)phenylarsonic acid], which would undergo a spectral shift to longer wave lengths when binding with antibody took place (Sehon, 1963). Through controlled assays and spectrophotometric determinations a forward reaction rate constant, $k_f = 2 \times 10^7 \text{ M}^{-1} \text{ sec}^{-1}$, and a reverse reaction rate constant, $k_r = 50 \text{ sec}^{-1}$, were obtained. The equilibrium constant was $K_0 = 4 \times 10^5 \text{ M}^{-1}$.

The instrumentation developed by Sturtevant in Singer's laboratory for rapid measurements was a thermostated stopped-flow recorder in which reactants could be mixed during flow in a special mixing chamber and brought to rest in a quartz observation tube, all in 0.003 sec (cf. L. Day, Sturtevant, and Singer, 1962, 1963). The reaction could then be followed fluorometrically or spectrophotometrically as a function of time after mixing and instantaneously recorded. One of the haptens that was used for which kinetically correlated and accurately measurable data could be obtained was 2-(2,4-dinitrophenylazo)-1-naphthol-3,6-disulfonic acid, in which marked spectral shifts would occur upon binding with antibody specific for dinitrophenyl groups (anti-DNP). A forward reaction rate constant, $k_f = 8.0 \times 10^7 \text{ M}^{-1} \text{ sec}^{-1}$, and a reverse reaction rate constant, $k_r = 1.4 \text{ sec}^{-1}$, were obtained, giving an equilibrium constant of $K_0 = 5.9 \times 10^7 \text{ M}^{-1}$. The reaction of antibody with DNP hapten was seen to be one of the fastest bimolecular reactions then on record in immunochemistry. Similar data were obtained for DNP-lysine and DNP-aminocaproate, the latter showing $k_f = 1.0 \times 10^8 \text{ M}^{-1} \text{ sec}^{-1}$, $k_r = 1.1 \text{ sec}^{-1}$, and $K_0 = 9.1 \times 10^7 \text{ M}^{-1}$.

Froese and Sehon (1964, 1965), in studying the reaction of anti-NP (rabbit antibodies to the mononitro determinant, p-nitrophenyl) with DHNDS-NP [4,5-dihydroxy-3-(p-nitrophenylazo)-2,7-naphthalene-disulfonic acid disodium salt], obtained $1.8 \times 10^8 \text{ M}^{-1} \text{ sec}^{-1}$ for k_f, 760 sec^{-1} for k_r, and $2.4 \times 10^5 \text{ M}^{-1}$ for K_0. Here was an example not only of an even faster forward reaction but also of a faster dissociation, resulting in an equilibrium constant of moderate value within the range set by Pauling. Froese (1968) studied analogs of the system in greater detail through the use of [1-hydroxy-4-(2,4-dinitrophenyl-azo)-2,5-naphthalene disulfonate] and [1-hydroxy-4-(4-nitrophenyl-azo)-2,5-naphthalene disulfonate], i.e., OHND-DNP and OHND-

NP. It was important to establish proper conditions for the antibody-hapten reactions both for equilibrium and kinetic data, in particular the pH dependence of the dye haptens, that had an effect on the pK of bound dye-hapten. Metzger, Wofsy, and Singer (1963) had previously pointed out and it was established here once more that antibody dye reactions could involve equilibrium states between antibody and protonated dye, DH, and between antibody and ionized dye, D⁻. Froese chose conditions at pH 6 in phosphate buffer and ionic strength of 0.1 to obtain binding data. As shown in Figure 6-12 the wavelength at 495 mμ was optimal at this pH and different antibody concentrations could be equated to optical density of dye emission (Fig. 6-13). The accumulation of binding data for this combination, when plotted in Langmuir form, revealed a considerably less heterogeneous reaction with the OHND-DNP hapten than with the OHND-NP hapten (Fig. 6-14). When a different antiserum was tested with OHND-DNP hapten the surprising result was a completely homogeneous reaction with a heterogeneity constant of 1.0 (Fig. 6-15). Kinetic data for antiserum #2 and antiserum #1 were obtained under the same conditions by temperature-jump relaxation experiments as shown in Figures 6-16 and 6-17. The tabulation of data (Table 6-3) showed that the forward rate constant was about the same as obtained before.

The greatest effect on the varying equilibrium constants was the dissociation rate of the complexes once formed. Froese concluded, "Thus, the binding constant of an antibody-hapten reaction appears to be governed mainly by the 'lifetime' of the complex and not by the rate at which the two reaction partners can combine. Therefore, it would appear that the forward rate constant of most antibody-hapten reactions is about $10^7 - 10^8$ M^{-1} sec^{-1}...." One would therefore be led to infer that, irrespective of the binding constant for these reactions, little or no conformational change is taking place in the antibody during the formation of the antibody-hapten complex.

4. Homogeneous binding

A. Hybrid haptens. A review of heterogeneity would appear to be in order at this juncture according to Singer's (1964) classification:

Class heterogeneity—heavy chain distinctions and distributions of activity among various immunoglobulins.

Intrachain heterogeneity—for a given immunoglobulin, variations in tertiary structures that are supportive of combining sites but that are not directly involved in the sites themselves.

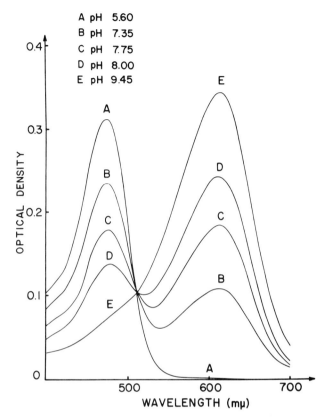

FIG. 6-12. Effect of pH on the absorption spectrum of OHND-DNP. (From Froese, 1968.)

Site heterogeneity—variations in combining sites themselves.

Singer added a fourth type of heterogeneity which had previously gone unrecognized: *structural heterogeneity*. He conceived of haptenic groups, themselves, not as homogeneous entities but as surface constituents capable of taking on a wide spectrum of structures depending on carrier environment. Some would protrude outwards from the surface; others, at the other extreme, would lie embedded in a protein surface in van der Waals contact with a constellation of amino acid residues. These embedded haptens with their amino acid vestments would form new antigenic determinants—*hybrid haptens* (Fig. 6-18). In the polypeptide-protein conjugate series, polyglutamyl groups would be expected to protrude because of their hydrophilic ionizable properties whereas polyleucyl and polyphenylalanyl groups would be more likely to form hybrid hap-

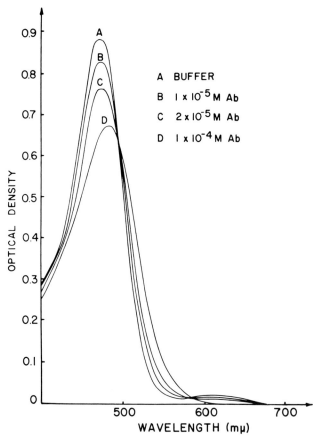

FIG. 6-13. Effect of various concentrations of anti-DNP on spectrum of OHND-DNP at pH 6.0, $\Gamma/2 = 0.1$. Antiserum #2 was used. (From Froese, 1968.)

tens because of their hydrophobic nature. Viewing the results of Stahmann, Lapresle, Buchanan-Davidson, and Grabar (1959) and those of Buchanan-Davidson, Dellert, Kornguth, and Stahmann (1959) with this picture in mind, Singer readily explained the discrepancies in their work. Immunization with polyglutamyl-bovine serum albumin resulted in antibodies that could be completely absorbed out by separate absorptions with bovine serum albumin and with polyglutamyl-rabbit serum albumin conjugate. However, immunization with polyleucyl- or polyphenylalanyl-bovine serum albumin resulted in antibodies of which 23–42% could *not* be absorbed out by separate absorptions with bovine serum albumin and with polyleucyl- or polyphenylalanyl-rabbit serum albumin. The remaining antibodies, easily absorbable by the homologous hapten

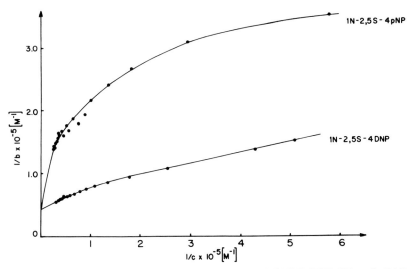

FIG. 6-14. Langmuir plot of antiserum #2 reaction with OHND-DNP (IN-2,5S-4DNP) and with OHND-NP (IN-2,5S-4pNP), pH 6.0, $\Gamma/2 = 0.1$, 23°C. (From Froese, 1968.)

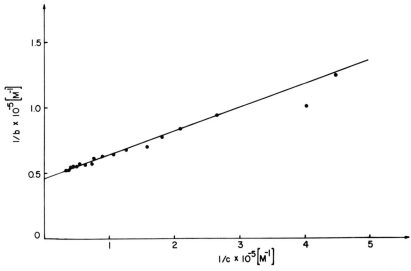

FIG. 6-15. Langmuir plot of antiserum #1 reaction with OHND-DNP, pH 6.0, $\Gamma/2 =$ 0.1, 23°C. (From Froese, 1968.)

protein conjugate, were very likely directed against hybrid antigens.

B. *Homogeneous binding defined.* To obtain a homogeneous preparation of antihapten antibody with limited or no heterogeneity appeared at the time to pose a number of difficult problems, but the search for nonhybridizable haptens was felt to be one approach.

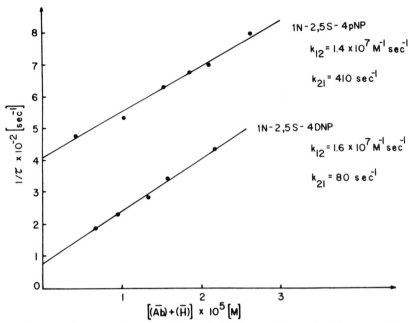

FIG. 6-16. Concentration dependence of $1/\tau$ for reactions of antiserum #2 with OHND-DNP (1N-2,5S-4DNP) and OHND-NP (1N-2,5S-4pNP). (From Froese, 1968.)

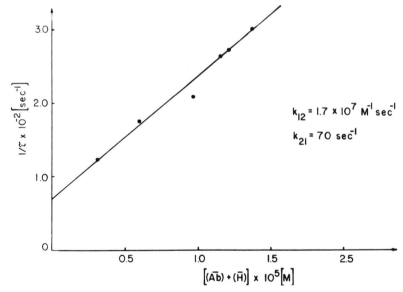

FIG. 6-17. Concentration dependence of $1/\tau$ for reactions of antiserum #1 with OHND-DNP. (From Froese, 1968.)

TABLE 6-3

Kinetic and Equilibrium Constants for Reactions of Anti-DNP Antibodies with Two Dye-Haptens That Are in Protonated State

Antibody	Hapten	k_1	k_2	$K_0 = k_1/k_2$	K_0 from Affinity Equation
anti-DNP #1	OHND-DNP	1.7×10^7 M^{-1} sec^{-1}	70 sec^{-1}	2.4×10^5 M^{-1}	2.4×10^5 M^{-1}
anti-DNP #2	OHND-DNP	1.6×10^7 M^{-1} sec^{-1}	80 sec^{-1}	2.0×10^5 M^{-1}	1.5×10^5 M^{-1}
anti-DNP #2	OHND-NP	1.4×10^7 M^{-1} sec^{-1}	410 sec^{-1}	3.4×10^4 M^{-1}	$\sim 1 \times 10^4$ M^{-1}

(From Froese, 1968.)

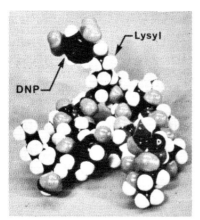 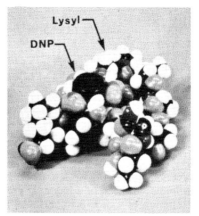

FIG. 6-18. Schematic view of a portion of the surface of a protein molecule with 2,4-DNP attached to the ϵ-NH$_2$ group of a lysyl residue of the protein. *Left*, protruding; *right*, embedded to form a hybrid determinant. (From Brenneman and Singer, 1970.)

It was Singer's (1964) belief that such preparations "may well be necessary for the ultimate determination of the detailed chemical structure of antibody molecules." This belief found fruition in the work of Brenneman and Singer (1968, 1970). One quotation from their 1970 paper is pertinent to the development of the present discussion.

> "Since something either is homogeneous or is not, we abjure the growing use of the term 'more homogeneous' in connection with what are properly 'less heterogeneous' antibodies."

The term "homogeneous binding" will be used in the present discussion to designate those antibody-antigen interactions that result in a Sipsian heterogeneity constant of 1.0 ± experimental error. Establishment of criteria for determining the nature and limits of complete homogeneity must be deferred until the existence of "homogeneous binding" itself is made credible. Equation 5.70 of Chapter 5 describes in an analytical way why one must distinguish between homogenous binding and overall homogeneity. One may conceivably have a heterogeneous population of both antigen and antibody molecules in which there is a one-to-one complementarity of uniform affinity between individual antigen and antibody pairs. The end result would be homogeneous binding with a constant equilibrium constant, and with a linear relationship between extent of reaction (jb or lq) and the free equilibrium concentration of binding sites ($1-jb$) and of antigenic determinants ($1-lq$). That such an event would appear to be rare speaks to the statistical unlikelihood of its occurrence; nevertheless, one could not, on the basis of homogeneous binding, tell the difference between this case and an overall homogeneous system. Does the example of homogeneous binding, reported by Froese (Fig. 6–15), constitute true or only apparent overall homogeneity? One cannot tell. Dandliker, Alonso, and Meyers (1967) in their investigation of human anti-penicillin antibodies through the use of fluorescence polarization of fluorescent penicilloyl haptens, determined that most human sera exhibited limited binding heterogeneity: 3.0×10^7 M^{-1} for the association constant in a case of penicillin serum sickness and 0.78 for the heterogeneity constant; 2.2×10^6 M^{-1} and 0.85 in another case with high hemagglutination titers; 2.3×10^7 M^{-1} and 0.90 in a case of anaphylactic shock; and 3.8×10^8 and 0.92 in a fourth case that had received a small dose of penicillin and had exhibited penicillin hypersensitivity one month later. Here homogeneous binding was approached. Was it due to restriction of antibody heterogeneity, of antigen heterogeneity, or of mere affinity heterogeneity? It is impossible to do more than speculate. One can, however, declare that a system cannot be over-homogeneous or super-uniform. To obtain Sipsian heterogeneity constants as high as 2.45 (Zimmering, Lieberman, and Erlanger, 1967) means that something is wrong with the technique (or, in this case, perhaps the computer). The Sipsian heterogeneity constant cannot be more than $1.0 \pm$ experimental error for that is the upper absolute limit.

   C. *The Klinman experiment—homogeneity and clonal selection.* The evidence for homogeneous binding was in view long before Klinman (1969) filled the credibility gap between homogeneous binding and homogeneous biosynthesis of antibody with his outstanding experiment. In a retrospective account such as this one it would seem more appropriate first to fill the gap and then to present the examples of homogeneity than to follow faithfully the historical development. Klinman stated the problem:

> "A single animal is capable of producing an extremely heterogeneous array of antibody against DNP-lysine (Eisen and Siskind, 1964) . . . This may be the result of the production of heterogeneous antibody by single clones, or it may be the result of stimulation by the haptenic group of several clones each producing homogeneous antibody . . . ."

Basing his hypothesis upon the statements of Burnet and Jerne that had been made at the Cold Spring Harbor Symposium on Antibodies in 1967, Klinman postulated that an antigen stimulates specific cells which possess genetic information for the production of the appropriate antibody. The outcome of this biological event would be 4-fold: (a) reactive cells would have limited genetic capacity to make antibody, (b) upon antigenic stimulation such cells would proliferate clones whose progeny would make identical molecules, (c) antibody molecules produced by a cell and its clonal progeny would be homogeneous in specific interaction with antigen, and (d) mixed antibody molecules from several clones would exhibit typical heterogeneity.

Klinman designed an experiment that would test (c) and (d), that would reflect upon (a) and (b), that would, in fact, test the clonal selection theory in a very rigorous fashion, and that would explain the meaning of binding site heterogeneity. Nossal and Lederberg (1958) had demonstrated antibody production by single cells; Jerne and Nordin (1963) had developed the agar-gel plaque technique for visualizing single antibody-producing cells; Nossal, Szenberg, Ada, and Austin (1964) had shown the production of 19S antibody by single cells; Mäkelä (1967) had shown the remarkable single ligand specificity of antibodies from single immunocytes; and Green, Vassill, Nussenzweig, and Benacerraf (1967) had also established that single cells, with a chance to make antibodies against two types of antigenic determinants, never made antibodies to both but always to one or the other.* Thus, there was enough data already accumulated to establish the biosynthetic unity of single cells and their clones. It only remained to work out a method that would collect enough synthesized antibody to test for binding affinity in a quantitative and unambiguous way.

---

* Cosenza and Nordin (1970) went on later to show that the frequency of double γM-γG producers never exceeded 1.2% and usually remained lower than 1%; Benjamin and Weigle (1970) further demonstrated that the chances of double specificity production of single cells could be no more than 1 out of 37, 568.

Klinman used a focus method of antibody production, similar to that employed earlier by Playfair, Papermaster, and Cole (1965). Local foci—colonies of homogeneous antibody-producing cells—could be developed in the spleens of irradiated mice by transferred cells from immunized nonirradiated mice. If the number of transferred cells were limited to 8×10^5, single focus formation in each 1-mm cube of irradiated spleen fragment could be assured when the time came (a day after transfer) to isolate the spleens, fragment them, and place in tissue culture as a clone for antibody production. Any focus with a rate of synthesis of 0.1–0.5 μg of antibody per day, would then produce enough globulin in 10–20 days to permit binding assays by microequilibrium dialysis. Antibodies in the experiment were raised against DNP-hemocyanin and were tested by the tritiated ligand, α, N-[^{3}H]-acetyl-DNP-lysine. When normal (as opposed to irradiated) spleen fragments were cultured from immunized mice after a secondary immune response the cells in the "secondary" fragments produced a very representative heterogeneous array of anti-DNP antibodies with an association constant of 2.3×10^7 M^{-1} and a Sipsian heterogeneity constant of 0.45. When two different foci from irradiated spleens were tested, one had an association constant of 2.7×10^7 M^{-1} and a heterogeneity constant of 0.98 (!) while the other had a much higher association constant, 1.3×10^8 M^{-1} but a heterogeneity constant that remained 0.98 (Fig. 6-19)! Klinman modestly concluded that his hypothesis was

> "...strongly favored by the finding that these two foci produce homogeneously reactive antibody of different affinities. In addition, the production of monospecific antibody to DNP by a cell stimulated with this hapten, in the face of many possible variations of specificity which exist for antibody against DNP strongly supports the notion that immunocompetent cells are unipotential. Finally, the demonstration that foci produce antibody with a homogeneous interaction with hapten suggests that a focus is the clonal product of a single cell induced to proliferate by the presence of antigen."

It can be seen that the slope of the highest binding portion of the normal fragments in Figure 6–19 has an intercept at $r = 1.0$. Since we know with a fair degree of certainty in this case that r is actually 2.0, we can calculate that the actual amount of antibody with high binding is one-half the total antibody in the preparation and has an association constant of about 3.3×10^8 M^{-1} (calculated from the slope). Furthermore, since we may assume that the

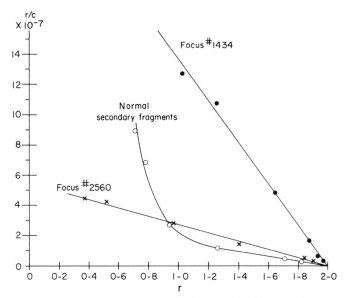

FIG. 6-19. Scatchard plots of focus-synthesized anti-DNP antibody in its interaction with α, N- [³H]-acetyl-DNP-lysine. (From Klinman, 1969.)

heterogeneity curve in Klinman's experiment is a composite of many homogeneous linear reactions we can be quite certain that the shape of the curve resulted from the pressure of increasing the concentration in mass action that first favored only high affinity antibody and then drove more and more hapten into the binding sites of low affinity antibody with increasing concentration of hapten. Finally all antibody was saturated and r became the antibody valence value of 2. The curve, in essence, describes the cumulative average affinity as one proceeds from relatively homogeneous high binding at low hapten concentrations to greater and greater heterogeneity and lower and lower average affinity at high hapten concentrations.

The accumulated evidence relating the structural and biosynthetic aspects of immunoglobulins makes possible the one-to-one assumption that biosynthetic homogeneity means structural homogeneity. Klinman's experiment completes the gap relating functional homogeneity to biosynthetic and thus to structural homogeneity, and represents, therefore, an adequate example of overall antibody homogeneity (and antibody diversity, one may add).

The reader may find additional information on monofocal antibody in the following papers: Klinman (1971a, b) and Klinman and Aschinazi (1971).

D. Crystalline antibodies and homogeneity. At the Cold Spring Harbor Symposium on Antibodies, Nisonoff, Zappacosta, and

Jareziz (1967) presented a case of acceptable complete homogeneity of an antibody immunoglobulin that was based upon it crystallizability. The very fact that immunoglobulins over the years have resisted crystallization under many attempts to bring it about makes a strong case for structural diversity. When one adds to the case the fact that the constant region, Fc, crystallizes so easily— in fact, receives its official international symbol from its crystallizing tendency—this all the more states how very diverse the variable regions must be. Northrop (1942) was the first to obtain a crystallized active antibody preparation. He treated diphtheria toxin-antitoxin with trypsin, fractionally precipitated the protein between $\frac{1}{3}$ and $\frac{1}{2}$-saturated ammonium sulfate, and twice crystallized the $(Fab_t)_2$ fragment (as we now would name it) from ammonium sulfate solution. Thin plates of an irregular quality formed (Fig. 6-20) that were 90% or more precipitable by antigen, homogeneous in the ultracentrifuge as a 5.7S protein with a molecular weight of 90,500, and homogeneous electrophoretically as well.

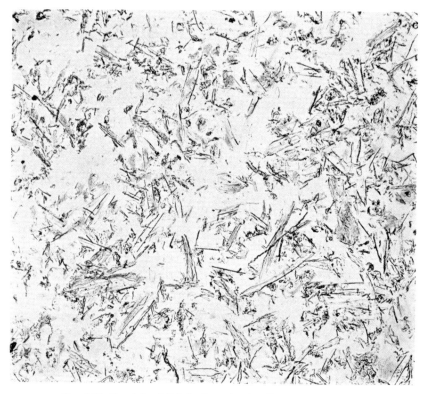

Fig. 6-20. Crystals of diphtheria antitoxin. (From Northrop, 1942.)

Homogeneity with respect to binding was, of course, not established since the work was carried out before criteria concerning binding were delineated. The crystals obtained by Nisonoff et al. were the first *whole* globulin to exhibit such structural homogeneity. A rabbit that had been immunized with p-azobenzoate was the source, and the antibodies, before crystallization, were specifically purified by precipitation with ovalbumin-p-azobenzoate, displaced from the precipitate by p-nitrobenzoate, and fractionated by DEAE-cellulose chromatography. The crystals formed in borate buffered saline at pH 8, $\Gamma/2$ = 0.1, and were recrystallized $\times 3$, a final yield of 150 mg resulting from 490 mg initial purified antibody protein. Upon equilibrium dialysis with ^{125}I-p-iodobenzoate, solutions of the crystals showed homogeneous binding. Disc electrophoretic patterns at pH 8.4 were, as expected, considerably more simple, the band widths much narrower. Allotypic analysis also revealed restriction—the serum from which the crystals were obtained was allotype a1, a2, whereas the crystallized antibody itself was homozygous for a1. The rarity of the event, together with the fact that by the time the crystals were obtained the rabbit was no longer available for clinical evaluation, may have left a lingering doubt in the minds of some that this proven case of homogeneity was a bona fide example of an ordinary immunological process that had somehow escaped the mechanics of heterogeneity and diversity. The subsequent experiments of Klinman certainly would dispel that doubt. Each clone that is stimulated to produce antibody must have the potential of producing crystallizable antibody, the rarity of the event stemming from the obvious fact that ordinary clonal selection by ordinary antigen is not a singular process but involves the selection of many structurally similar yet structurally diverse cross-reacting clones.

The valence of antibody obtained from the reciprocal of the extrapolated ordinate intercept of the Langmuir plot of figure 2 in the article by Nisonoff et al. (1967) was not 2 but only 1.55, an observation which puzzled the investigators and remained unresolved. It is possible that this was another instance of the persistence of unreleased hapten in the binding sites of purified antibody, mentioned previously (Section 2-M, this Chapter) from the work of Stevenson, Eisen, and Jones (1970). The values of $1/b$ (i.e., $1/r$) in the plot were determined on the basis of fully active antibody of 155,000 molecular weight where b (i.e., r) is the amount of radioactive hapten bound per total antibody in the system. If one assumes that $1/b$ (i.e., $1/r$) was actually $\frac{1}{2}$, then one must assume that only 77.5% of the antibody sites were available to bind the radioactive test antigen. Basing the value of $1/b$ upon a more likely molecular weight of 135,000 (Mamet-Bratley, 1970) for the bivalent 7S subunit raises the apparent valence from 1.55 to 1.78, but still leaves 11% of the crystallized antibody unavailable for binding of the test hapten. It is entirely possible that this 11% was already neutralized by hapten used for antibody purification and, moreover, that this portion, in a fully hapten-stabilized conformation, formed the nucleus for the crystallization process.

E. *Uniform amino acid composition and homogeneous binding.* Structural homogeneity need not be demonstrated by crystallization in order to be proved. In fact, crystallization *per se* does not prove absolute homogeneity either but only restricted heterogeneity. [A case in point is crystalline pepsin (Herriott, Desreux, and Northrop, 1940) which, if not carefully prepared, may contain a number of different pepsins, each distinguished by a different solubility. Another is Fc which may crystallize even when, by zone electrophoresis, it can be shown to separate into several distinct components (Gitlin and Merler, 1961; Putnam, 1965).] The structural homogeneity of two cross-reacting rabbit antibodies, with respect to their amino acid composition, has already been described in Chapter 4 (Koshland, Ochoa, and Fujita, 1970). In rabbits of restricted genotype, $a^1a^1b^4b^4$, anti-azophenylarsonate (anti-Rpz) and anti-azophenylphosphonate (anti-Fpz) antibodies were raised, purified, dissociated into light and heavy chain fractions, and shown to differ only by a single heavy chain tyrosine. When the antibodies were tested by equilibrium dialysis against homologous ligands (Fig. 6-21) homogeneous binding was obtained in each case. Anti-Rpz in its reaction with an acetamide of Rp had an association constant of 7.8×10^5 M^{-1} and a Sipsian heterogeneity constant of 1.0; anti-Fpz in its reaction with an acetamide of Fp had an association constant of 2.8×10^5 M^{-1} and a Sipsian heterogeneity constant of 1.0. The combination of homozygous, compositional, and binding homogeneity of each of the two antibodies makes it possible to conclude that in this instance, also, overall antibody homogeneity was demonstrated.

F. *Homogeneous binding in the face of structural heterogeneity.* To indicate, however, that binding homogeneity may be achieved even in the face of obvious and gross structural heterogeneity, the excellent and well controlled experiments of Hoffman and Campbell (1969) are a good example. Raising antibodies in ordinary bred New Zealand albino rabbits, pooling the sera from different bleedings and from different rabbits, and purifying the antibodies from an immunoadsorbent of hapten-protein conjugate entrapped in polyacrylamide gel, these investigators were able to obtain pure antibodies against aspirin.

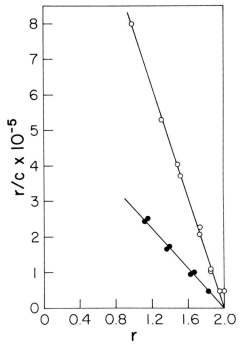

FIG. 6-21. Binding properties of arsonic and phosphonic antibodies. (O) Binding of p-acetamidophenylarsonic acid by arsonic antibody; (●) binding of p-acetamidophenylphosphonic acid by phosphonic antibody. (From Koshland, Ochoa, and Fujita, 1970.)

Aspirin   ε-Aspirylaminocaproate (aspiryl-ACA)

The pooled antibodies that were raised against aspiryl-hemocyanin conjugate and tested in equilibrium dialysis with the radioactive aspiryl-ACA ligand, aspiryl-carboxyl-^{14}C-ACA, had an association constant of $5.6 \pm 0.6 \times 10^5$ M^{-1} and a Sipsian heterogeneity constant of 1.0!. In the same experimental set up but with antibodies raised against aspiryl-bovine γG to form a similar pool the more usual binding heterogeneity was experienced with an average association constant of $2.2 \pm 0.6 \times 10^6$ and a Sipsian heterogeneity constant of 0.6. It is difficult to believe that a pool of structurally heterogeneous antibody molecules could fortuitously reach the pinnacle of homogeneous binding on the basis of unrestricted heterogeneous selection of cross-reacting clones within each rabbit and among several rabbits. It is much more likely that homogeneous binding was achieved because within and among rabbits there was already a built-in restriction of clonal selection for the aspiryl-hemocyanin conjugate and limited selectivity of cross-reacting types. The hapten carrier, though not a participant in binding, was important in the selection process and undoubtedly contributed much to clonal restriction. The work of Sela and Mozes (1966) on the importance of carrier portions of antigens to the control of the selection process with regard to net electrical charge has already been mentioned (Chapter 4). It would appear that carrier function may exert other types of control as well, and play a role in determining the extent of binding heterogeneity.

G. *Approach to binding homogeneity through light and heavy chain electrophoretic restriction.* Since the hapten carrier may play a role in the initial degree of clonal restriction and, hence, determine the degree of restriction in binding heterogeneity, and since the hapten carrier seems to have a greater effect upon restriction through light chain selection than directly through heavy chain selection, it is of interest to find out whether a correlation may be expected among light chain homogeneity, hapten specificity, and binding homogeneity. Herd and Cebra (1970) had a goat anti-rabbit light chain antibody that would distinguish two antigenic determinants in rabbit light chains in all rabbit sera regardless of allotype. In anti-DNP and anti-Rpz antibodies only one of the determinants—cyanogen bromide resistant—was present. This event is a long way from proof of homogeneity, but it does indicate restriction. Fraser and Edman (1970) compared the light chains of rabbit anti-Rpz antibodies to those of normal globulin by means of N-terminal sequenation and found considerable restriction by comparison:

anti-Rpz L-chain											Normal L-chain						
1	2	3	4	5	6	7	8	9	10		1	2	3	4	5	6	7
A	D	I	V	M	T	Q	T	P	A		A	V	I	V	V	T	G
D	V	V	M	T	Q	T	P	A	S		D	Y	V	T	Q	Q	V
	(E)					(P)						(Q)		(M)	(T)	(V)	(Q)
														(S)	(S)	(S)	(T)
																	(P)
																	(T)

(Minor amino acids found at each position are in parentheses.)

Again nothing is apparent in these data to indicate any correlation with the degree of binding site structural heterogeneity which depends upon the topography much further along the light chains, but again restriction itself is certainly indicated. Much more to the point are the experiments of Roholt, Seon, and Pressman (1970). Antibodies were raised in three individual rabbits of b^4b^4 genotype by hyperimmunization over a prolonged period of time with *p*-azo-

benzoate (Xpz) conjugated to bovine γG and were purified from immunoadsorbents. Light chains were analyzed by disc electrophoresis
(Fig. 6–22); antibodies were tested for binding homogeneity by
equilibrium dialysis with ^{125}I-labeled p-iodobenzoate ligand (Fig.
6–23). Antibody #2663 had a light chain disc pattern of considerable
simplicity compared with normal globulin and had a binding constant
of 1×10^4 M^{-1} with a heterogeneity constant of 1.0. Antibody #2717
also had a light chain disc pattern of considerable simplicity and
distinct in position from #2663. Its association constant was uniformly 5.1×10^5 M^{-1} with a heterogeneity constant of 1.0 also. Antibody #4174 had a much more complex light chain disc electrophoretic
pattern (although simpler than normal γG). Correlated with this
heterogeneous light chain pattern was a heterogeneous binding constant that averaged 1×10^5 M^{-1} but ranged over nearly 4 orders of
magnitude as indicated by its Sipsian heterogeneity constant of
0.4. Compositional correlations of light chain amino acid content with
degree of heterogeneity were also made with the finding that the
homogeneous antibodies deviated greatly from the average "normal"
composition whereas the heterogeneous antibody deviated only
slightly.

The series of experiments performed in Kabat's laboratory under
the title, "Studies on Human Antibodies" began with the observations of Edelman and Kabat (1964) upon the light chain electro-

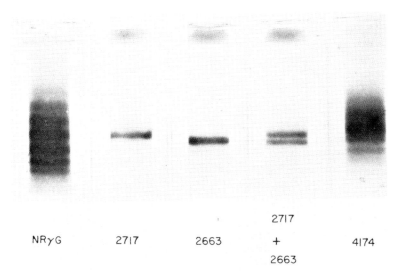

FIG. 6-22. Disc electrophoresis pattern of L chains from normal rabbit globulin and
from three purified rabbit anti-Xp antibodies. (From Roholt, Seon, and Pressman,
1970.)

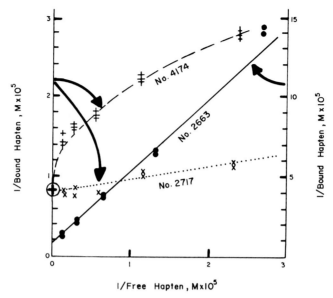

FIG. 6-23. Langmuir plots showing the interaction of three rabbit anti-Xp anti-bodies with *p*-iodobenzoate ligand. (From Roholt, Seon, and Pressman, 1970.)

phoretic patterns of purified anti-dextran antibodies. A considerably simpler pattern was obtained for anti-dextran as compared with "normal" globulin, the clonal selection apparently having been restricted by the nature of the polysaccharide with its composition based on a single sugar. Allen, Kunkel, and Kabat (1964) in the second paper of the series commented that the distribution of genetic factors seen in certain isolated human antibodies appeared to approach the selective occurrence in myelomas. In the third of the series (Bassett, Tanenbaum, Pryzwansky, Beiser, and Kabat, 1965), we have already seen in the Chapter 4 how compositional differences correlated with the four antibody specificities in a single individual. By the time the seventh experiment in Kabat's study appeared (Dorner, Yount, and Kabat, 1969) it was apparent that both antibody and myeloma globulins "represent fairly highly selected populations relative to normal γG immunoglobulin, with respect to their banding in acrylamide gel." The disc electrophoretic patterns of light chains and of heavy chains from six antibodies from a single individual are shown in separate and mixed analyses in Figure 6-24. Light and heavy chain patterns from a large number of myeloma proteins are shown in Figures 6-25 and 6-26.

H. Effect of degradation processes upon electrophoretic banding heterogeneity. There were indications from literature reports that some of the banding heterogeneity in myeloma proteins might re-

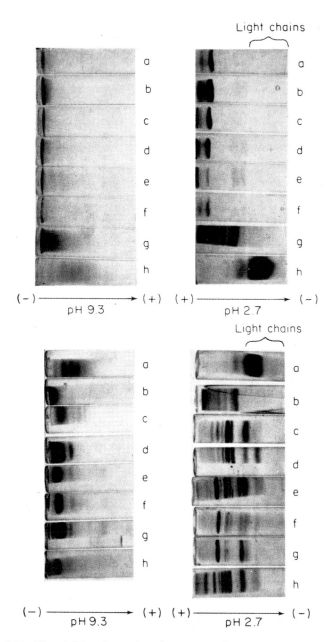

FIG. 6-24. (*Upper*) Disc electrophoretic patterns of 150–200 μg native antibodies of a subject at pH 9.3 and at pH 2.7: (*a*) anti-dextran, (*b*) anti-levan, (*c*) anti-teichoic acid, (*d*) anti-hog A, (*e*) anti-diphtheria toxoid, (*f*) anti-tetanus toxoid, (*g*) heavy chains of normal γG, (*h*) light chains of normal γG.

(*Lower*) Disc electrophoretic patterns of light chains (pH 9.3) and heavy chains (pH 2.7) of 150–200 μg protein: (*a*) light chains of normal γG, (*b*) heavy chains of normal γG, (*c–h*) reduced and alkylated antibodies of subject: (*c*) anti-dextran, (*d*) anti-levan, (*e*) anti-teichoic acid, (*f*) anti-hog A, (*g*) anti-diphtheria toxoid, (*h*) anti-tetanus toxoid. (From Dorner, Yount, and Kabat, 1969.)

235

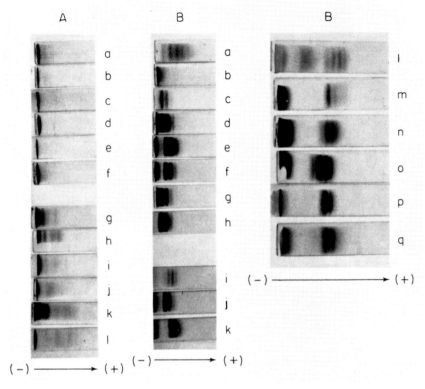

FIG. 6-25. Disc electrophoretic patterns of light chains of myeloma proteins, pH 9.3 of 150–200 µg protein. (A) Native (a–f) no banding; (g–l) very weak banding. (B) Reduced and alkylated, (c–h) two slow moving bands close to the beginning of small pore size gel (group 1); (i–k) bands move twice the distance of group 1 (group 2); (l–q) 2–4 fast moving bands, 3 times the distance of group 1 (group 3). (a) Light chains of normal γG; (b) heavy chains of normal γG. (From Dorner, Yount, and Kabat, 1969.)

flect degradative processes rather than synthetic ones and that the patterns might actually be much simpler than seen in the final patterns. Awdeh, Williamson, and Askonas (1969, 1970) proved that this indeed was the case. Taking as their subject the mouse plasma cell tumor #5563 they observed that as soon as 10 min after the start of incubation freshly synthesized γG$_{2a}$ had already become heterogeneous with respect to charge (Fig. 6-27). Conversion into differently charged components commenced soon after chain assembly into complete 7S molecules and continued to proceed extracellularly. Any enzymatic effects produced in serum (Awdeh, Askonas, and Williamson, 1967) would only complicate the disc patterns even further. The end result would also confirm the thoughts of Nisonoff et al. (1967) that the rarity of crystallized proteins among myelomas

A

B

Light chains

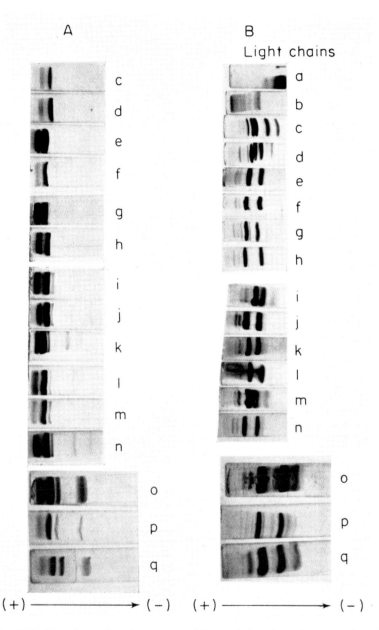

(+) ────────────→ (−)   (+) ────────────→ (−)

Fig. 6-26. Disc electrophoretic patterns of heavy chains of myeloma proteins, pH 2.7 of 150–200 μg protein. (A) Native (c-h) two bands; (i-n) three bands, (o-q) three bands, fastest is reasonably strong. (B) Same myeloma proteins, reduced and alkylated; (a) light chains of normal γG; (b) heavy chains of normal γG. (From Dorner, Yount, and Kabat, 1969.)

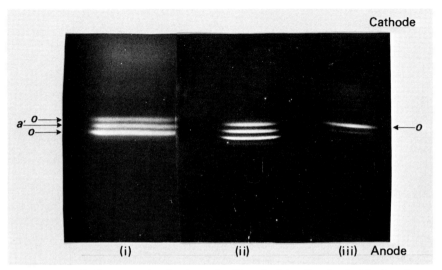

FIG. 6-27. Radioautograph of polyacrylamide-gel plate after isoelectric focusing. (i) Intracellular myeloma protein, 1-hr incubation with ^{14}C-labeled amino acids; (ii) extracellular protein after 1 hr; (iii) intracellular protein after 10 min. (From Awdeh, Williamson, and Askonas, 1970.)

might be accounted for by subtle degradative changes that would bring on a degree of imposed structural heterogeneity that would resist crystallization.

I. Homogeneous binding of ligands by myeloma proteins. For a long time the myeloma globulins that were produced in human and animal disease were considered to be devoid of any functional capacity and were classified along with normal globulins as non-specific and completely lacking in binding capacity. This belief was logically derived during the instructionist period, but was left without support when the selectionist period began. With the advent of clonal selection, homogeneous myeloma proteins essentially became antibodies in search of a ligand. When Eisen, Little, Osterland, and Simms (1967) announced at the Cold Spring Harbor Symposium on Antibodies their finding of a myeloma protein with antibody activity, the clonal selection theory was vindicated on yet another front. After screening 87 multiple myeloma proteins for possible hyperchromic shifts at 400–500 mμ when exposed to ϵ-DNP-lysine and obtaining nothing but hypochromic nonspecificity, this group found an 88th that was positive. Purification by DEAE-cellulose chromatography led to a protein which exhibited, upon equilibrium dialysis with the ligand, [3H]-ϵ-DNP-L-lysine, an affinity constant of 2.3×10^4 M^{-1}, a heterogeneity constant of 1.0, and a valence of 2.0. As predicted for a single clone of immunoglobulin secretors, their biosynthetic product exhibited binding homogeneity in keeping with its structural specificity.

The next myeloma globulin to show binding with [³H]-ε-DNP-L-lysine was a γA mouse protein, MOPC-315 (Eisen, Simms, and Potter, 1968). Homogeneous binding was demonstrated and a uniform equilibrium constant of 1.6×10^7 was obtained at all concentrations of ligand, but a valence of only 1.2 for the 7S monomer was obtained. This led to considerable consternation and erroneous speculation about a possible univalent γA until Underdown, Simms, and Eisen (1970) solved the problem. A reinvestigation of the binding properties of the protein led to the discovery that at low γA concentrations denaturation occurred to some extent. By repeating the assays at a higher antibody concentration or at low concentrations in the presence of normal γG, a normal valence of 2 was obtained. Jaffe, Eisen, Simms, and Potter (1969) reported another homogeneous γA mouse myeloma protein with homogeneous binding properties for ε-DNP-L-lysine that had an affinity constant of 3×10^5 M^{-1}, a heterogeneity constant of 1.0, and a valence of 2 ± 0.1 (Fig. 6-28). In the same manner Terry, Ashman, and Metzger (1970) obtained a human γA1 myeloma, BOY, that also exhibited homogeneous binding, an association constant of 2.65×10^4 M^{-1}, and a valence of 2.12. The protein existed in both monomeric and polymeric forms, but both bound ligand uniformly and to the same extent (Fig. 6-29).

Ashman and Metzger (1969) obtained nitrophenyl binding with γM immunoglobulin from a case of Waldenstrom macroglobulinemia, WAR (cf. Chapter 3). Homogeneous binding was obtained whether

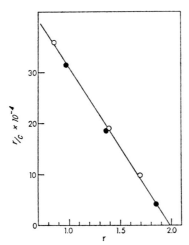

FIG. 6-28. Homogenous binding of [³H]-ε-DNP-L-lysine by mouse myeloma γA MOPC 460 in equilibrium dialysis. (From Jaffe, Eisen, Simms, and Potter, 1969.)

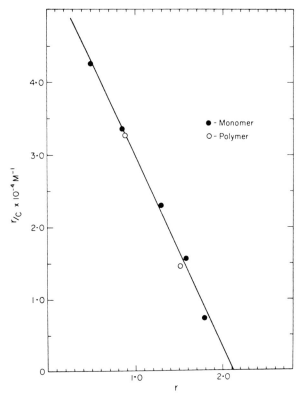

FIG. 6-29. Homogeneous binding of [³H]-ε-DNP-aminocaproate by human my-eloma γA BOY in equilibrium dialysis; (●) monomer; (○) polymer. The value of r taken as ligand bound per 161,500 molecular weight units. (From Terry, Ashman, and Metzger, 1970.)

the protein was the intact pentamer, 7S subunit, $5S(Fab')_2$, or Fab (Fig. 6-30) such that the data could be plotted in terms of moles of ligand bound per mole of heavy-light chain pair. A valence of 9.8 was obtained for γM, 2.0 for γM_s, 2.0 for $(Fab')_{2\mu}$, and 0.91 for Fab; association constants were 3.8, 3.9, 3.7, and $3.8 \pm 0.1 \times 10^4$ M^{-1}.

J. Design of antigens of restricted heterogeneity. Richards and Haber (1967) and Richards, Sloane, and Haber (1967) decided to try to design an antigen of restricted heterogeneity with the character-istics of a small strong antigenic determinant (DNP) located in the milieu of a poor immunogenic background (poly-D,L-alanine). The model compound had a defined sequence of alternating D- and L-alanine to prevent α-helix formation and also lacked β structure as shown by optical rotatory dispersion. The DNP determinants were placed 30 Å apart in fully extended form in order to meet the de-mands of the Sage model (cf. Chapter 4) which set 25 Å as the

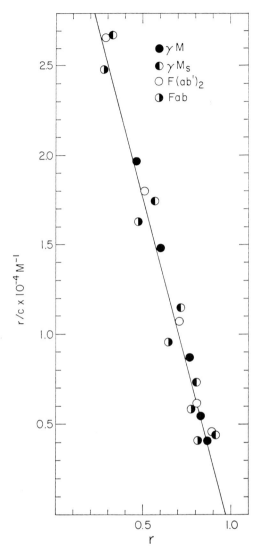

FIG. 6-30. Results of equilibrium dialysis of γM, γM_s (cysteine-produced subunit), $F(ab')_{2\mu}$, and $Fab\mu$ with [^{3}H]-ϵ-DNP-aminocaproate. The data are expressed as moles of hapten bound per mole of heavy-light chain pair in each molecular species, r, at varying concentrations of free hapten (c). The line was drawn by the method of least squares, using all the data. The myeloma protein was from human WAR myeloma. (From Ashman and Metzger, 1969.)

maximum width of a combining site. The entire polymer averaged 10,100 in molecular weight, was water soluble, and had the formula [(D-ala-L-ala)$_5$-ϵ-DNP-L-lys]$_{10.2}$. Immunization of 19 rabbits with the defined sequence polymer resulted in the production of high af-

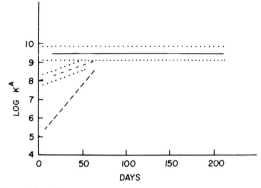

FIG. 6-31. Plot of log K_A vs. time in days following immunization. Values for 19 rabbits injected with 1.0 mg of defined-sequence polymer, 42 data points from 17 to 196 days are represented by solid line (—); values for 7 rabbits injected with 1.0 mg of "random" N-carboxyanhydride polymer, 14 data points 17–93 days are represented by dotted lines (· · · ·); and values for rabbits injected with 5.0 mg of dinitrophenyl-ated bovine γ-globulin, 9 data points (recalculated from Eisen and Siskind, 1964) are represented by dashed lines (----). All K_A values were determined by equilibrium dialysis against [³H] DNP-lysine of specific radioactivity 9000 Ci/mole or in suitable dilution. All data lines, one standard deviation from the mean, are calculated on the PDP9 or IBM 360 computer using a FORTRAN LV/CYTOS system, to determine best fit by least-squares analysis. (From Richards et al., 1969.)

finity antibody as soon as any could precisely be measured by equilibrium dialysis (Fig. 6-31). At 17 days the binding constant was 10^4 higher than DNP-bovine γG would produce at that time and the constant remained level in all 19 rabbits for the 200 days studied. An intermediate effect was obtained with a random N-carboxyan-hydride polymer (Richards, Pincus, Bloch, Burnes, and Haber, 1969). Haber, Richards, Spragg, Austen, Vallotton, and Page (1967) in referring to this experiment concluded: "While the molecular heterogeneity of antibody to the uniform sequence synthetic peptide has not as yet been examined, it seems apparent that at least one factor contributing to the heterogeneity of the immune response has been modified."

In another approach to defined antigenic sequences Haber's group designed a large structural antigen with a determinant that would fill an antibody combining site and behave, not as a collection of in-dividual amino acids, but as an integral whole. Bradykinin appeared to be a distinct possibility as a nonapeptide, RPPGFSPFR. Spragg, Austen, and Haber (1966) coupled the amino terminus of bradykinin to poly-L-lysine by means of toluene diisocyanate such that there was 1 bradykinin chain per 5 lysine residues, and immunized rabbits with the polymer:

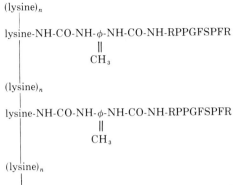

Branched Chain Copolymer of Bradykinin (RPPGFSPFR) and Poly-L-lysine

The high binding affinity of bradykinin and the relatively low specific activity of ³H-acetylated peptide made binding curves difficult to construct, so a related branched polymer with angiotensin was prepared. The octapeptide, NRVYVHPF, was attached to the ε-amino groups of polylysine through its carboxyl terminus with carbodiimide reagent:

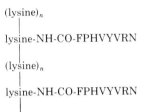

Branded Chain Copolymer of Angiotensin (FPHVYVRN) and Poly-L-lysine

Antibodies were raised to angiotensin-polylysine branched chain polymer and were tested in binding experiments with ¹³¹I-angiotensin (iodinated through its tyrosine residue). At the Cold Spring Harbor Symposium on Antibodies, Haber, Richards, Spragg, Austen, Vallotton, and Page (1967) were able to report the successful finding of homogeneous binding: an association constant of $2.64 \times 10^9 \ \text{M}^{-1}$, a valence of 2 and a Sipsian heterogeneity constant of 1.02!.

K. Homogeneous antibodies to pneumococcal ligands. Another ligand just large enough to occupy an average antibody-combining site completely is the octasaccharide obtained by enzymatic digestion of the capsular polysaccharides of types III and VIII pneumococci (Pappenheimer, Reed, and Brown, 1968). Depolymerase activity against S-VIII, for example, results in two fractions which can be separated by passage through Bio-Gel P-2 columns. One of these, 8-S-VIII, is the octasaccharide which can be reduced with tritium gas to form the radioactive [³H]-8-S-VIII. The label appears on the reduced terminal 4,5-dehydroglucuronide residues. Pappenheimer *et al.* tested the ligand for binding in equilibrium dialysis with different preparations of horse and rabbit antisera against S-VIII, against the antibodies of anti-S-III that would cross-react with S-VIII, and against the antibodies of S-VIII that would cross-react with S-III (the cross-reacting antigenic determinants due to cellobiuronic acid). Scatchard and Sips plots of the various antisera (Figs. 6-32 and 6-33) revealed homogeneous binding: horse #741, $K_0 = 2.2 \times 10^5$ M^{-1}, $a = 1.005$ at 25°C; rabbit #6, $K_0 = 1.25 \times 10^5$, $a = 1.045$ at 25°C; rabbit #7 mgh, genotype b⁵, $K_0 = 8 \times 10^4$ M^{-1}, $a = 1.05$ at 4°C.

Similar studies (Katz and Pappenheimer, 1969) were carried out with two different hexasaccharides derived from S-III that were reduced with tritiated sodium borohydride to form ligands 3A6 and 3D6:

$$3A6: \left\{\text{→ 3)-}\beta\text{-D-glcA(1→4)-}\beta\text{-D-glc(1}\right\}_3 - [^3\mathrm{H}]$$
$$3D6: \left\{\text{→ 4)-}\beta\text{-D-glc(1→3)-}\beta\text{-D-glcA(1}\right\}_3 - [^3\mathrm{H}]$$

Antibodies were raised in homozygous a¹b⁴ rabbits and in untyped rabbits against formalinized type III pneumococcal vaccine. The reactions between antibodies from rabbit #300 and the two ligands are shown in Figure 6-34. Both intact γG and Fab were tested. With

$$r/c = (n - r)K$$

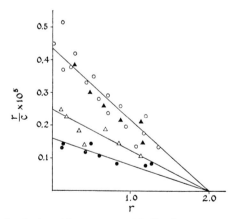

FIG. 6-32. Scatchard plot of homogeneous binding between anti-S-VIII antibodies and [³H]-8-S-VIII. (○) Horse #741, anti-SVIII-III at 25°C; (▲) at 4°C; (△) rabbit #6, anti-S-VIII at 25°C; (●) rabbit #7 mgh, genotype b⁵, anti-S-VIII at 4°C. (From Pappenheimer, Reed, and Brown, 1968.)

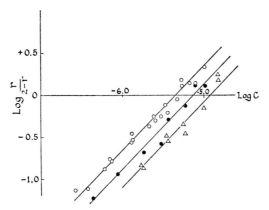

FIG. 6-33. Sips plot of homogeneous binding between anti-S-VIII antibodies and [³H]-8-S-VIII. (O) Horse #741, anti-S-VIII-III at 25°C and 4°C; (●) rabbit #6, anti-SVIII at 25°C; (Δ) rabbit #7 mgh, anti-S-VIII at 4°C. (From Pappenheimer, Reed, and Brown, 1968.)

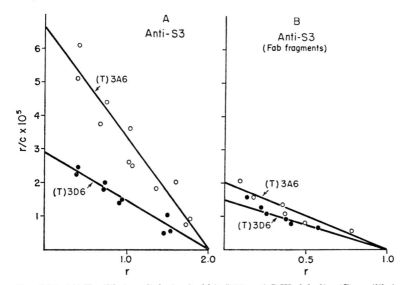

FIG. 6-34. (A) Equilibrium dialysis of rabbit #300 anti-S-III globulin; (B) equilibrium dialysis of purified Fab fragments from the same serum; (O) against [³H]-3A6 as ligand; (●) against [³H]-3D6 as ligand.

[³H]-3A6 γG and Fab had association constants of 3.2 and 2.0 × 10⁵ M^{-1}, $a = 0.99$ in both cases, with [³H]-3D6 the two entities had affinities of 1.4 and 1.55 × 10⁵ M^{-1} and Sipsian constants of 0.96 and 0.98, respectively. Katz and Pappenheimer (1969) concluded: "It thus seems likely that homogeneity of binding sites will prove the rule, rather than the exception, in the case of antibodies directed against antigens containing linearly arranged and evenly spaced simple repeating determinant groups."

As was emphasized at the beginning of the discussion on homogeneous binding, the demonstration of uniform binding properties of an antibody preparation does not establish the structural homogeneity of the preparation. Considerable restriction is evident, of course, when compared with the extremes of heterogeneity described in the first portion of this chapter, but not necessarily enough restriction. The difference between the two types of homogeneity was shown very well by Pincus, Haber, Katz, and Pappenheimer (1968) who demonstrated considerably polydisperse electrophoretic patterns in antipneumococcal polysaccharide antisera that had homogeneous binding characteristics. Pincus, Jaton, Bloch, and Haber (1970a) summarized their experience in trying to achieve restriction of structural heterogeneity: 8/116 rabbit antisera to S-III and 11/116 rabbit antisera to S-VIII showed a marked increase in γG content *and* restriction in electrophoretic mobility. There was a distinct correlation between restriction and the appearance of a sharp high peak in the electrophoretic pattern of the immune sera, very much like that of a myeloma protein. A typical human myeloma hypergammaglobulinemic serum pattern, taken from Korngold's (1961) definitive study is shown in Figure 6-35, in comparison with a normal serum pattern (albumin to the right, γ-globulin to the left). The cellulose acetate electrophoretic patterns of one of the eleven rabbits undergoing the immune process of raising anti-S-VIII antibodies in large quantity and electrophoretic restriction are shown in Figure 6-36. The similarity between the two figures needs no further elaboration.

Jaton, Waterfield, Margolies, and Haber (1970) investigated the light chain amino acid sequences of some of the antibodies that showed electrophoretic mobility restriction. To do so they devised a method of purification utilizing immunoadsorbents. In the pioneering days of immunochemistry Avery and Goebel (1931) had already shown how one could couple pneumococcal polysaccharide S-III to equine serum albumin (which they had used for immunization as well as purification). Jaton *et al.* used the same procedure to couple S-III and S-VIII to bovine serum albumin (BSA) which was then reacted with bromoacetylcellulose (BAC) to form the complete immunoadsorbents S-III-BSA-BAC and S-VIII-BSA-BAC. Anti-S-VIII antibodies in 90–95% yield, that were fractionated via S-VIII-BSA-BAC, still had 3 electrophoretic components but when a subsequent fractionation was carried out via S-III-BSA-BAC, the

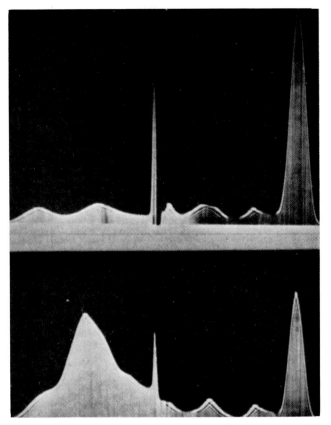

Fɪɢ. 6-35. Moving-boundary electrophoresis of normal serum (*top*) and hypergam-maglobulinemic serum (*bottom*). Descending limb. (From Korngold, 1961.)

slowest moving component was exclusively adsorbed and could be purified in 90–100% yield by subsequent elution from the adsorbent. The light chains from the 3-component anti-S-VIII antibody produced a 5-band pattern in disc electrophoresis; light chain from the 2 components remaining after S-III adsorption contained 4 bands; the cross-reacting anti-S-VIII-S-III component had the fifth and slowest band. Thus there was charge heterogeneity among the three components associated mainly with light chains with anti-S-VIII-S-III associated with the slowest mobility. Edman sequenation of this purified component gave a light chain amino acid pattern that had a single sequence for the first 11 residues:

D-V-V-M-T-Z-T-P-A-T-V

The mixture from the whole rabbit had the following:

D	V	V	M	T	Z	T	P	A	T	V	
66	100	100	54	83	79	73	54	38	50	60	%
A			V	L	T	V	L	P	V	T	
34			19	17	21	15	32	27	27	29	%
			L		L	V	L	A	L		
			15		12	14	18	22	11		%
			T				V				
			12				17				%

Further evidence of structural homogeneity of the purified antibody was obtained from peptide maps of the light chains: the purified anti-S-VIII-S-III antibody light chains had unique peptides that were not present in a nominal pool of light chains with the same allotype. In these most important experiments can be seen the outline for immunochemical progress of the 1970s—the structural delineation and topographical detailing of specific binding sites for specific

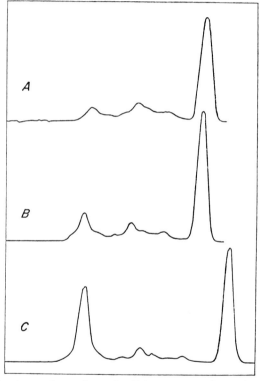

FIG. 6-36. Densitometric tracings of cellulose acetate electrophoresis patterns of serum obtained from rabbit #325 after the first (A), second (B), and third (C) course of immunization with type VIII pneumococci. (From Pincus, Jaton, Bloch, and Haber, 1970b.)

ligands. For the first time a method is available that can raise and purify antibodies in as large a quantity and with the same degree of homogeneity as myeloma proteins. The additional feature not present in the myeloma studies is the ability to know before hand the specific structures of the antigenic determinants that are most intimately involved in complementation. With this method the "insertion-deletion theory" of Wu and Kabat (1970) is now subject to complete and definitive testing.

L. *Homogeneous antibodies to streptococcal ligands.* Other haptens are needed to explore the diverse number of binding site structures as far as possible, and other haptens are available. In fact, another example of homogeneous antibody was being structured parallel in time with that of Haber's group. Krause (1963) had given a detailed review of the immunochemical and biochemical nature of the cell walls of hemolytic streptococci, and McCarty (1964) and McCarty and Morse (1964) had reviewed in particular their concepts of the immunochemistry and biochemistry of the carbohydrate of group A streptococci. The group A streptococci schematically were visualized as shown in Figure 6-37; the group A carbohydrate, in Figure 6-38. The experiments in McCarty's laboratory established that the immunodominant residues are the terminal β-N-acetylglucosaminide (NAcGlu) moieties and that when 11 of the 17 NAcGlu groups are removed through the action of β-N-acetylglucosaminidase, a relatively inert polymer, predominantly rhamnose, remains.

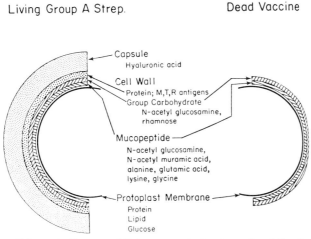

FIG. 6-37. Schematic diagram of living group A streptococci and the dead vaccine prepared from it. (From Krause, 1970.)

The variant group A and the group C structures have the same backbone but different proportions of NAcGlu termini; group C has NAc galactosamine in place of NAc glucosamine; group A variant none:

Group A,
NAcGlu 30%
Rhamnose 60%
CHO backbone

Group A variant,
NAcGlu 4%
Rhamnose 85%
CHO backbone

Group C,
NAcGlu 5%
Rhamnose 42%
NAcGal 40%
CHO backbone

Osterland, Miller, Karakawa, and Krause (1966) determined through densitometric scans of electrophoretic patterns of anti-group specific antisera in rabbits that markedly elevated γG of singular mobility many times arose during the immune response. The pattern shown in Figure 6-36 for anti-pneumococcal polysaccharide antisera was, in fact, demonstrated much earlier by this group for the anti-streptococcal polysaccharide. One rabbit produced 55 mg γG/ml serum which was homogeneous in gel electrophoresis, which gave a single-banded light chain electrophoretic pattern, and which contained

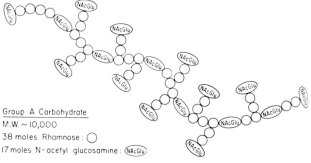

Group A Carbohydrate
M.W. ~ 10,000
38 moles Rhamnose : ○
17 moles N-acetyl glucosamine : (NAcGlu)

FIG. 6-38. Schematic diagram of the chemical structure of the group A carbohydrate antigen extracted from the streptococcal cell wall. (From Krause, 1970.)

specificity for group A streptococci. Miller, Osterland, Davie, and Krause (1967) continued the pursuit of restricted electrophoretic homogeneity; Fleischman, Braun, and Krause (1968) showed how the restriction became more evident after secondary immunization; and Davie, Osterland, Miller, and Krause (1968) even encountered a two-peak cryoglobulin in one rabbit which composed 90% of the γG and which was distributed in specificity between group B activity in the slower peak and cell-wall agglutinability in the faster one. Light chain patterns revealed 5 bands for the slower component, 2 bands for the faster. Hood, Lackland, Eichmann, Kindt, Braun, and Krause (1969) next demonstrated the amino acid sequence restriction in the light chains of group A and group C specific rabbit antibodies. Preimmune N-terminal sequences of γG from rabbit 22–85 for example were highly mixed, immune globulins much less so.

In assessing the immune response to streptococcal vaccines Braun, Eichmann, and Krause (1969) stated that "in rabbits with hyper-γ-globulinemia following primary immunization, group-specific precipitins predominate. They are electrophoretically monodisperse, possess individual antigenic specificities, resemble M-proteins, and sometimes are not seen until the secondary response." Indeed Eichmann, Lackland, Hood, and Krause (1970) found one rabbit anti-streptococcal antibody whose whole and light chain electrophoretic behavior and N-terminal light chain sequence could not be readily distinguished from myeloma proteins. The one important difference was the knowledge of antigenic specificity in the case of the rabbit antibody! Basing their experiments upon the experiences stemming from Krause's laboratory Rodkey, Choi, and Nisonoff (1970) were able to isolate from heterozygous rabbit globulin antibodies with specificity for *Streptococcus pyogenes*. When the ^{125}I-labeled antibodies were mixed with ^{131}I-labeled nonspecific γG and subjected to isoelectric focusing the charge homogeneity was beautifully demonstrated (Fig. 6-39). By the method of refocusing another technique then became available for the purification of homogeneous antibody. Light chains could also be focused, after separation from refocused specifically purified antibody, with preservation of the very narrow isoelectric band. The distribution of allotypic specificities during the purification process describes the drive toward homogeneity in clear-cut terms (Table 6-4).

Kindt, Todd, Eichmann, and Krause (1970) also determined that electrophoretically restricted, myeloma-like anti-streptococcal antibody exhibited allotypic exclusion, and even obtained one antibody which, after purification, lacked any group a allotypic marker on its heavy chains.

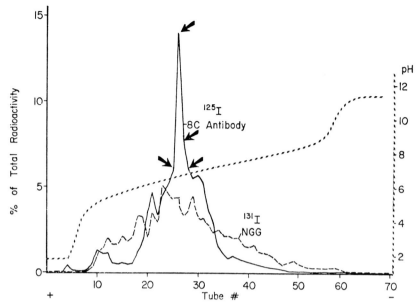

Fɪɢ. 6-39. Isoelectric focusing profile (pH 5–9) of ^{125}I-labeled specifically purified antistreptococcal polysaccharide antibody from rabbit GC in the presence of ^{131}I-nonspecific γG. (From Rodkey, Choi, and Nisonoff, 1970.)

Krause (1970) summarized the characteristics of homogeneity in the antibodies to group-specific carbohydrates as follows:

(a) Monodisperse by zone electrophoresis.
(b) Individual antigenic specificity.
(c) Single class and single subgroup.
(d) Selective absence of allotypic markers.
(e) Homogeneous binding characteristics.
(f) Monodisperse light chains by disc electrophoresis.
(g) Amino acid sequence analysis.

He also listed two reasons for the failure of all rabbits to respond in this way. As Braun (1969) had pointed out there was great variability among rabbits in the magnitude of the immune response—brisk, high level, poor. Braun attributed the variation to: (a) prior exposure to antigen and (b) genetic differences in the immune response. He went on to say that "what is intriguing is the possibility that an immune response characterized by antibodies with uniform properties may be under genetic control." He concluded:

"By a judicious selection of those microbes which possess chemically well-defined superficial carbohydrate antigens,

TABLE 6-4

Distribution of Allotypic Specificities in Fractions of Anti-streptococcal and Nonspecific Immunoglobulins

Nonspecific γG from Rabbit Allotype a¹b⁴b⁵	b4	b5
	%	%
Whole γG	52	38
Focus, pH 6.1 peak	52	34
Focus, pH 6.5 peak	52	32
Focus, pH 7.0 peak	54	33
Refocus, pH 6.1 peak	51	32
Refocus, pH 6.5 peak	53	34
Refocus, pH 7.0 peak	53	32

Rabbit 8C, Anti-streptococcal	b4	b5
	%	%
Nonantibody γG	61	29
Precipitated Ab γG	34	71
×2 focused Ab γG	13	92
Focused light chains from ×2 focused Ab γG	1	99

Rabbit 10C, Anti-streptococcal	a2	a3
	%	%
Preimmune γG	37	48
Precipitated Ab	63	30
×2 focused Ab	84	5

(From Rodkey, Choi, and Nisonoff, 1970.)

it may become possible to procure, within reasonable limits, antibodies to the determinant of your choice.''

By way of example he mentioned a personal communication from T. Feizi and E. Gotschlich (1970) that N-acetyl-*O*-acetyl-mannosamine-PO₄ from group A meningococci also give rise to rabbit antibodies with uniform properties.

M. Electrophoretic restriction of anti-DNP antibodies to DNP-papain. Whereas ligand binding characteristics were established in the case of anti-pneumococcal antibodies none was in evidence in the case of anti-streptococcal antibodies. Yet the evidence for an approach to restricted heterogeneity was overwhelming in the latter, and by analogy to the former presumably will exhibit many examples of homogeneous binding once a suitable test ligand is available. In the same way the experiments of Singer's group can be expected to yield additional examples. By reacting the one lone —SH group per mole of active papain with α-N-iodoacetyl-ε-N-dinitrophenyl-L-lysine these investigators were able to produce a univalent hapten-protein conjugate. Immunization of mice with the conjugate produced antihapten antibodies with electrophoretically homogeneous light chains (Brenneman and Singer, 1968, 1970). With the method of isoelectric focusing (pH 4–8) Trump and Singer (1970) obtained ascitic fluid from 88/232 immune mice with 2 μg antibody/ml or greater by the 10th day; 66 of these were in the 2–5 μg range, 10 were in the 5–10 μg range; 10, 15–25 μg; and 2 greater than 50 μg/ml. Selection for anti-DNP antibody with a large net negative charge was based upon the relative positive charge of the carrier protein (isoelectric point of 8.8); thus, ⅓ of the antibody proteins were accountably homogeneous at pH 5.0 while the remainder spread themselves heterogeneously between pH 5 and 8.

N. Folic acid, vasopressin, and digoxin. Five examples of homogeneous binding remain to be discussed. Two of these involve multivalent antigenic structures of tobacco mosaic and influenza viruses and will be taken up in the next chapter. Three involve univalent ligands and belong to this chapter: folic acid, vasopressin, and digoxin.

The experiments of Rubinstein and Little (1970) with folic acid have already been discussed in connection with the use of the ligand as an electron acceptor and, hence, as a compound useful in determining the quenchability of specific antibody fluorescence. [³H]-folate, in equilibrium dialysis with antifolate antibodies, approached homogeneous binding with an average association constant of 4.1×10^6 M^{-1} in early antisera, 3.2×10^6 M^{-1} in late antisera, and with a Sipsian heterogeneity constant of 0.92. The importance of achieving complete structural homogeneity of antibodies against this and similar compounds stems from the similarity that the antibody binding site might have in common with folate-binding enzymes. Topology comparisons may be very important in investigating the further details of dihydrofolic reductase activity.

Wu and Rockey (1969) chose the neurohypophyseal nonapeptide hormone, vasopressin, as another example of a ligand with dimensions very close to binding site regions (Fig. 6–40). The nonapeptide, like angiotensin previously discussed, also had a tyrosine residue that could be iodinated and used as a tracer ligand. For immunization it was coupled to equine γGab-globulins with carbodiimide reagents in the ratio of 7–8 moles peptide per mole globulin and injected into rabbits. Extent of binding was determined by the technique of radioimmunoprecipitation by which the soluble immune complexes of ^{125}I-vasopressin and rabbit antibody at various concentrations were precipitated by sheep-anti-rabbit γG antibodies. The Scatchard and Sips plots of the binding data are shown in Figure 6–41. Reproduci-

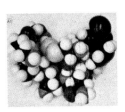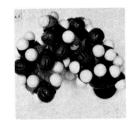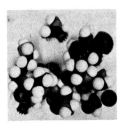

FIG. 6-40. Space-filling three-dimensional Corey-Pauling-Koltun molecular models of radioiodinated Lys-vasopressin (A) and performic acid oxidized Lys-vasopressin (B). Two views of the native hormone are presented in A1 and A2. The dimensions of the native molecule are 19 × 4 × 11 Å. A model of the S-carbamidomethyl group of reduced and alkylated vasopressin also is shown in B. The lysine nonapeptide from the pig has the sequence, CYFQNCPKG. Bovine vasopressin has an arginine at position 8: CYFQNCPRG. Oxytocin has a related sequence, CYIQNCPLG, with leucine at position 8. The vasopressins cause pressure increase in the peripheral and coronary arteries and also act as diuretics. Oxytocin causes milk ejection and contraction of uterine muscles in mammals, lowered blood pressure in birds. (From Wu and Rockey, 1969.)

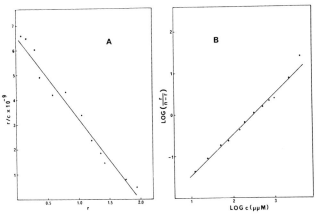

FIG. 6-41. Radioimmunoprecipitation vasopressin binding curves constructed with radioiodinated vasopressin and rabbit 17 anti-vasopressin serum. (A) Binding data presented in terms of r and c, where r = moles of hapten bound/mole of antibody, and c = free hapten concentration ($r/c = (n - r)K_0$, $n = 2$). Average intrinsic association constant, $K_0 = 3.2 \times 10^9$ M^{-1}. (B) Binding data expressed in terms of the Sips distribution function, $\log(r/(n - r)) = a \log c + a \log K_0$. Data fitted to a linear curve by the method of least squares. Index of heterogeneity, a, is 1.04. (From Wu and Rockey, 1969.)

ble binding curves could be constructed even at very low antibody concentrations since the binding constants were so high. As shown in the figure for a *typical* antiserum, an association constant of 3.2×10^9 M^{-1} could be obtained and a Sipsian constant of 1.04.

The digitalis glycoside digoxin can be conjugated to human serum albumin by a mechanism such as that shown in Figure 6–42. Smith,

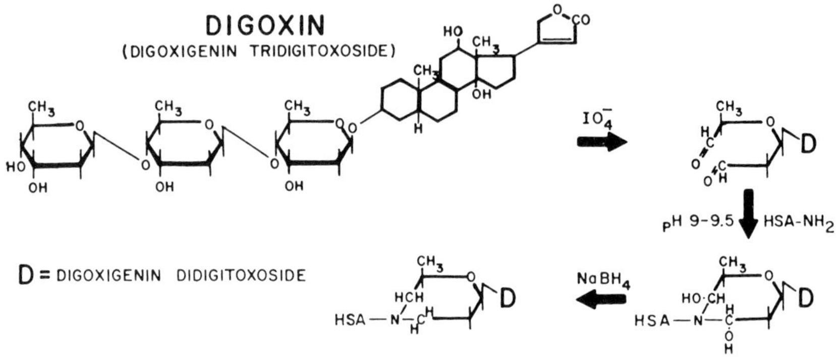

FIG. 6-42. Proposed mechanism for the conjugation of digoxin to human serum albumin. (From Smith, Butler, and Haber, 1970.)

Butler, and Haber (1970) immunized rabbits with the conjugate and raised antibodies of extremely high affinity and specificity. One rabbit produced a hypergammaglobulinemic titer of 5.8 mg antibody/ml. For binding measurements digoxin was tritiated in the 12α position and tested in equilibrium dialysis. Antibodies with an association constant of 1.7×10^{10} M^{-1} and with a Sipsian heterogeneity constant of 0.95 were produced in one rabbit (Figs. 6–43 and 6–44). Two other antisera gave association constants of 1.2×10^9 M^{-1} and 1.1×10^{10}, respectively, and Sipsian constants of 0.99 and 0.60. The binding was of such high affinity that as little as 3×10^{-13} moles digoxin/ml could be detected in physiological fluids. Digitoxin, which differs from digoxin only in a single hydroxyl group at the C_{12} position of the steroid nucleus (Fig. 6–45), competed very poorly with digoxin, and had a binding constant of 5.3×10^8 M^{-1} and heterogeneity constant of 0.83 when tested with the same antiserum as shown in Figure 6–43. Deslanoside, which differs from digoxin by having an additional glucose residue coupled to the terminal digitoxose (Fig. 6–45), competed freely with digoxin in inhibition tests (Fig. 6–46).

O. High affinity and homogeneity. Up until now the importance of homogeneous binding has been stressed in one example after another in this Chapter without much comment about the affinity achieved. In fact, some structural homogeneous examples were offered without specification of the strength of binding. Now it is time to stress affinity itself. Selection depends upon it. The higher the affinity the more dilute the ligand or antigen may be that reacts with antibody whether *in vitro* or *in vivo*. Obviously, an antibody as high in affinity as the one just discussed need be produced in only very minute quantities indeed to be useful (or harmful). From the point of

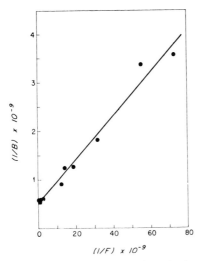

FIG. 6-43. Langmuir plot of bound (B) and free (F) molar hapten concentrations as determined by equilibrium dialysis of tritiated digoxin with 0.025 μl of antiserum 46/97. The line, determined by least-squares regression analysis, has a correlation coefficient of 0.99 and the experimental points shown extend over a range from 14 to 90% saturation of antibody combining sites. (From Smith, Butler, and Haber, 1970.)

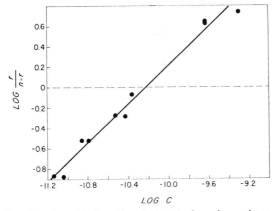

FIG. 6-44. Sips plot of equilibrium dialysis data for homologous hapten digoxin with antiserum 46/97. Range of antibody saturation 12 to 85%; correlation coefficient 0.99. $K_0 = 1.7 \times 10^{10}$ M^{-1}; $a = 0.95$. (From Smith, Butler, and Haber, 1970.)

view of binding site topology it also stands to reason that to probe the very intimate details of the binding site one needs more than homogeneous antibody of just any affinity; one needs *high affinity* homogeneous antibody. The problem of designing the proper determinant of one's choice does not end, therefore, with the achieve-

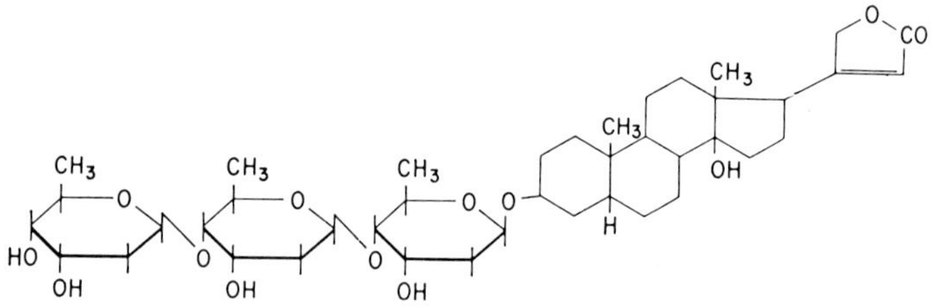

DIGITOXIN

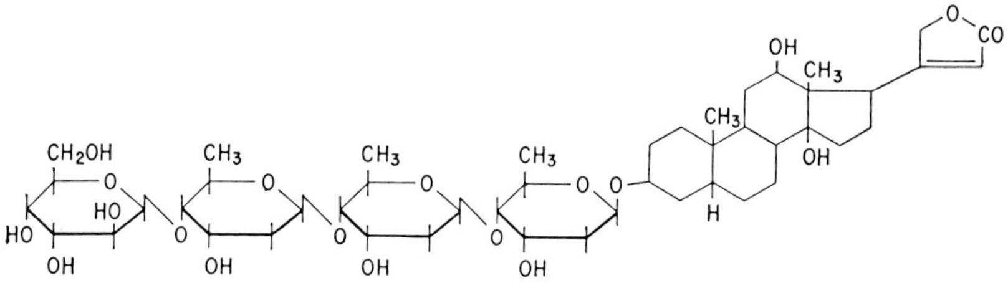

DESLANOSIDE

FIG. 6-45. Structural formulas of steroid glycosides closely related to digoxin. Digitoxin differs only in the absence of the C-12 OH group, whereas deslanoside has an additional glucose residue coupled to the terminal digitoxose. (From Smith, Butler, and Haber, 1970.)

ment of complete homogeneity. One must reach for the high affinity such as that displayed by antibodies to digoxin.

The search does not end there either. The subject of the multivalent antigen which will be discussed in the next chapter will reveal the nuances achieved by extending beyond univalency. The techniques for probing the nature of binding between macromolecular multivalent antigens and multivalent antibodies are not so extensive as in hapten research, and in many ways are completely lacking. This deficiency does not for a moment, however, detract from the high priority that the problem should be given during the 1970s and the 1980s. The nature of the transition from univalent haptens to multivalency is best stated, perhaps, in the simple equation which Singer (1965) has used to convert from intrinsic affinity constants to extrinsic ones:

$$K' = fK/2$$

where K is intrinsic, K' is extrinsic, f is antigen valence, and 2 is antibody valence. Singer concludes:

"Therefore, for antigens with large values of f, such as viruses, the observed equilibrium (Ag + Ab $\rightleftharpoons$ AgAb) may

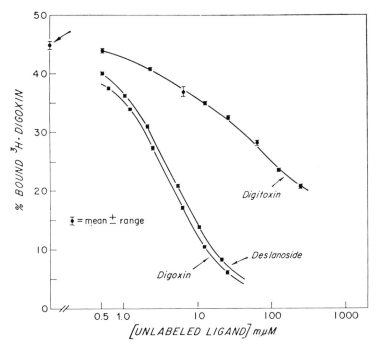

FIG. 6-46. Hapten inhibition curves from antiserum 46/97 plotting on semilogarithmic scale the extent to which the steroid glycosides digoxin, deslanoside, and digitoxin displace tritiated digoxin from the antibody combining site. The control value with no unlabeled ligand added is indicated by the *arrow* on the ordinate. (From Smith, Butler, and Haber, 1970.)

be far to the side of complete reaction even though the *intrinsic* equilibrium constant is no larger than the usual value."

REFERENCES

Allen, J. C., Kunkel, H. G., and Kabat, E. A. (1964). Studies on human antibodies. II. Distribution of genetic factors. J. Exp. Med. *119:* 453–465.

Ashman, R. F., and Metzger, H. (1969). A Waldenstrom macroglobulin which binds nitrophenyl ligands. J. Biol. Chem. *244:* 3405–3414.

Avery, O. T., and Goebel, W. F. (1931). Chemoimmunological studies on conjugated carbohydrate-proteins. V. The immunological specificity of an antigen prepared by combining the capsular polysaccharide of type III pneumococcus with foreign protein. J. Exp. Med. *54:* 437–447.

Awdeh, Z. L., Askonas, B. A., and Williamson, A. R. (1967). The homogeneous γG-immunoglobulin produced by mouse plasmacytoma 5563 and its subsequent heterogeneity in serum. Biochem. J. *102:* 548–553.

Awdeh, Z. L., Williamson, A. R., and Askonas, B. A. (1969). Heavy and light chains of a homogeneous immunoglobulin-G. Fed. Eur. Biochem. Soc. Letters *5:* 275–278.

Awdeh, Z. L., Williamson, A. R., and Askonas, B. A. (1970). One cell–one immunoglobulin. Origin of limited heterogeneity of myeloma proteins. Biochem. J. *116:* 241–248.

Bassett, E. W., Tanenbaum, S. W., Pryzwansky, K., Beisen, S. M., and Kabat, E. A. (1965). Studies on human antibodies. III. Amino acid composition of four antibodies from one individual. J. Exp. Med. *122:* 251–261.

Benjamin, D. C., and Weigle, W. O. (1970). Frequency of single spleen cells from hyperimmune rabbits producing antibody of two different specificities. J. Immunol. *105:* 537–540.

Berson, S. A., and Yalow, R. S. (1959). Quantitative aspects of the reaction between insulin and insulin-binding antibody. J. Clin. Invest. *38:* 1996–2016.

Bowman, J. D., and Aladjem, F. (1963). A method for the determination of heterogeneity of antibodies. J. Theor. Biol. *4:* 242–253.

Braun, D. G. (1969). Homogeneous antibody populations in rabbits following the immunization with streptococcal vaccines. Behringwerk-Mitteil. *49:* 105–120.

Braun, D. G., Eichmann, K., and Krause, R. M. (1969). Rabbit antibodies to streptococcal carbohydrates. Influence of primary and secondary immunization and of possible genetic factors on the antibody response. J. Exp. Med. *129:* 809–830.

Brenneman, L., and Singer, S. J. (1968). The generation of antihapten antibodies with electrophoretically homogeneous L chains. Proc. Natl. Acad. Sci. *60:* 258–264.

Brenneman, L. D., and Singer, S. J. (1970). On homogeneous antigens and antibodies. III. The preparation and properties of the univalent hapten-protein conjugate papain-S-DNPL. Ann. N.Y. Acad. Sci. *169:* 72–92.

Buchanan-Davidson, D., Dellert, E., Kornguth, S., and Stahmann, M. (1959). Immunochemistry of synthetic polypeptides and polypeptidyl proteins. II. Quantitative studies on the modified proteins. J. Immunol. *83:* 543–551.

Burnet, F. M. (1967). The impact on ideas of immunology. Symp. Quant. Biol. *32:* 1–8.

Cosenza, H., and Nordin, A. A. (1970). Immunoglobulin classes of antibody-forming cells in mice. III. Immunoglobulin antibody restriction of plaque-forming cells demonstrated by the double immunofluorescent technique. J. Immunol. *104:* 976–983.

Dandliker, W. B., Alonso, R., and Meyers, C. Y. (1967). The synthesis of fluorescent penicilloyl haptens and their use in investigating 'penicillin' antibodies by fluorescence polarization. Immunochemistry *4:* 295–302.

Davie, J. M., Osterland, C. K., Miller, E. J., and Krause, R. M. (1968). Immune cryoglobulins in rabbit streptococcal antiserum. J. Immunol. *100:* 814–820.

Day, L. A., Sturtevant, J. M., and Singer, S. J. (1962). The direct measurement of the rate of a hapten-antibody reaction. J. Am. Chem. Soc. *84:* 3768–3770.

Day, L. A., Sturtevant, J. M., and Singer, S. J. (1963). The kinetics of the reactions between antibodies to the 2,4-dinitrophenyl group and specific haptens. Ann. N. Y. Acad. Sci. *103:* 611–625.

Dorner, M. M., Yount, W. J., and Kabat, E. A. (1969). Studies on human antibodies. VII. Acrylamide gel electrophoresis of purified human antibodies and myeloma proteins, their heavy and light chains. J. Immunol. *102:* 273–281.

Edelman, G. M., and Kabat, E. A. (1964). Studies on human antibodies. I. Starch gel electrophoresis of the dissociated polypeptide chains. J. Exp. Med. *119:* 443–452.

Eichmann, K., Lackland, H., Hood, L., and Krause, R. (1970). Induction of rabbit antibody with molecular uniformity after immunization with group C streptococci. J. Exp. Med. *131:* 207–221.

Eigen, M., and De Maeyer, L. (1962). Relaxation methods. In *Techniques of Organic Chemistry*, Ed. 2, Vol. 8, Weissburger, A., ed., Interscience (New York, 1582 pp.), pp. 895–1054.

Eisen, H. N., and Karush, F. (1949). The interaction of purified antibody with homologous hapten. Antibody valence and binding constant. J. Am. Chem. Soc. 71: 363–364.

Eisen, H. N., Little, J. R., Osterland, C. K., and Simms, E. S. (1967). A myeloma protein with antibody activity. Symp. Quant. Biol. 32: 75–81.

Eisen, H. N., and Pearce, J. H. (1962). The nature of antibodies and antigens. Ann. Rev. Microbiol. 16: 101–126.

Eisen, H. N., Simms, E. S., Little, J. R., and Steiner, L. A. (1964). Affinities of anti-2,4-dinitrophenyl (DNP) antibodies induced by ε-41-mono-DNP-ribonuclease. Fed. Proc. 23: 559 incl.

Eisen, H. N., Simms, E. S., and Potter, M. (1968). Mouse myeloma proteins with antihapten antibody activity. The protein produced by plasma cell tumor MOPC-315. Biochemistry 7: 4126–4134.

Eisen, H. N., and Siskind, G. W. (1964). Variations in affinities of antibodies during the immune response. Biochemistry 3: 996–1008.

Epstein, S. I., Doty, P., and Boyd, W. L. (1956). A thermodynamic study of hapten-antibody association. J. Am. Chem. Soc. 78: 3306–3315.

Feizi, T., and Gotschlich, E. (1970). Personal communication to Krause, R., as reported in Krause, R., Fed. Proc. 29: 59–65.

Fleischman, J. B., Braun, D. G., and Krause, R. M. (1968). Streptococcal group-specific antibodies: occurrence of a restricted population following secondary immunization. Proc. Natl. Acad. Sci. 60: 134–139.

Fraser, K. J., and Edman, P. (1970). N-terminus of light chains from rabbit arsonic antibody. Fed. Eur. Biochem. Soc. 7: 99–100.

Froese, A. (1968). Kinetic and equilibrium studies on 2,4-dinitrophenyl hapten-antibody systems. Immunochemistry 5: 253–264.

Froese, A., and Sehon, A. H. (1964). Kinetics of antibody-hapten reactions. Ber. Bunsenges Physik. Chem. 68: 863–864.

Froese, A., and Sehon, A. H. (1965). Kinetic and equilibrium studies of the reaction between anti-p-nitrophenyl antibodies and a homologous hapten. Immunochemistry 2: 135–143.

Froese, A., Sehon, A. H., and Eigen, M. (1962). Kinetic studies of protein-dye and antibody-hapten interactions with the temperature-jump method. Can. J. Chem. 40: 1786–1797.

Fujio, H., and Karush, F. (1966). Antibody affinity. II. Effects of immunization on antihapten antibody in the rabbit. Biochemistry 5: 1856–1863.

Gitlin, D., and Merler, E. (1961). A comparison of the peptides released from related rabbit antibodies by enzymatic hydrolysis. J. Exp. Med. 114: 217–230.

Green, I., Vassill, P., Nussenzweig, V., and Benacerraf, B. (1967). Specificity of the antibodies produced by single cells following immunization with antigens bearing two types of antigenic determinants. J. Exp. Med. 125: 511–526.

Haber, E., and Richards, F. F. (1966). The specificity of antigenic recognition of antibody heavy chain. Proc. Roy. Soc. Lond. 166: 176–187.

Haber, E., Richards, F. F., Spragg, J., Austen, K. F., Vallotton, M., and Page, L. B. (1967). Modifications in the heterogeneity of the antibody response. Symp. Quant. Biol. 32: 299–310.

Hauglund, R. P., Stryer, L., Stengle, T. R., and Baldeschweiler, J. D. (1967). Nuclear magnetic resonance studies of antibody-hapten interactions using a chloride ion probe. Biochemistry 6: 498–502.

Haurowitz, F., and Breinl, F. (1933). Chemische Untersuchung der spezifischen Bindung von Arsanil-Eiweiss und Arsanilasaure an Immunserum. Hoppe Seylers Z. Physiol. Chem. *214:* 111–120.

Herd, Z. L., and Cebra, J. J. (1970). Selection of a single antigenic type of rabbit light chains by the 2,4-dinitrophenyl hapten. Immunochemistry *7:* 7–13.

Herriott, R. M., Desreux, V., and Northrop, J. H. (1940–1941). Fractionation of pepsin. I. Isolation of crystalline pepsin of constant activity and solubility from pepsinogen or commercial pepsin preparations. II. Preparation of a less soluble fraction. III. Solubility curves of mixtures of the soluble and insoluble fractions. IV. Preparation of highly active pepsin from pepsinogen. J. Gen. Physiol. *24:* 213–246.

Hoffman, D. R., and Campbell, D. H. (1969). Model system for the study of drug hypersensitivity. I. The specificity of the rabbit anti-aspiryl system. J. Immunol. *103:* 655–661.

Hood, L., Lackland, H., Eichmann, K., Kindt, T. J., Braun, D. C., and Krause, R. M. (1969). Amino acid sequence restriction in rabbit antibody light chains. Proc. Natl. Acad. Sci. *63:* 890–896.

Jaffe, B. M., Eisen, H. N., Simms, E. S., and Potter, M. (1969). Myeloma proteins with anti-hapten antibody activity: ϵ-2,4-dinitrophenyl lysine binding by the protein produced by mouse plasmacytoma MOPC-460. J. Immunol. *103:* 872–874.

Jaton, J.-C., Waterfield, M. D., Margolies, M. N., and Haber, E. (1970). Isolation and characterization of structurally homogeneous antibodies from anti-pneumococcal sera. Proc. Natl. Acad. Sci. *66:* 959–974.

Jerne, N. K., and Nordin, A. A. (1963). Plaque formation in agar by single antibody-producing cells. Science *140:* 405 incl.

Karush, F. (1956). The interaction of purified antibody with optically isomeric hapten. J. Am. Chem. Soc. *78:* 5519–5526.

Karush, F. (1957). The interaction of purified anti-β-lactoside antibody with haptens. J. Am. Chem. Soc. *79:* 3380–3384.

Karush, F. (1958). Structural and energetic aspects of antibody-hapten interactions. Conf. Protein Metab. (Rutgers) *4:* 40–55.

Karush, F. (1962). Immunologic specificity and molecular structure. Adv. Immunol. *2:* 1–40.

Karush, F., and Sonenberg, M. (1949). Interaction of homologous alkyl sulfates with bovine serum albumin. J. Am. Chem. Soc. *71:* 1369–1376.

Katz, M., and Pappenheimer, A. M., Jr. (1969). Quantitative studies of the specificity of anti-pneumococcal antibodies types III and VIII. IV. Binding of labeled hexasaccharides derived from S3 by anti-S3-antibodies and their Fab fragments. J. Immunol. *103:* 491–495.

Kindt, T. J., Todd, C. W., Eichmann, K., and Krause, R. M. (1970). Allotype exclusion in uniform rabbit antibody to streptococcal carbohydrate. J. Exp. Med. *131:* 343–354.

Kitagawa, M., Grossberg, A. L., Yagi, Y., and Pressman, D. (1967). Antibodies directed to singly and doubly charged forms of the *p*-azobenzenearsonate group. Immunochemistry *4:* 197–202.

Klinman, N. R. (1969). Antibody with homogeneous antigen binding produced by splenic foci in organ culture. Immunochemistry *6:* 757–759.

Klinman, N. R. (1971a). Regain of homogenous binding activity after recombination of chains of "monofocal" antibody. J. Immunol. *106:* 1330–1337.

Klinman, N. R. (1971b). Purification and analysis of "monofocal" antibody. J. Immunol. *106:* 1345–1352.

Klinman, N. R., and Aschinazi, G. (1971). The stimulation of splenic foci *in vitro*. J. Immunol. *106:* 1338–1344.

Klinman, N. R., and Karush, F. (1967). Equine anti-hapten antibody. V. The non-precipitability of bivalent antibody. Immunochemistry *4:* 387–405.

Klinman, N. R., Rockey, J. H., Frauenberger, G., and Karush, F. (1966). Equine anti-hapten antibody. III. The comparative properties of γG- and γA- antibodies. J. Immunol. *96:* 587–595.

Klinman, N. R., Rockey, J. H., and Karush, F. (1964). Valence and affinity of equine non-precipitating antibody to a haptenic group. Science *146:* 401–403.

Korngold, L. (1961). Abnormal plasma components and their significance in disease. Ann. N. Y. Acad. Sci. *94:* 110–130.

Koshland, M. E., Ochoa, P., and Fujita, N. J. (1970). Amino acid differences between highly cross-reactive antibodies. Biochemistry *9:* 1880–1886.

Krause, R. M. (1963). Antigenic and biochemical composition of hemolytic streptococcal cell walls. Bacteriol. Rev. *27:* 369–380.

Krause, R. M. (1970). Factors controlling the occurrence of antibodies with uniform properties. Fed. Proc. *29:* 59–65.

Landsteiner, K. (1921). Uber heterogenetisches Antigen und Hapten XV. Mitteilung uber Antigene. Biochem. Z. *119:* 294–306.

Little, J. R., Border, W., and Freidin, R. (1969). The binding reactions of antibodies specific for the 2,6-dinitrophenyl group. J. Immunol. *103:* 809–817.

Little, J. R., and Counts, R. B. (1969). Affinity and heterogeneity of antibodies induced by ϵ-2,4-dinitrophenylinsulin. Biochemistry *8:* 2729–2736.

Little, J. R., and Eisen, H. N. (1966). Preparation and characterization of antibodies specific for the 2,4,6-trinitrophenyl group. Biochemistry *5:* 3385–3395.

Mäkelä, O. (1967). The specificity of antibodies produced by single cells. Symp. Quant. Biol. *32:* 423–430.

Mamet-Bratley, M. D. (1970). Molecular weight of a rabbit antibody. Biochim. Biophys. Acta *207:* 76–91.

Mancino, D., Paul, W. E., Benacerraf, B., Siskind, G. W., and Ovary, Z. (1970). Binding properties of anti-dinitrophenylated-bacitracin A antibodies produced in guinea pigs. J. Immunol. *104:* 224–229.

Marrack, J., and Smith, F. C. (1932). Quantitative aspects of immunity reactions: the combination of antibodies with simple haptenes. Brit. J. Exp. Pathol. *13:* 394–402.

Mattioli, C. A., Yagi, Y., and Pressman, D. (1968). Production and properties of mouse anti-hapten antibodies. J. Immunol. *101:* 939–948.

McCarty, M. (1964). In *The Streptococcus, Rheumatic Fever, and Glomerulonephritis*, Uhr, J. W., ed. Williams & Wilkins (Baltimore, 419 pp.), p. 3.

McCarty, M., and Morse, S. I. (1964). Cell wall antigens of Gram-positive bacteria. Adv. Immunol. *4:* 249–286.

Metzger, H., Wofsy, L., and Singer, S. J. (1963). A specific antibody-hapten reaction with novel spectral properties. Arch. Biochem. Biophys. *103:* 206–215.

Miller, E. J., Osterland, C. K., Davie, J. M., and Krause, R. M. (1967). Electrophoretic analysis of polypeptide chains isolated from antibodies in the serum of immunized rabbits. J. Immunol. *98:* 710–715.

Moreno, C., and Kabat, E. A. (1969). Studies on human antibodies. VIII. Properties and association constants of human antibodies to blood group A substance purified with insoluble specific adsorbents and fractionally eluted with mono- and oligosaccharides. J. Exp. Med. *129:* 871–896.

Nisonoff, A., and Pressman, D. (1958a). Heterogeneity and average combining constants of antibodies from individual rabbits. J. Immunol. *80:* 417–428.

Nisonoff, A., and Pressman, D. (1958b). Heterogeneity of antibody sites in their relative combining affinities for structurally related haptens. J. Immunol. *81:* 126–135.

Nisonoff, A., Zappacosta, S., and Jareziz, R. (1967). Properties of crystallized rabbit anti-p-azobenzoate antibody. Symp. Quant. Biol. *32:* 89–93.

Northrop, J. H. (1942). Purification and crystallization of diphtheria antitoxin. J. Gen. Physiol. *25:* 465–485.

Nossal, G. J. V., and Lederberg, J. (1958). Antibody production by single cells. Nature *181:* 1419–1420.

Nossal, G. J. V., Szenberg, A., Ada, G. L., and Austin, C. M. (1964). Single cell studies on 19S antibody production. J. Exp. Med. *119:* 485–502.

Osterland, C. K., Miller, E. J., Karakawa, W., and Krause, R. M. (1966). Characteristics of streptococcal group-specific antibody isolated from hyperimmune rabbits. J. Exp. Med. *123:* 599–614.

Pappenheimer, A. M., Jr., Reed, W. P., and Brown, R. (1968). Quantitative studies of the specificity of anti-pneumococcal polysaccharide antibodies, types III and VIII. III. Binding of a labeled oligosaccharide derived from S8 by anti-S8 antibodies. J. Immunol. *100:* 1237–1244.

Parker, C. W., Godt, S. M., and Johnson, M. C. (1967). Fluorescent probes for the study of the antibody-hapten reaction. II. Variation in the antibody combining site during the immune response. Biochemistry *6:* 3417–3427.

Parker, C. W., Yoo, T. J., Johnson, M. C., and Godt, S. M. (1967). Fluorescent probes for the study of antibody-hapten reaction. I. Binding of the 5-dimethylaminonaphthalene-1-sulfonamido group by homologous rabbit antibody. Biochemistry *6:* 3408–3416.

Pauling, L. (1940). A theory of the structure and process of formation of antibodies. J. Am. Chem. Soc. *62:* 2643–2657.

Pincus, J. H., Haber, E., Katz, M., and Pappenheimer, A. M., Jr. (1968). Antibodies to pneumococcal polysaccharides: relation between binding and electrophoretic heterogeneity. Science *162:* 667–668.

Pincus, J. H., Jaton, J.-C., Bloch, K. J., and Haber, E. (1970a). Antibodies to type III and type VIII pneumococcal polysaccharides: evidence for restricted structural heterogeneity in hyperimmunized rabbits. J. Immunol. *104:* 1143–1148.

Pincus, J. H., Jaton, J.-C., Bloch, K. J., and Haber, E. (1970b). Properties of structurally restricted antibody to type VIII pneumococcal polysaccharide. J. Immunol. *104:* 1149–1154.

Playfair, J. H. L., Papermaster, B. W., and Cole, L. J. (1965). Focal antibody production by transferred spleen cells in irradiated mice. Science *149:* 998–1000.

Putnam, F. W. (1965). Structure and function of the plasma proteins. In *The Proteins*, Ed. 2, Vol. 3, Neurath, H., ed., Academic Press (New York, 585 pp.), pp. 153–267.

Richards, F. F., and Haber, E. (1967). Antibodies to relatively homogeneous haptens: the temporal pattern of their antigen-binding energies. Biochim. Biophys. Acta *140:* 558–560.

Richards, F. F., Pincus, J. H., Bloch, K. J., Barnes, W. T., and Haber, E. (1969) The relationship between antigenic complexity and heterogeneity in the antibody response. Biochemistry *8:* 1377–1384.

Richards, F. F., Sloane, R. W., Jr., and Haber, E. (1967). The synthesis and antigenic properties of a macromolecular peptide of defined sequence bearing the dinitrophenol hapten. Biochem. *6:* 476–484.

Rockey, J. H., Klinman, N. R., and Karush, F. (1965). Equine antihapten antibody. I. 7S β_{2A}- and 10S γ_1-globulin components of purified anti-β-lactoside antibody. J. Exp. Med. *120:* 589–609.

Rodkey, L. S., Choi, T. K., and Nisonoff, A. (1970). Isolation of molecules of restricted allotype from antistreptococcal polysaccharide antibody. J. Immunol. *104:* 63–71.

Roholt, O. A., Seon, B. K., and Pressman, D. (1970). Antibodies of limited heterogeneity: L chains of a single mobility. Immunochemistry *7:* 329–340.

Rubinstein, W. A., and Little, J. R. (1970). Properties of the active sites of antibodies specific for folic acid. Biochemistry *9:* 2106–2114.

Saha, K., Karush, F., and Marks, R. (1966). Antibody affinity. I. Studies with a large haptenic group. Immunochemistry *3:* 279–298.

Schneider, H., and Sehon, A. H. (1961). Determination of the lower limits for the rate constants of a hapten-antibody reaction by polarography. Trans. N. Y. Acad. Sci. *24:* 15–22.

Sehon, A. H. (1963). Kinetics of antibody-hapten interactions. Ann. N. Y. Acad. Sci. *103:* 626–629.

Sela, M., and Mozes, E. (1966). Dependence of the chemical nature of antibodies on the net electrical charge of antigens. Proc. Natl. Acad. Sci. *55:* 445–452.

Singer, S. J. (1964). On the heterogeneity of anti-hapten antibodies. Immunochemistry *1:* 15–20.

Singer, S. J. (1965). Structure and function of antigen and antibody proteins. In *The Proteins*, Ed. 2, Vol. 3, H. Neurath, ed., Academic Press (New York, 585 pp.), pp. 269–357.

Smith, T. W., Butler, V. P., Jr., and Haber, E. (1970). Characterization of antibodies of high affinity and specificity for the digitalis glycoside digoxin. Biochemistry *9:* 331–337.

Spragg, J., Austen, K. F., and Haber, E. (1966). Production of antibody against bradykinin: demonstration of specificity by complement fixation and radioimmunoassay. J. Immunol. *96:* 865–871.

Stahmann, M., Lapresle, C., Buchanan-Davidson, D. J., and Grabar, P. (1959). Immunochemistry of synthetic polypeptides and polypeptidyl proteins. I. Qualitative studies on the modified proteins. J. Immunol. *83:* 534–542.

Stevenson, G. T., Eisen, H. N., and Jones, R. H. (1970). The problem of hapten persistently bound to antibody. Biochem. J. *116:* 151–153.

Stryer, L., and Griffith, O. H. (1965). A spin-labeled hapten. Proc. Natl. Acad. Sci. *54:* 1785–1791.

Talmage, D. W. (1960). The kinetics of the reaction between antibody and bovine serum albumin using the Farr method. J. Infect. Dis. *107:* 115–132.

Terry, W. D., Ashman, R. F., and Metzger, H. (1970). Human IgA-myeloma protein which binds nitrophenyl ligands. Immunochemistry *7:* 257–260.

Trump, G. N., and Singer, S. J. (1970). Electrophoretically homogeneous anti-DNP antibodies with restricted isoelectric points elicited in mice by immunization with the antigen papain-S-DNPL. Proc. Natl. Acad. Sci. *66:* 411–418.

Underdown, B. J., Simms, E. S., and Eisen, H. N. (1970). Myeloma proteins with anti-hapten activity. Fed. Proc. *29:* 437 incl.

Velick, S. F., Parker, C. W., and Eisen, H. N. (1960). Excitation energy transfer and the quantitative study of the antibody hapten reaction. Proc. Natl. Acad. Sci. *46:* 1470–1482.

Winkelhake, J. L., and Voss, E. W., Jr. (1970). Recognition of carrier residues adjacent to hapten by anti-trinitrophenyl antibodies. Biochemistry *9:* 1845–1853.

Winkler, M. (1962). A molecular probe for the antibody site. J. Mol. Biol. 4: 118–120.

Wu, T. T., and Kabat, E. A. (1970). An analysis of the sequences of the variable regions of Bence Jones proteins and myeloma light chains and their implications for antibody complementarity. J. Exp. Med. 132: 211–250.

Wu, W.-H., and Rockey, J. H. (1969). Antivasopressin antibody. Characterization of high-affinity rabbit antibody with limited association constant heterogeneity. Biochemistry 8: 2719–2728.

Yoo, T.-J., and Parker, C. W. (1968). Fluorescent enhancement in antibody-hapten interaction. 1-Anilinonaphthalene-8-sulfonate as a fluorescent molecular probe for anti-azonaphthalene sulfonate antibody. Immunochemistry 5: 143–153.

Zimmering, P. E., Lieberman, S., and Erlanger, B. F. (1967). Binding of steroids to steroid-specific antibodies. Biochemistry 6: 154–164.

7

ANTIBODY REACTIONS WITH MULTIVALENT ANTIGENS
I. The Virus Model

1. Tobacco mosaic virus (TMV) and homogeneous binding

As the first virus to be identified and crystallized (Stanley, 1935), TMV became a reference material for a number of different studies in biology and biochemistry. The first electron microscope views of an antibody reaction, for example, utilized TMV as the antigen (Anderson and Stanley, 1941), and a relatively early detailed physicochemical study of antigen-antibody interaction utilized TMV as the multivalent structure of choice (Rappaport, 1959). Interest heightened further when the virus coat protein was sequenced and its subunit arrangement was established (cf. reviews by Anderer, 1963; Caspar, 1963; Fraenkel-Conrat, 1965). A model of the subunit arrangement, based upon X-ray scattering data, is shown in Figure 7-1; the coat protein sequence, in Table 7-1. Anderer and Schlumberger (1965, 1966) prepared antisera to synthetic antigens bearing the C-terminal di-, tri-, tetra-, penta-, and hexapeptides and showed that the antibodies reacted with and neutralized the virus, particularly if made against the homologous C-terminal dipeptide (alanine-threonine in TMV *vulgare*; alanine-serine in TMV *dahlemense*). Antibodies against the C-terminal peptides did not bind as strongly, however, as antibody against the whole virus, and Benjamini, Young, Shimizu, and Leung (1964) showed why. The tryptic peptide #8, IIEVENQANPTTAETLDATR (residues 93–112), lay at the heart of one type of immunochemical specificity. Some antibodies to the whole protein had specificity for the tryptic peptide (Benjamini, Young, Peterson, Leung, and Shimizu, 1965); a solid-phase synthetic decapeptide analog had cross-reactive properties (Young, Benjamini, Stewart, and Leung, 1967); and through use of octanoyl-DATR, octanoyl-ATR, and octanoyl-TR, it was found that at least part of the active center involved the

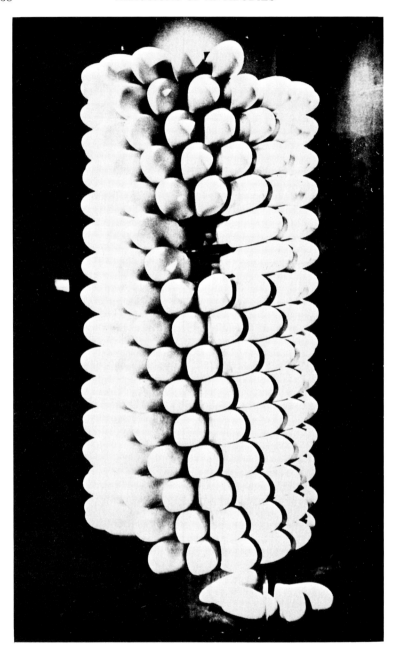

FIG. 7-1. Model of subunit arrangement in TMV based on X-ray scattering data of Franklin, Caspar, and Klug (1959) and presented by Fraenkel-Conrat (1965). The virus consists of an RNA core and 2130 identical polypeptide units in its protein coat.

TABLE 7-1

Amino Acid Sequences of Two Strains of TMV Coat Proteins

Strain	Sequence						Residue Positions
TMV *vulgare*	SYSIT	TPSQF	VFLSS	AWADP	IELIN	LCTNA	(1–30)
TMV *dahlemense*	SYSIT	SPSQF	VFLSS	VWADP	IELLN	VCTSS	
vulg.	LGNQF	QTQQA	RTVVQ	RQFSQ	VWKPS	PQVTV	(31–60)
dahl.	LGNQF	QTQQA	RTTVQ	QQFSE	VWKPF	PQSTV	
vulg.	RFPDS	DFKVY	RYNAV	LDPLV	TALLG	AFDTR	(61–90)
dahl.	RFPGD	VYKVY	RYNAV	LDPLI	TALLG	TFDTR	
vulg.	NRIIE	VENQA	NPTTA	ETLDA	TRRVD	DATVA	(91–120)
dahl.	NRIIE	VENQQ	SPTTA	ETLDA	TRRVD	DATVA	
vulg.	IRSAI	NNLIV	ELIRG	TGSYN	RSSFE	SSSGL	(121–150)
dahl.	IRSAI	NNLVN	ELVRG	TGLYN	QNTFE	SMSGL	
vulg.	VWTSG	PAT					(151–158)
dahl.	VWTSA	PAS					

(Sequences are those of Anderer, Wittman-Liebold, and Wittman, as given in Dayhoff, 1969, pp. D174-D175.)

tripeptide, ATR (residues 110–112). The octanoylated dipeptide was not reactive with antibodies to the whole virus coat protein, the octanolylated tri- and tetrapeptides were both specifically reactive (Benjamini, Shimizu, Young, and Leung, 1968a). In spite of the apparent importance of this antigenically active center in the development of subsequent investigations (Benjamini, Shimizu, Young, and Leung, 1969), the group were most acutely aware of the danger of drawing sweeping conclusions (1968b):

> " . . . the definition of an antigenic area or areas of a protein antigen and of the complementary antibody-reactive site should be derived cautiously not only because generalizations derived from randomly bred animals are difficult but also because the populations of antibodies derived from the same animal, at various time intervals following immunization, may change with respect to their quantity and areas with which they bind."

Since the C-terminal end of each polypeptide chain in TMV is readily attacked by carboxypeptidase (Harris and Knight, 1955) it is certain that these termini serve as apical antigenic determinants in the manner described by Anderer and Schlumberger (1965, 1966) but with considerably more tertiary and conformational structure involved.

Whatever the nature of the total immunogen may be in each determinant of the virus coat, Mamet-Bratley (1966) chose this protein for her elegant study in homogeneous binding. Here was an

immunogen with a genetically controlled uniform amino acid sequence that was repeated 2130 times in each virus particle and that
represented among complex multivalent antigens a relatively simple design. Antibodies were raised to TMV, were cleaved into Fab
fragments, incubated in different proportions with TMV, and
evaluated for binding by a well designed and carefully tested
ultracentrifuge method. The results were expressed in terms of
moles of antigen sites bound per mole of Fab, it having been accepted that the total number of antigen sites per virus particle
was equal to the number of subunits, 2130. The experiments were
carried out in regions less than half-saturation of virus, i.e., less
than 1000 Fab fragments per TMV particle. Under these conditions
homogeneous binding was predicted and homogeneous binding
was obtained (Figs. 7-2 and 7-3). It is significant that this work
stands as the first real demonstration of homogeneous binding,
recognized as such by Haber *et al.* (1967), and yet represents an
approach to the problem through multivalent antigens and univalent Fab rather than univalent haptens and multivalent antibody.
The technique has not, however, been used to any great extent.
It is obvious that for investigations of conformational antigens that
depend upon tertiary structures of macromolecules the method
of Mamet-Bratley is ready made. Out of it would easily come determinations of binding-site homogeneity to macromolecular antigens.

The data of Table 7-2 show that homogeneous binding was demonstrated with four antisera, one of them pooled from the sera of 12
rabbits. An ideal valence of 1.00 for Fab was not obtained, according to the author, because of a certain amount of activity loss
expected from the Fab preparation. It is also possible that the antigenic valence, *s*, may be less than the known number of subunits
2130. In any event it is of extreme interest that the valence that
Rappaport (1959) reported for TMV, based upon binding studies
with intact bivalent γG (1959), is 950, whereas the minimum valence
obtained by Mamet-Bratley with univalent Fab (using the value
for rabbit #83 in Table 7-2) is 2130 × 0.86/0.93 or no less than 1970.
Steric factors had been assumed by Rappaport to prevent additional
antibody binding, an assumption based upon the close packing of
old model cigar-shaped antibody molecules. The antibodies had
been assumed to bind under such conditions only at one univalent
end. It is now evident that monogamous bivalent binding was the
reason for Rappaport's lower valence value for TMV. With the
present Y-model of γG established it is conceptually more satis-
fying to visualize each mole of bivalent antibody accounting for two

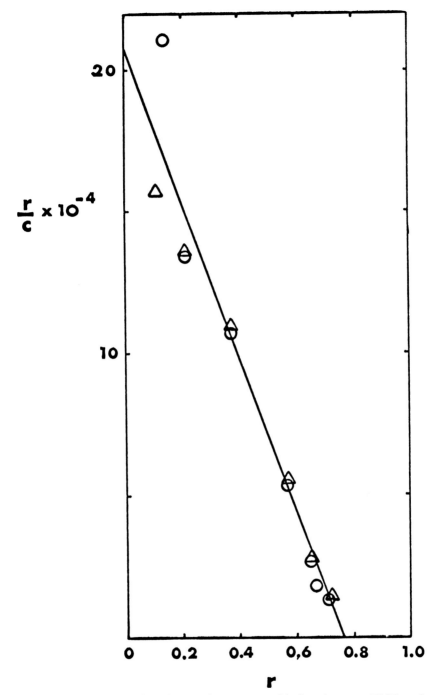

Fig. 7-2. Scatchard plot showing homogeneous binding between TMV and anti-TMV Fab. r = moles of virus subunits per mole Fab. c = moles of viral subunits not covered. 2130 subunits per virus particle assumed. Molecular weight of virus = 39.4×10^6; molecular weight of Fab = 4.3×10^4. Two separate experiments given. (From Mamet-Bratley, 1966.)

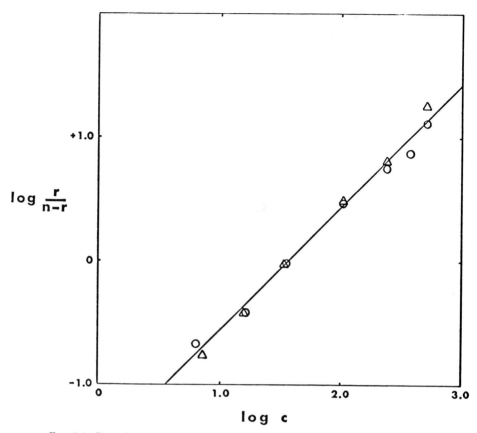

Fig. 7-3. Sips plot showing homogeneous binding between TMV and anti-TMV Fab. Same data as in Figure 7-2. $a = 0.99$; $K_0 = 2.7 \pm 0.1 \times 10^5$ M^{-1} at 4°C; $n = 0.76$. At 26°C, $K_0 = 2.8 \pm 0.1 \times 10$ M^{-1}, $\Delta H° = 0$, $\Delta S° = 25$ eu/mole. (From Mamet-Bratley, 1966.)

TABLE 7-2
Binding Properties of Anti-TMV Fab with TMV

Anti-TMV Source	$10^5 K_0$	a	n	Precipitability before Fab Preparation
	M^{-1}		sites/mole	%
Serum pool, 4°C	2.7 ± 0.1	0.99 ± 0.01	0.76	92
Serum pool, 26°C	2.8 ± 0.1	0.99 ± 0.01	0.78	92
Rabbit 83	2.4 ± 0.2	0.98 ± 0.05	0.86	93
Rabbit 424	2.4 ± 0.2	0.98 ± 0.05	0.47	65
Rabbit 76	2.3 ± 0.3	0.95 ± 0.05	0.78	81

(From Mamet-Bratley, 1966.)

TMV subunit determinants. On this basis the antigenic valence obtained by Rappaport would actually be $2 \times f = s$ or $2 \times 950 = 1900$, very close to that value reported by Mamet-Bratley. The discussion will return to the fact of monogamous bivalent binding later in the chapter with supportive data from the experiments of Hornick and Karush (1969).

Although Mamet-Bratley based her binding experiments upon the standard Scatchard equation for univalent hapten binding to antibody,

$$r/c = nK - rK = K - rK \qquad (7.1)$$

where

r = univalent TMV determinants bound per Fab
c = unbound TMV determinants
n = 1 for Fab
K = association constant,

the equation of choice would actually be the one obtained from Chapter 5 (Equation 5.14a)

$$f/d = sK - nfK = 2130K - fK \qquad (7.2)$$

where

f = univalent Fab bound per total added virus particles
d = unbound Fab
s = 2130, the accepted (or sought for) TMV valence
n = valence of Fab = 1
K = association constant as above.

Each equation is equivalent. The latter, however, need not assume a valence for the antigenic particle; instead may be used to seek it.

2. Influenza virus, equilibrium filtration, and the question of homogeneity

Equilibrium filtration is as effective in determining the extent of reaction between multivalent unfilterable virus particles and filterable antibodies as equilibrium dialysis is in determining the extent of reaction between multivalent undialyzable antibody molecules and dialyzable haptens. In the latter case it has already been shown how the Scatchard equation

$$r/c = nK - srK \qquad (7.3)$$

applies. In the former case it would follow that the equation

$$f/d = sK - nfK \tag{7.4}$$

would apply (as long as monogamous bivalent binding is assumed such that $f = jbA/P = bA/P$ and $d = (1 - jb) A = (1 - b) A = aA$). Thus,

f = antibody molecules bound per total virus particles in system
d = antibody molecules passing the filter
s = valence of virus particles
n = valence of antibody molecules
K = intrinsic equilibrium constant.

The parallel nature of the two essentially equivalent expressions of the "law of mass action" has already been described in Chapter 5.

Fazekas de St. Groth and Webster (1961; 1963a, b; 1966a, b), Fazekas de St. Groth (1961, 1962, 1967a, 1969), Webster and Laver (1966, 1967), Webster (1966), and Fazekas de St. Groth, Webster, and Davenport (1969) were the group who conceived, developed, and made extensive use of equilibrium filtration (and an equivalent ultracentrifugal technique) as a means of describing the interaction between influenza virus and antibody. In order to reach an understanding of the nature of antigenic determinants among the large variety of hypermutable virus strains—their specificities and cross-reactivities—a quantitative method based upon sound physico-chemical principles was required. Likewise, in order to understand the immune responses of individuals to "original antigenic sin" of a "senior" virus strain and subsequent exposures to "junior" cross-reacting strains, it was necessary to be able to dissect an individual's heterogeneous antibody population into specificities and cross-reactivities. Extent of reaction, i.e., the product of binding affinity and free equilibrium concentration of antibody, was recognized as the only real measure of influenza virus impact not only upon the individual but also upon the whole population.

The late Dr. Thomas Francis, Jr., in his James D. Bruce Memorial Lecture on Preventive Medicine (1953) referred to influenza as "the newe acquayantance" out of which grew the idea of "original antigenic sin." Francis, Davenport, and Hennessy (1953) at the same time expanded the idea. Shortly before his death, Francis along with his colleagues (Davenport, Minuse, Hennessy, and Francis, 1969), at a World Health Organization meeting on the Hong-Kong influenza pandemic, referred to influenza as an "old antigenic acquaintance" and declared:

> "Large and ordered gaps in the age distribution of anti-
> bodies oriented to strains of remote periods of past preva-
> lence favour the spread of 'old antigenic acquaintances'

once they arise. Hence, given the appropriate variant by genetic limitations, recycling is encouraged . . .

"Whatever the source or sources of pandemic strains, the antibody spectrum of the human population, which is remarkably similar throughout the world, acts as a limiting influence on the spread of strains antigenically like their predecessors."

It was obvious in this paper and in others of the meeting how important the work of Fazekas de St. Groth and Webster had really been in disclosing the nature of the disease. Others had given rich clinical and epidemiological flavor to the description of influenza, but Fazekas de St. Groth and Webster had provided the precise and unequivocal substance of physical measurement. It is important, therefore, to come to grips with the data of these Australian workers and to understand their expressions for the equilibrium parameters of antisera to influenza viruses.

The Cold Spring Harbor Symposium on Antibodies in 1967 not only was the stage for the expression of new thought concerning antibody structure and homogeneous binding but also of cross-reactivity among multivalent antigens as presented by Fazekas de St. Groth (1967a, b). In setting the stage for immunochemical investigations of the 1970s and 1980s his paper was as important as, if not more than, any other. The problem in comprehending and appreciating his quantitative message is that his data are presented in unfamiliar terms. One must either convert one's habit of thinking to his form or convert his system into one's own more familiar frame of reference. Since the Scatchard and Langmuir forms of mass action are now prevalent in the literature in presenting hapten binding data and since the affinity constant is habitually presented in terms of association, k_1/k_2, rather than in terms of its reciprocal dissociation, k_2/k_1, it would appear reasonable to view the data of Fazekas de St. Groth and Webster in the Scatchard and Langmuir forms and in terms of association.

The basic equilibrium between antibody molecules and antigen sites on particles of influenza virus, as given by Fazekas de St. Groth and Webster (1963b), is

$$K = \frac{[sV(1 + n) - y][A - y]}{y} \tag{7.5}$$

where

K = intrinsic *dissociation* constant
y = concentration of antigen-antibody complexes
s = number of antigenic sites per virus particle

$V(1 + n)$ = total concentration of virus particles of which V are
                infective and nV are noninfective

A = concentration of antibody molecules

The value y is then expressed as a fraction α of all antibody molecules
in the system that are bound to virus such that

$$y = \alpha A \tag{7.6}$$

Equation (7.5) is then written as

$$K = \frac{[sV(1 + n) - \alpha A][A - \alpha A]}{\alpha A} \tag{7.7}$$

For purposes of plotting data the equation is simplified by elimination
of terms and rearranged to give

$$K = [sV(1 + n) - \alpha A]\frac{(1 - \alpha)}{\alpha} \tag{7.8}$$

$$\frac{K}{A} = \frac{sV(1 + n)(1 - \alpha)}{\alpha A} - (1 - \alpha) \tag{7.9}$$

$$(1 - \alpha) = \frac{s}{A} \cdot \frac{V(1 + n)(1 - \alpha)}{\alpha} - \frac{K}{A} \tag{7.10}$$

The value $V(1 + n)$ is changed to an expression of the original virus
particle concentration V_0 and the dilution factor d that stands for
the fixed amount dV_0 used in any particular assay. The final analytical equation that is used in evaluating the equilibrium constants
becomes

$$(1 - \alpha) = \frac{sV_0}{A} \cdot \frac{d(1 - \alpha)}{\alpha} - \frac{K}{A} \tag{7.11}$$

By plotting $(1 - \alpha)$ vs. $d(1 - \alpha)/\alpha$ one obtains a line whose slope is
related to antigenic valence, s, and whose intercept is related to the
dissociation constant, K. By knowing the total number of antibody
molecules A in a preparation by labeling them with radioactive iodine
one can easily evaluate α as the radioactive fraction passing a filter
and $1 - \alpha$ as the radioactive fraction remaining behind. With V_0 and
d also given one has all the parameters needed. A detailed assay is
given for influenza virus for strain SW and rabbit anti-SW by Fazekas
de St. Groth (1961) which is described in his subsequent papers as
typical (Table 7-3 and Fig. 7-4). For convenience the data are given
in logarithmic terms in the table but are used in natural form in the
figure. The original virus preparation contained 1.63×10^{11} par-

TABLE 7-3

Evaluation of Equilibrium Filtration Test: Experimental Results

Equal volumes of a hyperimmune rabbit serum against SW-virus (diluted 1:10 in saline) and of dilutions of SW-virus stock were mixed, kept at 20°C for 30 min, and filtered through a gelatin-treated Millipore VM membrane. The antibody content of the original serum and of all filtrates was assayed in duplicate as antihemagglutinin against 4 agglutinating doses of SW-virus.

Dilution of Virus (d)	Antibody Titer of Filtrate ($\log_{10}$ units/ml)	Fraction of Antibody Free* ($\log [1 - \alpha]$)
1/6	1.90	−1.65
	2.00	−1.55
1/7	2.08	−1.47
	2.08	−1.47
1/8	2.29	−1.26
	2.20	−1.35
1/9	2.38	−1.17
	2.38	−1.17
1/10	2.50	−1.05
	2.47	−1.08
1/11	2.65	−0.90
	2.65	−0.90
1/12	2.68	−0.87
	2.68	−0.87
1/13	2.77	−0.78
	2.80	−0.75
1/14	2.80	−0.75
	2.80	−0.75
1/15	2.89	−0.66
	2.98	−0.57
1/20	3.01	−0.54
	3.01	−0.54
Controls (no virus):		
Filtered	3.55	≡0.00
	3.55	
Unfiltered	3.55	
	3.55	

* $\log_{10}$ filtrate units/ml − $\log_{10}$ control units/ml = $\log_{10}$ (filtrate units/ml)/(control units/ml) = $\log_{10}$ fraction free antibody.
(From Fazekas de St. Groth, 1961.)

ticles/ml and the original serum preparation contained 3.27×10^{14} antibody molecules/ml. The virus was diluted by an equal volume of serum for equilibrium tests so that V_0 became 8.15×10^{10} particles/ml; antibody was diluted 1/10 for use and became 1/20 when mixed with virus, i.e., $A = 1.635 \times 10^{13}$. The value sV_0/A, actually the number of antigenic sites per total antibody molecules in the system,

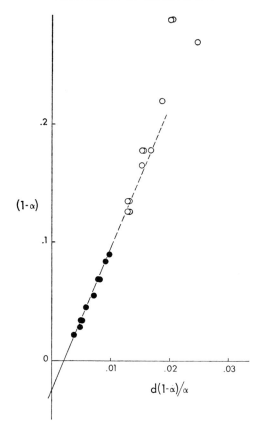

Fig. 7-4. Strain SW-influenza virus interaction with rabbit antibody as measured by equilibrium filtration. Estimation of parameters by Equation 7.11. The data of Table 7-3 falling in the most reliable range are represented by *closed circles*, the rest by *open circles*. The straight line is fitted by eye to the first 10 entries of Table 7-3. (From Fazekas de St. Groth, 1961.)

was found by least squares evaluation to be 11.307 ± 0.459 and the antigenic valence was $11.307 \times 1.635 \times 10^{13}/8.15 \times 10^{10} = 2268$. The equilibrium constant was determined from the intercept on the ordinate which by a least squares evaluation of the plot was -0.02293. The value for K was 3.75×10^{11} molecules/ml which by statistical evaluation ranged from 2.53×10^{11} to 4.95×10^{11}. For purposes of tabulation such as in the Cold Spring Harbor presentation (Fazekas de St. Groth, 1967a) it was found most convenient to express the results of an assay in logarithmic terms. Three values were of interest, equilibrium constant, antibody content of the serum, and a "heterogeneity" factor. The values in the assay just given would have been tabulated in the Cold Spring Harbor presentation as

Dissociation constant K: 11.574 or (log 2.75 $\times 10^{11}$)
Original serum antibody A: 14.515 or (log 3.27 $\times 10^{14}$)
"Heterogeneity" factor: ± 1.058 or (standard error of the slope $\times$ student's t value for $n - 2$ degrees of freedom at the 5% level, i.e., 0.459 $\times 2.306$).

To convert the dissociation constant K, which is in cgs terms (molecules/ml) to the more familiar association constant in molar terms one must use the Avogadro number, $N = 6.020 \times 10^{23}$ molecules/mole/liter:

$$K_{21} \text{ (in molecules/ml)} = \frac{K_{21}}{N \times 10^{-3}} \text{ (in M)}$$

$$K_{12} \text{ (in M}^{-1}) = 60.20 \times 10^{19}/K_{21} \text{ (in cgs)}$$

Thus when $K_{21} = 3.75 \times 10^{11}$ molecules/ml in cgs terms, $K_{12} = 1.61 \times 10^9$ M^{-1}. To convert the Fazekas de St. Groth equation to the Scatchard form of equation (7.4) for equilibrium filtration (assuming monogamous bivalent binding) one finds that

$$f = \alpha A/V$$
$$d = (1 - \alpha)A$$
$$f/d = \alpha/(1 - \alpha)V$$

and equation (7.4) becomes

$$\frac{\alpha}{(1 - \alpha)V} = sK_{12} - \frac{n\alpha A K_{12}}{V} \tag{7.12}$$

Fazekas de St. Groth took the value of antibody valence as $n = 1$ (Fazekas de St. Groth, 1961):

> " ... antibody is treated as univalent—this simplification, contrary to the well-established experimental evidence, can be maintained only in the case of dilute systems where the mean free path of antibody is negligible compared to the average distance between viruses ... Even if the latter condition were not strictly fulfilled, no substantial error can arise from the assumption of univalence as long as the system is far from saturation."

One can see, however, that if one wishes to determine the antigenic valence by extrapolation at $\alpha(1 - \alpha)V = 0$, one obtains, as

$$\alpha/(1 - \alpha)V \to 0$$
$$sK_{12} = n\alpha A K_{12}/V$$
$$s = n\alpha A/V \tag{7.13}$$

The antigenic valence s depends upon the value for n. If univalency is assumed one obtains a value $\frac{1}{2}$ that if bivalency is assumed. The equilibrium constant also depends on antibody valence; if univalency is accepted, a value twice as large is obtained than if bivalency is assumed.

The data from Table 7-3 are converted to the Scatchard form in Table 7-4 and are plotted in Figure 7-5 in the form $\alpha/(1 - \alpha)V$ vs. $\alpha A/V$. The data represented by *filled circles* in Figure 7-4 and used to obtain the straight line in that figure are faithfully designated as such in the converted table and figure. The data represented by *open circles* are the data which Fazekas de St. Groth left out of his straight-line evaluation. By way of explanation he stated that "the last four points show definite curvature towards the ordinate and also wider scatter, as could be expected from the emergence of complications in this region and from the increasing uncertainty of the estimate of α."

It can be seen in the Scatchard plot that a typical case of hetero-

TABLE 7-4

Conversion of Equilibrium Data from Fazekas de St. Groth (Table 7-3) to Scatchard Form

$10^{10}V^*$	$10^{13}A^*$	α	$1 - \alpha$	$\alpha A/V$	$\alpha/10^{19}(1 - \alpha)V$	Type of Data†
0.489	1.962	0.712	0.288	2856	5.050	O
0.489	1.962	0.712	0.288	2856	5.050	O
0.652	1.962	0.731	0.269	2199	4.165	O
0.652	1.962	0.781	0.219	2351	5.480	O
0.699	1.962	0.822	0.178	2308	6.615	O
0.699	1.962	0.822	0.178	2308	6.615	O
0.752	1.962	0.822	0.178	2145	6.148	O
0.752	1.962	0.834	0.166	2176	6.681	O
0.815	1.962	0.865	0.135	2082	7.863	O
0.815	1.962	0.865	0.135	2082	7.863	O
0.889	1.962	0.874	0.126	1929	7.807	O
0.889	1.962	0.874	0.126	1929	7.807	O
0.978	1.962	0.917	0.083	1839	11.275	●
0.978	1.962	0.911	0.089	1828	10.464	●
1.087	1.962	0.932	0.068	1683	12.683	●
1.087	1.962	0.932	0.068	1683	12.683	●
1.223	1.962	0.955	0.045	1532	17.429	●
1.223	1.962	0.945	0.055	1516	14.063	●
1.397	1.962	0.966	0.034	1357	20.468	●
1.397	1.962	0.966	0.034	1357	20.468	●
1.630	1.962	0.972	0.028	1170	21.157	●
1.630	1.962	0.978	0.022	1177	26.934	●

* No. of particles and antibody molecules in 1.20 ml, the assay volume.

† Open circles and closed circles as used by Fazekas de St. Groth (Fig. 7-4) to indicate poor and good data. (From Fazekas de St. Groth, 1961.)

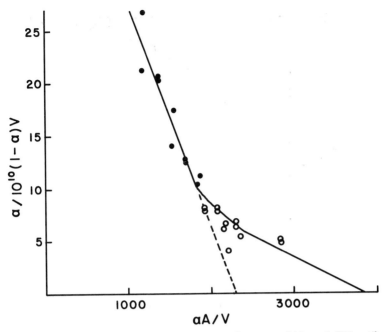

FIG. 7-5. Scatchard plot of equilibrium binding between rabbit anti-SW antibody and strain SW-influenza virus. *Closed circles* used by Fazekas de St. Groth in his regression line (Fig. 7-4). Extrapolated line in this figure to $\alpha A/V = 2268$ is exactly equivalent to that regression line. Extrapolation to 3850 is most probable route. Antigenic valence is twice the extrapolated value in either case.

geneous binding is obtained when all the data are considered and that Fazekas de St. Groth's regression line represents only the highest affinity reactions. Under no circumstances can the extrapolated value represent the total valence of the virus particle any more than the extrapolated values of high binding in Klinman's graph (Fig. 6-19 in Chapter 6) represent total antibody valence. Moreover, the extrapolated value can only be ½ the antigenic valence if one is to assume, as is most probable, that the effective antibody valence is 2. To arrive at an actual value for antigenic valence is difficult but the method of Fritz, Lassiter, and Day (1967) offers an approximation. When αA and V are plotted against each other (Fig. 7-6), the data take the form of a quantitative precipitin reaction and when $\alpha A/V$ vs. V are plotted a Heidelberger-type plot is obtained (Fig. 7-7). Fritz, Lassiter, and Day utilized the form, $\log (\alpha A/V)$ vs. V, to obtain a linear relation for extrapolation of nonlinear Heidelberger plots to $V = 0$. The intercept on the ordinate can be taken as an approximation to one-half the antigenic valence according to the principles set forth in Chapter 5. As shown in Figure 7-8, both the *open* and *closed*

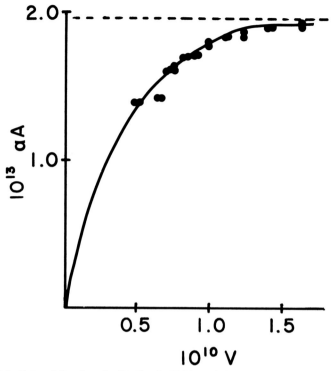

FIG. 7-6. Data of Fazekas de St. Groth (Table 7-4) in the form of a quantitative precipitin curve. *Dashed horizontal line* is the total amount of antibody added in the system.

circle data of Fazekas de St. Groth become quite acceptable as a linear relation; extrapolation to $V = 0$ gives a value of 3847 for the least-squares evaluation of the data. Taking $2 \times 3847 = 7694$ as the most reasonable value of s, one can now calculate a Sipsian heterogeneity constant from the relation

$$\frac{\alpha A}{sV - n\alpha A} = [(1 - \alpha)AK_{12}]^a \qquad (7.14)$$

$$\log \frac{\alpha A}{sV - n\alpha A} = a \log [(1 - \alpha)A] + a \log K_{12} \qquad (7.15)$$

$$\log \frac{\alpha A}{7694V - 2\alpha A} = a \log [(1 - \alpha)A] + a \log K_{12} \qquad (7.16)$$

The data from Table 7-4 were converted to the form of Equation 7.16, a least-squares linear relationship between $\log (\alpha A)/(7694V - 2\alpha A)$ vs. $\log [(1 - \alpha)A]$ was calculated, and the heterogeneity constant a was found to be 0.568. The equilibrium constant was then calculated from the same equation and found to be 8.5×10^7 M^{-1}. (In the terms of dissociation and cgs units used by Fazekas de St. Groth the constant would be $K_{21} = 7.08 \times 10^{12}$ molecules/ml and $\log K_{21} = 12.850$.) The Langmuir plot of the data without correction for heterogeneity is shown in Figure 7-9. The Nisonoff-Langmuir plot with the correction for Sipsian heterogeneity is shown in Figure 7-10.

The average intrinsic equilibrium constant is obtained not when $\alpha A/V = s/2$ but when $\alpha A/V = s/3$ since then

$$\frac{\alpha A}{sV - 2\alpha A} = \frac{(1/3)s}{s - (2/3)s} = 1 \qquad (7.17)$$

$$a \log [(1 - \alpha)A] + a \log K_{12} = 0 \qquad (7.18)$$

$$\log [(1 - \alpha)A] = - \log K_{12} \qquad (7.19)$$

$$K_{12} = 1/(1 - \alpha)A \qquad (7.20)$$

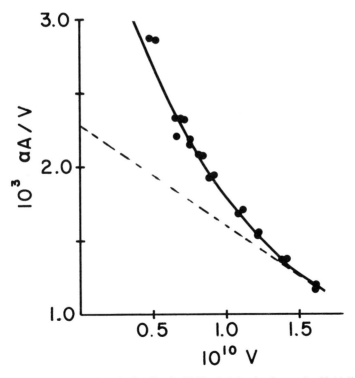

FIG. 7-7. Data of Fazekas de St. Groth (Table 7-4) in the form of a Heidelberger precipitin plot. *Dashed line* extends from equivalence to a value of 2268.

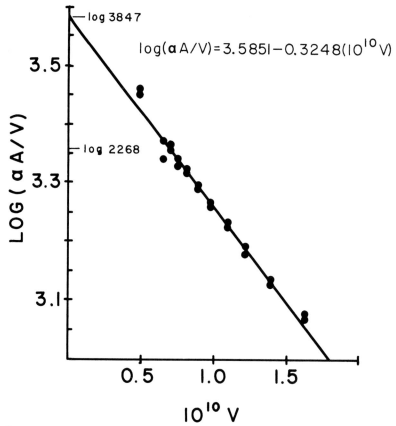

FIG. 7-8. Data of Fazekas de St. Groth (Table 7-4) in the form of a Fritz-Lassiter-Day precipitin plot. Equation is derived by the method of least-squares and has an ordinate intercept of 3.5851, the log of 3847.

and the equilibrium constant is free from the confines of hetero-geneity at that point. With s = 7694 and $s/3$ = 2565 the average equilibrium constant K_0 = 1.03 × 10^8 M^{-1}

A similar treatment has been given (Table 7-5) to the SW-virus-anti-SW-serum data of Fazekas de St. Groth and Webster (1963b) which were obtained equally well by equilibrium filtration and, as shown here, by an ultracentrifugal method (Fig. 7-11). The Scatchard plot of the SW-anti-SW data from Figure 7-11 reveals heterogeneity as given by the shape of the curve in Figure 7-12. The SW *regression line* of Figure 7-11, when converted to the Scat-chard form, becomes the *dashed line* in Figure 7-12. As can be seen, it crosses the Scatchard curve of heterogeneity in two places and makes the best linear plot of homogeneity for essentially hetero-geneous data.

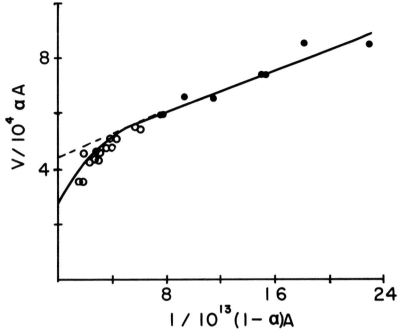

FIG. 7-9. Data of Fazekas de St. Groth (Table 7-4) in the form of a Langmuir plot. Extrapolations represent the values given by Fazekas de St. Groth (*dashed line*) and Fritz-Lassiter-Day (*solid line*).

By the same process as used in the first presentation of Fazekas de St. Groth data, the data (Table 7-5) for this second presentation were put in the form log $(\alpha A/V)$ vs. V and extrapolated to $V = 0$ (Fig. 7-13) from which an ordinate intercept of 3565 for f_0 was obtained and a valence of 7130 for $s = 2f_0$ was calculated. Sipsian treatment produced a heterogeneity constant of 0.543, an association constant from the Sipsian plot of $K_s = 2.39 \times 10^8$ M^{-1}, an average association constant at one-third saturation of 7130 antigen sites of $K_0 = 4.15 \times 10^8$ M^{-1}, and an association constant for high binding antibody of $K_H = 4.54 \times 10^9$ M^{-1}. The Nisonoff-Langmuir plot of the Sipsian linear relation is given in Figure 7-14.

A summary of the equilibrium parameters as obtained by the various methods of analytical treatment are given in Table 7-6. On the basis that 7130 represents the full valence of SW-virus for this particular heterogeneous antibody population, it can be seen that a population of homogeneous high binding antibodies represents 45% of the total and that the population taken by Fazekas de St. Groth and Webster for average analytical treatment involved perhaps 62%.

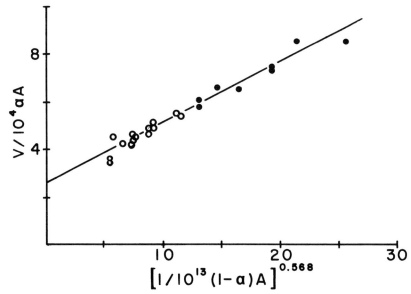

FIG. 7-10. Data of Fazekas de St. Groth (Table 7-4) in the form of a Nisonoff-Langmuir plot with the correction for Sipsian heterogeneity (a = 0.568).

The ambiguity concerning the virus valence in this type of assay could easily be dismissed through the use of univalent Fab rather than bivalent antibody.

Fazekas de St. Groth and Webster (1963b) drew the following conclusions from their data:

> "It is interesting to note that the surface of a spherical particle of 0.080 μ diameter (i.e., 0.021 μ^2) could accommodate at close packing about 2500 circular areas of the dimensions of an antibody molecule (minor axis 14 Å). Thus, it seems, that the experimentally determined number of sites comes very close to the maximum possible, and that the antibody molecules can be expected to attach by their tips and be arranged normal to the surface of the virus."

The two assays of heterogeneity presented here for SW-strain influenza virus would appear to show the involvement of between 3500 and 4000 antibody molecules per virus particle and the coverage of between 7000 and 8000 determinants at saturation. Even if one were to preserve the concept of a univalent antibody, which originated from the collision theory of Fazekas de St. Groth, Watson, and Reid (1958) and which was presented in detail by Fazekas de St. Groth (1962), the data would indicate double the number of 2000 assumed sites. Since the concept of the rigid effectively univalent

TABLE 7-5

Equilibrium Data of SW-strain Influenza Virus and Rabbit anti-SW Antiserum System Converted to Various Analytical Forms for Use in Figures 7-11, 7-12, and 7-13

Figure 7-11 Fazekas de St. Groth		Figure 7-12 Fritz-Lassiter-Day		Figure 7-13 Scatchard		Figure 7-14 Nisonoff-Langmuir	
$(1 - \alpha)$	$d(1 - \alpha)\alpha$	$\log(\alpha/d)$	d	$\alpha/d(1 - \alpha)$	α/d	d/α	$\dfrac{[1/}{(1 - \alpha)]^{0.543}}$
0.178	0.0650	0.438	0.30	15.4	2.74	0.365	2.55
0.178	0.0650	0.438	0.30	15.4	2.74	0.365	2.55
0.135	0.0547	0.393	0.35	18.3	2.47	0.405	2.96
0.135	0.0547	0.393	0.35	18.3	2.47	0.405	2.96
0.112	0.0505	0.346	0.40	19.8	2.22	0.451	3.28
0.112	0.0505	0.346	0.40	19.8	2.22	0.451	3.28
0.068	0.0329	0.316	0.45	30.4	2.07	0.483	4.32
0.079	0.0386	0.311	0.45	25.9	2.05	0.489	3.96
0.063	0.0336	0.272	0.50	29.8	1.87	0.533	5.02
0.063	0.0336	0.272	0.50	29.8	1.87	0.533	5.02
0.042	0.0241	0.241	0.55	41.4	1.74	0.574	5.60
0.042	0.0241	0.241	0.55	41.4	1.74	0.574	5.60
0.032	0.0198	0.208	0.60	50.4	1.61	0.620	6.50
0.032	0.0198	0.208	0.60	50.4	1.61	0.620	6.50
0.030	0.0201	0.174	0.65	49.8	1.49	0.672	6.70
0.025	0.0167	0.176	0.65	60.0	1.50	0.667	7.42

Antibody concentration $A = 1.07 \times 10^{15}$ molecules/ml. Virus concentration $V = 1.41 \times 10^{10}$ particles/ml. The values d for virus dilution factor and α for fraction of antibody molecules bound were obtained from Fazekas de St. Groth and Webster (1963a, b).

antibody must now be discarded, with the advent of the current Y-shaped antibody and its flexible arms, the number of antigenic determinants would most likely approach 8000. *There would then be at least four types of antigenic determinants for each protein-coat subunit.* In the TMV virus we have already seen how the C-terminal peptide acted as one type while an internal sequence acted as another, and we have been cautioned to expect others.

One would presume that there must be at least two populations of high binding antibody in the anti-SW antisera which in the first assay (Table 7-4) covered about 4500 determinants and in the other (Table 7-5), 3200. Some overlap obviously must have occurred in the second serum which prevented a full complement of 4000–4500 determinants from reacting. From an analysis of the cross-reaction data of Fazekas de St. Groth (1967a, 1969) one would guess that at least one of these populations was against a subunit cross-reaction determinant, the other against a subunit determinant of strain specificity. These would be analogous in TMV (a) to the internal peptides, resi-

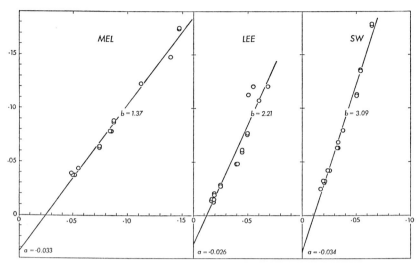

Fig. 7-11. Estimation of equilibrium parameters for three virus-antibody systems. Ultracentrifugal separation: The data (Table I in the reference) are plotted according to $d(1 - \alpha)/\alpha$ on the abscissa and $(1 - \alpha)$ on the ordinate. The straight lines were fitted by the method of least squares; estimated values of the slopes (b) and intercepts (a) are shown on the graphs. (From Fazekas de St. Groth and Webster, 1963b.)

dues 110–112, which are known determinants, which are identical in the *vulgare* and *dahlemense* strains, and which are thus cross-reactive; (b) to the known antigenic C-terminal peptides, residues 156–158, which are different and thus individual specific; and (c) to the internal peptides, residues 99–101, which are in the antigenically active tryptic peptide, which are also different, and which are also possibly involved in strain-specific antigenicity.

Haber (1967) must have had this view in mind when he commented upon Fazekas de St. Groth's paper at Cold Spring Harbor:

> *E. Haber:* "The heterogeneity of the immune response which you have demonstrated is not at all surprising in view of the multideterminant nature of your immunogen. To be sure, influenza virus is composed of repeating subunits, yet the size of each subunit is substantial, allowing for a large number of overlapping antigenic sites."
>
> *S. Fazekas de St. Groth:* "...this is in no way incompatible with what we might call serological simplicity. The virus particle has about 2000 demonstrably identical stubs on its surface, exposing antigenic areas almost exactly the same size as the tip area of an antibody molecule. The gap between the stubs is only 20 Å, too narrow for an antibody mol-

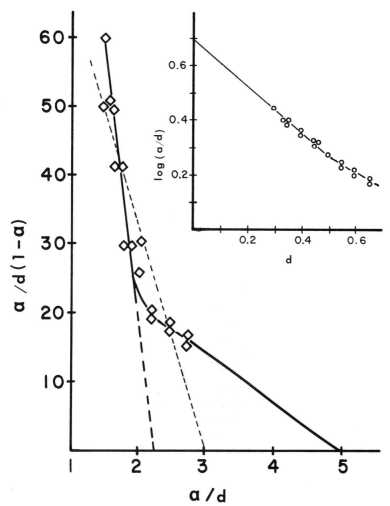

FIG. 7-12. Data of Fazekas de St. Groth (Table 7-5) in Scatchard form. The SW regression line of Figure 7-11 becomes the *light dashed line* in this figure that crosses the Scatchard curve in two places. The *heavy dashed line* is an extrapolation of high binding antibody. Every unit of α/d is equal to 713 antibody molecules per virus particle.

FIG. 7-13 (*inset*). Data of Fazekas de St. Groth (Table 7-5) in Fritz-Lassiter-Day form. Intercept at 0.699 gives a value of 5.00 for α/d and an antibody/virus ratio of 3565 which corresponds to a determinant valence on the virus of 7130.

ecule to squeeze into, and too wide for effective bridging. And even if several kinds of antibody were produced against the internal components of the virus (which, by the way is not the case), these would be irrelevant to our results since the test antigen was always the intact virus particle."

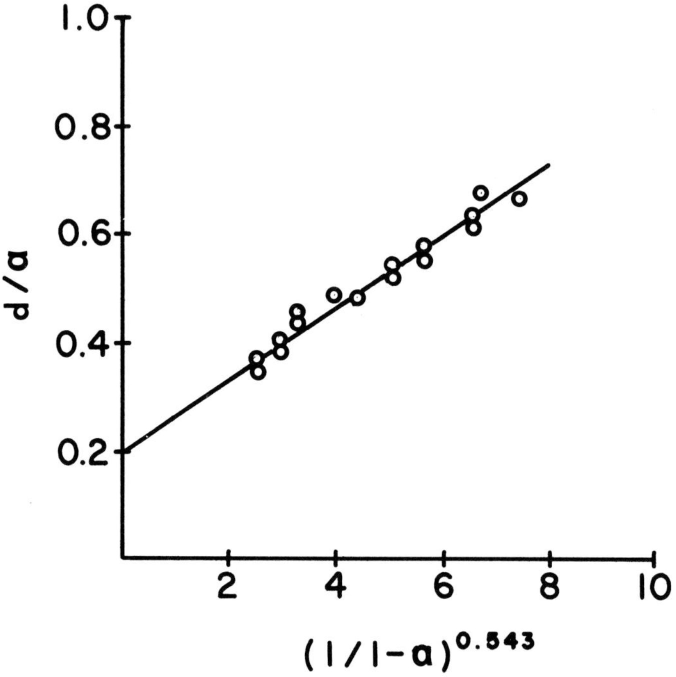

FIG. 7-14. Nisonoff-Langmuir plot of the SW-anti-SW-influenza system (Table 7-5) of Fazekas de St. Groth and Webster (1963b). A Sipsian heterogeneity constant of 0.543 was used.

TABLE 7-6
Equilibrium Parameters as Given by Fazekas de St. Groth and Webster (1963a, b) and by Scatchard-Sipsian Treatment of the Same Data

Parameter	Relation			
	Fazekas de St. Groth and Webster	Sipsian	Scatchard, High Affinity	Scatchard, ⅓ Saturation*
Antibody valence	1	2	2	2
Dissociation constant	1.82×10^{11} molecules/ml	2.52×10^{12} molecules/ml	1.32×10^{11} molecules/ml	1.45×10^{12} molecules/ml
Antibodies/particle	2208	3565	1604	3565
Virus valence	2208	7130	7130	7130
Association constant	3.36×10^{9} M^{-1}	2.39×10^{8} M^{-1}	4.54×10^{9} M^{-1}	4.15×10^{8} M^{-1}
Percentage of total antibody†	62	100	45	100

* See Equation 7.17.
† On the basis of $n = 2$ and $s = 7130$.

It is now abundantly clear that the very large amount of elegant quantitative data published by Fazekas de St. Groth and Webster, when combined with current concepts of heterogeneity, antibody structure, and binding affinity produce a contrary picture such that as many as 8000 determinants of an influenza virus particle can at once be covered by antibody binding sites at a single moment in equilibrium. The nature of these determinants, their conformational exposure, and their reactivity must await additional structural studies on the viral protein coat; meanwhile, it is clear that the squeeze is not so difficult and the bridging between subunits not so impossible.

3. Phage neutralization with antibody; role of antibody bivalence

In his Ph.D. dissertation Lafferty (1960) proposed that antibody bivalence was important to the neutralization of influenza virus and that both binding sites were bound to the same virus particle. He based his argument upon the fact that papain fragmentation of antiviral antibody into univalent Fab led to a reduction in neutralizing capacity. His proposed reaction mechanism was published in 1963 (Lafferty, 1963). Fazekas de St. Groth (1962) in his lengthy review in *Advances in Virus Research* dismissed Lafferty's proposal on a number of counts: (a) distortion of antibody tertiary structure would be required; (b) stabilization is proportionate to the number of already formed virus-antibody complexes and doesn't require the additional stability of bivalent binding (a reversal requiring breakage of two virus-antibody bonds); (c) stabilized virus-antibody complexes will agglutinate free virus, thus showing that free antibody binding sites are available in the complexes; (d) the kinetics of stabilized virus-antibody union are incompatible with Lafferty's model and require a multihit process like that of Fazekas de St. Groth and Webster. In essence Lafferty's proposal was incompatible with Fazekas de St. Groth's notion of antibody univalency. In section II. A.1.C. of his review, Fazekas de St. Groth (1962) wrote:

> "In the case of viruses the bivalency of antibodies is of little concern, except in very special circumstances. This will be evident on considering that an antibody molecule already attached to a virus particle will be slowed down, and its chance of colliding with a free antigenic site lowered by the factor $\sqrt{2(1+M/m)}$ (where M is the mass of the virus particle, and m the mass of the antibody molecule). In the case of influenza this factor is about fiftyfold, and even for the smallest virus about tenfold. Hence, antibodies can be expected to behave as univalent in their reaction with viruses up to the level where the concentration of antigen-antibody complexes greatly exceeds the concentration of free antibody."

It now appears that Lafferty was right after all and that Fazekas de

St. Groth was in error. The definitive experiments of Klinman, Long, and Karush (1967) and Hornick and Karush (1969) on phage neutralization provide the evidence.

Coliphage R-17 belongs to that group of simple ribonucleic acid (RNA) phages, along with MS-2, M-12, and f2, that specifically infect F+ strains of *Escherichia coli*. Their capsids have icosahedral symmetry with a protein coat composed of a quaternary arrangement of 18S repeating capsomeric subunits. Each subunit has a molecular weight of about 15,000 and is distinguished by a single amino acid difference between any two strains (Table 7-7). Neutralization kinetics of phage with antibody can be followed through the relationship

$$K = -\frac{ln(P/P_0)}{CT} \tag{7.21}$$

where

P = plaque count at time T
P_0 = plaque count at time 0
C = concentration of γG, molecules/ml
T = minutes
K = molecules^{-1} ml min^{-1}

A typical neutralization assay is given in Figure 7-15 taken from the work of Rowlands (1967) on the antibody neutralization of f2. Klinman, Long, and Karush (1967) raised antibodies to R17 phage and then prepared various recombinants between antibody and normal

TABLE 7-7
Amino Acid Sequences of RNA Bacteriophage Coat Proteins

Strain	Sequence of Residues						Position of Residues
f2	ASNFT	QFVLV	NDGGT	GNVTV	APSNF	ANGVA	(1–30)
R17	ASNFT	QFVLV	NDGGT	GNVTV	APSNF	ANGVA	
f2	EWISS	NSRSQ	AYKVT	CSVRQ	SSAQN	RKYTI	(31–60)
R17	EWISS	NSRSQ	AYKVT	CSVRQ	SSAQN	RKYTI	
f2	KVEVP	KVATQ	TVGGV	ELPVA	AWRSY	LNLEL	(61–90)
R17	KVEVP	KVATQ	TVGGV	ELPVA	AWRSY	LNMEL	
f2	TIPIF	ATNSD	CELIV	KAMQG	LLKDG	NPIPS	(91–120)
R17	TIPIF	ATNSD	CELIV	KAMQG	LLKDG	NPIPS	
f2	AIAAN	SGIY					(121–129)
R17	AIAAN	SGIY					

Note that f2 and R17 differ at position 88. f2 sequence, that of Weber and Konigsberg; R17 sequence, of Weber, as given by Dayhoff (1969, p. D177 and D228).

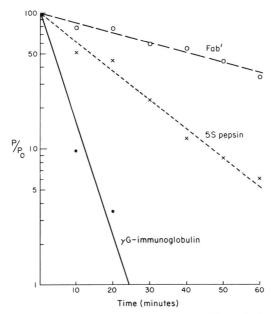

FIG. 7-15. Comparison of kinetics of neutralization of bacteriophage f2 by equal molar quantities of γG (O), 5S pepsin fragments ($\times$), and Fab' fragments ($\bullet$). $K = 2.12 \times 10^{-12}$ molecules^{-1} ml min^{-1} for γG; 0.44×10^{-12} for 5S (Fab')$_2$; and 0.16×10^{-12} for Fab'. (From Rowlands, 1967.)

halves of γG, and between various antibody and normal halves of (Fab')$_2$, to form both bivalent 7S γG, monovalent 7S γG, bivalent 5S (Fab')$_2$, monovalent 5S (Fab')$_2$, and monovalent 3S Fab'. Neutralization kinetics were studied and neutralization constants were obtained (Table 7-8). The results were unequivocal. Goodman and Donch (1964, 1965) had shown that a decrease occurred in phage neutralization activity of 5S and 3S fragments; and Stemke and Lennox (1967) had shown that only 10–20% phage neutralizing activity was left in rabbit antibody after papain digestion, a remarkably similar result to Lafferty's with influenza virus; but the work of Klinman et al. demonstrated that the effect was not some odd participation of Fc, suggested by Fazekas de St. Groth, but a true binding site phenomenon.

It is interesting in this regard that the number of molecules of antibody per phage particle obtained by Rowlands (1967) was slightly over 90 (Fig. 7-16). On the basis of bivalent binding this would mean that slightly over 180 antigenic determinants were covered, the same number as there are subunits on the phage. Rohrmann and Krueger (1970) also obtained a value of 90 for the "valence, f" of phage MS-2, another indication, it would appear, of bivalent binding. Krueger

(1970) calculated that either f2 or MS-2 could accommodate as many as 180 antibody molecules on the basis of 30 Å diameter per γG, but reiterated that a valence of 90 appeared to be maximal. He did not comment upon the possibility of monogamous bivalent binding of antibody, but the phenomenon appears certain. There are other reasons to believe so from the work of Hornick and Karush (1969) on

TABLE 7-8

Antibody Bivalence in Bacteriophage Neutralization of f2

Antibody	K^*
7S bivalent antibody, untreated	1123 ± 11
7S bivalent antibody, mildly reduced and alkylated	672 ± 18
7S bivalent antibody, acidified	1046 ± 14
5S bivalent antibody	1775 ± 3
7S monovalent antibody	19 ± 3
5S monovalent antibody	22 ± 41
3S monovalent antibody	14 ± 31

*In terms of mg^{-1} ml min^{-1}; to get molecules^{-1} ml min^{-1}, multiply by 10^3 mol. wt./N; thus at K of 1123 mg^{-1} ml min^{-1}, for 7S 150,000 mol. wt. $Ab = 2.5 \times 10^{-12}$ molecules^{-1} ml min^{-1}.

(From Klinman, Long, and Karush, 1967.)

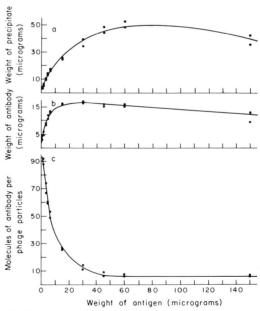

Fig. 7-16. Precipitin curve of bacteriophage f2 and rabbit γG antibody (*a*) total precipitate, (*b*) antibody in precipitate, and (*c*) antibody molecules per bacteriophage particles. (From Rowlands, 1967.)

modified phage.

4. Neutralization of modified phage by antibody

The contention of Burnet, Keogh, and Lush (1937) was that antibody-phage reactions, unlike the neutralization reactions of animal viruses, were not reversible. Dulbecco, Vogt, and Strickland (1956) 20 years later claimed that animal virus neutralizations were irreversible also. Fazekas de St. Groth and Reid (1958) argued for dissociation reactions in animal virus-antibody complexes and have now won the argument on the basis of an overwhelming amount of equilibrium evidence and virus reactivation after complete neutralization. Reversibility was suggested by Jerne and Avegno (1956) to explain reactivation in completely neutralized T2 phage, but Bowman and Patnode (1964) still could find no evidence for dissociation in ϕX174 phage-rabbit antibody complexes. Krummel and Uhr (1969) finally were able to resolve the problem: guinea pig antibody complexes with ϕX174 did dissociate, but the rate of dissociation was so much lower than the rate of association that it could be neglected in the mathematical solution of complex kinetics.

The probability velocity function, based on Maxwell mechanics of collisions between particles, was used by Krummel and Uhr (1969) in the same manner as Fazekas de St. Groth (1962) and also failed to take into account antibody valency. That the mathematical model did, in fact, prove true in practice said a very important thing: bivalent binding of antibody takes place as if it were a single two-body collision. The binding of the two antibody sites must be simultaneous or very rapidly consecutive with energy considerations favoring the second bond once the first is formed. Krummel and Uhr (1969) used two standard techniques and a third one of their own to investigate the kinetics of complex formation (Fig. 7-17): direct plating, decision tube, and complex inactivation. By the last method a homogeneous reaction should be obtained from the equation if $A_0 >> nP_0$ or, for a large n, if $(P_0/A_0)Kt << 1$.

$$\frac{P}{P_0} = \left[\frac{A_0 \exp \left((A_0 - nP_0)\dfrac{k_a t}{n} \right) - nP_0}{A_0 - nP_0} \right]^{-n} \quad (7.22)$$

where

P = ϕX174 phage, particles/ml
P_0 = phage at zero time
A_0 = antibody concentration at time zero, molecules/ml
n = average maximum number of antibody molecules that will bind to phage

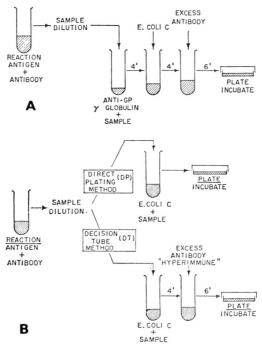

Fɪɢ. 7-17. Schemes for complex inactivation (CI) (A) and direct plating (DP) and decision tube (DT) (B). (From Krummel and Uhr, 1969.)

k_a = reaction rate association constant
t = time
K = antibody activity, $k_a A_0$

As shown in Figure 7-18, with $P_0 = 4 \times 10^5$, homogeneity of binding was beautifully demonstrated. Additional populations of antibody other than those reacting with the 10^5 phage population were present, but were discretely different and could be differentiated as such.

The importance to immunochemists of understanding phage kinetics is made immediately apparent in the work of Mäkelä (1966) who coupled 3-iodo-4-hydroxy-5-nitrophenyl acetic acid chloride (NIP) to T2 phage and showed by phage inactivation kinetics that anti-NIP antibodies gave a first order reaction until over 99% of the phage was inactivated (Fig. 7-19). When incubated with phage for 6 hr, a concentration of antiserum as low as 10^{-7} (1.9×10^{-5} μg/ml) or less caused measurable inactivation (Fig. 7-20).

Haimovich and Sela (1966) in the same year demonstrated the inactivation of poly-ᴅʟ-alanyl bacteriophage T4 with specific anti-poly-ᴅʟ-alanine antibodies and used the decision technique as well

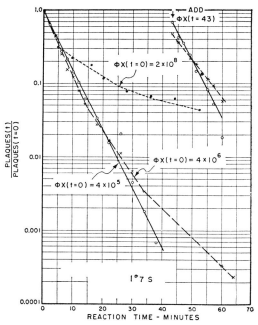

FIG. 7-18. Homogenous reaction of guinea pig 7S antibodies with ϕX174 phage using the complex inactivation (CI) method. (From Krummel and Uhr, 1969.)

as direct plating to show the fate of phage survivors. In their decision technique phage survivors were allowed to adsorb to bacteria while any unadsorbed phage was irreversibly inactivated by strong anti-phage serum. Any deviations from first order kinetics would then have to be due to the reversibility of reaction between alanylated phage and antipolyalanyl antibody. Haimovich, Sela, Dewdney, and Batchelor (1967) extended this type of assay to the detection of antipenicilloyl antibodies with penicilloylated T4 phage, using rabbit anti-6-aminopenicillanic acid I as the neutralizing antibody. Shortly thereafter Carter, Yo, and Sehon (1968), using 2,4-DNP-T2 phage, showed that less than 2 nanograms of antihapten antibody could be detected. Additional conjugates continue to be added to the list, for example Rp-poly-6-tyrosyl phage which can be inactivated with anti-Rp antibodies (Becker, Conway-Jacobs, Wilchek, Haimovich, and Sela, 1970).

With the use of the modified-phage neutralization technique Hornick and Karush (1969) proposed to ask the question of bivalent binding of antibody. Choosing conditions to obtain less than 100% in-activation they were able to determine that the forward rate reaction constant was 3.7×10^7 M^{-1} sec^{-1} and that under equilibrium conditions *an affinity constant of 3.5×10^{11} M^{-1} described the*

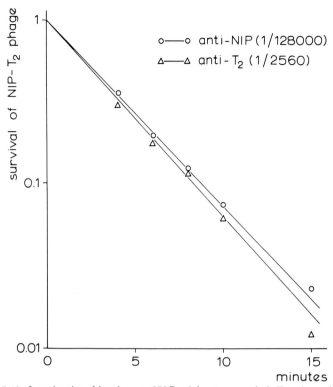

F<small>IG</small>. 7-19. Inactivation kinetics at 37°C of hapten-coupled T2 phage by anti-hapten (anti-NIP-chicken globulin) or by anti-T2 antibody. (O) Anti-NIP (1/128,000) and (Δ) anti-T2 (1/2560). (From Mäkelä, 1966.)

reaction of antibody and virus—at an antibody concentration of 1.5×10^{-11} M, 84% neutralization could be obtained! Because single hit kinetics were operative it could be concluded that this high affinity constant represented the binding of a single anti-DNP molecule at the critical site of bacteriophage. Both the rate constant and the single hit kinetics were very much in keeping with phage neutralization kinetics such as described for f2 phage by Dudley, Henkens, and Rowlands (1970). Equilibrium dialysis experiments with the same antibody against DNP-lysine produced an average affinity constant of $K_0 = 6 \times 10^6$ M^{-1}. A 10^4-fold difference was found between the affinity of antibody complexed to DNP-ϕX174 and that to DNP-lysine hapten. Yet DNP-lysine could be used to reverse equilibrium conditions in modified phage from which the calculation of 1.1×10^{11} M^{-1} for K_0 was obtained. Haimovich, Novik, and Sela (1969) also reported this type of affinity difference between equilibrium dialysis and hapten phage neutralization. The decisive factor in explaining the energy difference, according to Hornick and

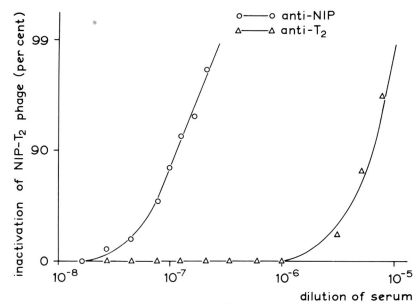

FIG. 7-20. Inactivation of hapten-coupled T2 phage by varying low concentrations of anti-hapten or of anti-T2 antibody during a period of 6 hr at 37°C. Phage concentration 2.5 × 10³ PFU/ml. Anti-hapten and anti-T2 antibodies are those of Figure 7-19. (O) Anti-NIP and (Δ) anti-T2. (From Mäkelä, 1966.)

Karush, was very clearly the multivalence of bacteriophage contrasted to the monovalence of DNP-lysine. By means of a *monogamous bivalent* interaction with simultaneous reaction of both binding sites of an antibody, enhancement of the effective binding constant is obtained.

"The energetic gain due to bivalency, coupled with the structural flexibility of the antibody molecule, suggests that this combination of properties has evolved because of an important biological advantage it confers with respect to immunity. Since infectious agents, e.g., bacteria and viruses, contain a multiplicity of identical antigenic determinants, the flexibility of the antibody would facilitate its bivalent interaction. The enhanced association constant this provides, relative to a monovalent antibody, means that lower levels of antibody will suffice to provide an effective immune response to infective agents and to maintain immunity against the disease they cause."

Not only haptens but proteins can now be used in the preparation of protein-phage conjugates which are effective in detecting antibody down to the 0.5–2.0 nanograms/ml level (Haimovich and Sela, 1969b). By combination with an inhibition assay for free protein threshold

concentrations, as little as 0.4 nanogram of lysozyme and 0.05 nanogram of rabbit γG are within measurable range (Haimovich, Hurwitz,
Novik, and Sela, 1970). Monovalent Fab' coupled to phage makes the
detection of 6 nanograms of anti-Fab antibody/ml possible (Taussig,
1970).

The modified-phage system is particularly useful currently in the
measurement of γM antibody, the latter often requiring detection at
very low serum concentrations. Surprisingly γM is not always more
efficient than γG, γG having the advantage in neutralizing T4 and
penicilloyl-phage conjugate, γM the advantage in poly-D-alanyl-
phage (Haimovich and Sela, 1969a). With TNP-phage γM also
appears more effective than γG from the *same* pool of early antibody
(Barber and Rittenberg, 1970).

One of the most important uses of the modified-phage technique
for detecting antibodies has been in the disclosure of the antibody
nature of "normal" immunoglobulins in normal sera. In much the
same way that myeloma proteins were tested for possible reaction
with a variety of haptens at a relatively gross microgram level, normal
rabbit sera were screened by Haimovich, Tarrab, Sulica, and Sela
(1970) for reactivity with a number of modified phage conjugates
(Table 7-9). In those positive reactions neutralization was described
as the extent of inhibition of plaque-forming units (PFU). As shown
in Table 7-10, specific haptens could interfere with PFU inhibition.
But 2-mercaptoethanol, principally a γM inactivator, also eliminated
PFU inhibition. The probability of γM antibodies in the normal
serum was therefore suspect. The appearance of such "non-in-
structed" antibodies at very low concentrations in normal serum was
yet another in the now extensive list of reasons for accepting the
"clonal selection theory" as current dogma.

The virus, as a model of a multivalent antigen, has had the advantage of a functional repeating subunit structure by which bivalent
antibody could act monogamously and attach both binding sites to a

TABLE 7-9
Antibody Detection in 28 Normal Rabbit Sera by Modified Phage Inactivation

Modified Phage	Positive/Total
Lysozyme-T4	0/28
Insulin-T4	1/28
Unmodified-T4	11/28
DNP-T4	28/28
Penicilloyl-T4	20/20

(From Haimovich, Tarrab, Sulica, and Sela, 1970.)

TABLE 7-10
Extent of PFU Inhibition of Modified Phage by Normal Rabbit Sera

Modified Phage	Serum Treatment	Extent of PFU Inhibition (PFU in serum/PFU in buffer)
DNP-T4	None	12/405
	DNP-AC added	432/400
	2-ME added	491/411
Penicilloyl-T4	None	162/444
	Penicilloyl-AC added	446/460
	2-ME added	581/590

(From Haimovich, Tarrab, Sulica, and Sela, 1970.)

particle. Similar conditions prevail in other systems: in solid synthetic immunoadsorbents, in mammalian cell systems such as erythrocyte membranes, and in monomolecular layers of antigenic macromolecules on barium stearate films. The only criteria are that repeating determinants lie close enough together for bivalent monogamous bridging, and that antibody molecules have enough flexibility to form binding site anchors of the bridge at the determinant sites.

5. Monogamous bivalent binding in non-viral systems

During the 15 years before Porter opened the new era of immunochemistry with his description of papain cleavage of γG, a number of enzyme cleavage experiments had taken place, mainly with horse antitoxin against diphtheria. In previous chapters we have mentioned the cleavage work of Parfentjev and of Pope and have seen the crystalline $(Fab_t)_2$ of Northrop, all with the horse antitoxin immunoglobulin. Generalization to other immunoglobulins was prevented, however, during that earlier period because in many ways horse immunoglobulin had reaction characteristics, particularly in the precipitin reaction, that set it apart from the more usual antibody reactants. For example, it would form flocculents with toxin rather than true precipitins. Since it was a pseudoglobulin rather than a euglobulin there was additional question as to whether it should be included in the category of general antibody reactants at all. The reason for intensive interest in the antitoxin was its clinical role in diphtheria control, and it had been hoped that enzymatic fragmentation would result in an antitoxin with full retention of potency but with less horse globulin antigenicity when injected into humans. The Parfentjev and the Pope processes accomplished this goal.

Pappenheimer and his colleagues investigated the properties of the horse antitoxin in depth. Partial digestion of antitoxin with pepsin according to the Parfentjev process resulted in nearly twice as many units of specific antibody nitrogen per milligram of toxin-antitoxin precipitate as undigested antitoxin (Pappenheimer and Robinson, 1937). Utilizing the Langmuir-Schaeffer method of monomolecular adsorption of substances on stearate films, Porter and Pappenheimer (1939) showed that when diphtheria toxin was adsorbed first, giving a thickness of 33 Å, a layer of antitoxin with a thickness of 49 ± 2 Å would adsorb to the toxin layer. However, the antitoxin layer would not adsorb toxin to form a third layer even though it would adsorb toxin if layered first on the stearate film. This was contrary to their experience with pneumococcal polysaccharides (Ps) and horse anti-Ps antibodies (IgM) in which reactions took place regardless of layering order and multiple layers of antigens and antibodies could be formed.

From this evidence it was concluded "that the antitoxic groups are distributed in an unsymmetrical manner on the antitoxin molecule and that a large inactive portion of the molecule is split off by treatment with the enzymes," and, further, "that the antitoxic groups may lie fairly close together on one side only of the antitoxin molecule, in contrast to other precipitating antibodies, and therefore the formation of a lattice leading to precipitation is impossible, from steric considerations, in regions of antitoxin excess where toxin molecules are saturated with antitoxin" (Pappenheimer, Lundgren, and Williams, 1940).

The model of the antitoxin molecule thus was remarkably similar to the current Y-model of immunoglobulins in general while the cigar-shaped model of γG, with its binding sites at opposite ends of the rigid ellipsoid, provided the comfortable contrast to explain differences in properties. With the advent of the current structural model of immunoglobulins, the structural contrast between antitoxin molecules and ordinary precipitating antibodies has again been lost. Klinman and Karush (1967) finally provided the explanation.

Anti-Lac antibodies were raised in a horse, purified by adsorption-elution procedures, separated into γG and γT fractions by diethylaminoethyl (DEAE)-cellulose column chromatography, and labeled with tritiated [³H]-acetic anhydride.

A. γG antibody precipitated with Lac-HSA (lactoside hapten coupled to human serum albumin) while γT antibody failed to form any precipitate over a wide range of antigen concentrations. Thus, the γT was established as typical of the behavior of diphtheria antitoxin; γG, as ordinary precipitating immunoglobulin.

B. Equilibrium dialysis experiments with [³H]-Lac-dye hapten established that both antibodies were *bivalent* and that K_0 = 1.8×10^7 M^{-1} for γT, $K_0 = 8 \times 10^6$ M^{-1} for γG.

C. Sedimentation analysis of Lac-HSA complexes with γG anti-Lac and γT anti-Lac revealed in ultracentrifugal patterns that soluble 16S complexes were unique to the γG antibody.

D. γG and γT antibodies bound equally well to Lac-HSA immunoadsorbent (*broken lines* in Fig. 7-21) as indicated by equivalent uptake of the radioactive [³H]-γG and [³H]-γT.

E. After γG and γT were adsorbed to the immunoadsorbents, γG could adsorb 10% of labeled [³H]-Lac-HSA from solution, indicating the presence of many free binding sites on the adsorbed antibody, while γT adsorbed only a fifth as much (Fig. 7-21, *continuous lines*). Monovalent γG Fab had the full capacity to bind to the column also and, of course, could not at the same time bind additional free hapten from solution (Fig. 7-21, *line close to abscissa*).

The γG antibody thus showed a markedly greater capacity to cross-link multivalent antigen molecules than did γT, whereas γT

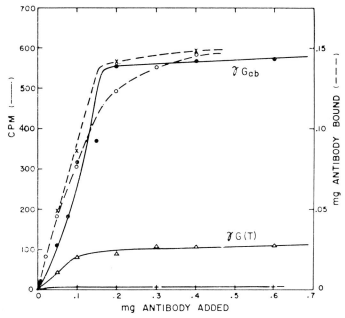

FIG. 7-21. *Broken lines:* binding of [³H]-γT (O) and [³H]-γG (×) antibodies against Lac hapten by Lac-HSA immunoadsorbent (ordinate on right). *Continuous lines:* binding from solution of [³H]-lac-HSA on column-adsorbed γT (Δ), γG (●), and γG Fab″ (+, very near abscissa). (From Klinman and Karush, 1967.)

had a marked tendency for monogamous bivalent binding of both binding sites to the same antigen molecule. Nevertheless, in multivalent
antigen excess both γG and γT exhibited the property of binding
only one multivalent antigen molecule and both appeared to do so in
a bivalent monogamous way. And in monovalent antigen excess both
exhibited the property of bivalency. In *either antigen or antibody
excess both γT and γG tended to have both sites occupied* either
by one antigen molecule or two. Thus, although γG had 5 times more
free binding sites available than γT on the column of immunoadsorbent yet it, too, had by far the bulk (90%) of its binding sites already
filled and unavailable for binding of free hapten. The early model
of Fazekas de St. Groth, for example, would have had 50% of the sites
available. It could be concluded that neither γG nor γT antibody
would generally be found in complex with many free sites still available. The thermodynamic basis for the advantage of monogamous bivalent binding as opposed to cross-linking would stem from an
entropy-driven consideration—that given proper conformation and
geometrical relationships the occupancy of the second site to the
same antigen as the first site would have considerable energetic favor.

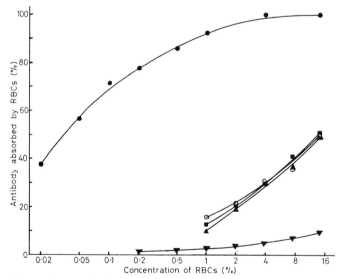

FIG. 7-22. Avidity of bivalent and univalent 5S and 3.5S antibody (serum 101).
(●) Bivalent 5S; univalent 5S; (■) 3.5S (reduced 5S which did not recombine; (▲)
3.5S (reduced alkylated 5S). Antibodies were anti-A; red cells were type A₁;
red cells of type O (▼) were used to measure nonspecific uptake. (From Greenbury,
Moore, and Nunn, 1965.)

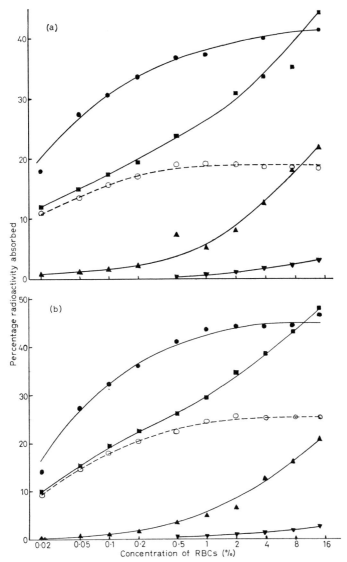

FIG. 7-23. Avidity of recombined bivalent 5S antibody; (a) serum 112, (b) serum 101. (●) 7S antibody; (■) recombined 5S antibody; (○) calculated uptake of bivalent 5S antibody; (▲) 3.5S antibody (reduced 5S which did not recombine); (▼) mean O cell uptake. Antibodies were anti-A; red cells were type A_1; red cells of type O were used to measure nonspecific uptake. (From Greenbury, Moore, and Nunn, 1965.)

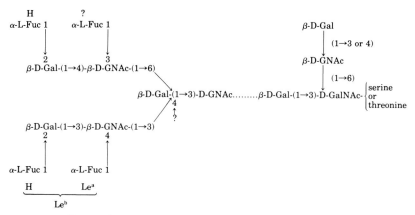

F<small>IG</small>. 7-24. Proposed composite structure for a blood group H megalosaccharide. (From Kabat, 1970.)

Support for this idea also comes from the electron microscopy of Almeida and Waterson (1969) who found that viruses, in extreme antibody excess, had no cross-linking between particles; "each virus is enclosed in an antibody halo and any clumping that occurs is due to entanglement of the antibody molecules." Almeida and Waterson were not convinced of the Y-model morphology of γG structure because they saw *too many* linking antibodies near equivalence and too few bivalent binding molecules on a single virus. The ideas of Klinman and Karush would appear to satisfy that argument also and to remove any reservation from acceptance of the Y-model.

Greenbury, Moore, and Nunn (1965) have shown, in fact, that rabbit γG antibody against blood group A substance also exhibits monogamous bivalent binding on red cells with considerable increase in "avidity," that is, ability to be adsorbed at low concentrations of red cells. As shown in Figure 7-22, bivalent 5S (Fab'')$_2$ was very much more active than 3.5S Fab''. Recombinants from 3.5S Fab'' fragments had restoration of "avidity" (Fig. 7-23). The authors concluded that the antibodies must be flexible enough to permit binding of both sites on a single red cell and they derived a formula for calculating an association constant on the basis of such monogamous bivalency.

Perhaps the best way to conclude this chapter is to reproduce the Y-shaped determinant that Kabat (1970) presented in the discussion following Morgan's paper on blood group specificity at the Karl Landsteiner Centennial Symposium. A proposed composite structure for a blood group H megalosaccharide was shown (Fig. 7-24) indicating the H, Le^a, Le^b groupings. The A determinants would have Gal NAc and the B determinants would have galactose linked $\alpha - (1 \rightarrow 3)$

to the galactose at the left of the formula. Kabat speculated as follows:

"... it's interesting to think how these two determinants would react with this flexible bivalent γG globulin molecule [if both were A_2 or both A_1]. Is it possible that each determinant on the Y could fit so that you had a very tight linkage of the type which he [Dr. Karush] spoke about?"

REFERENCES

Almeida, J. D., and Waterson, A. P. (1969). Morphology of virus-antibody interaction. Adv. Virus Res. 15: 307–338.

Anderer, F. A. (1963). Recent studies on the structure of tobacco mosaic virus. Adv. Protein Chem. 18: 1–35.

Anderer, F. A., and Schlumberger, H. D. (1965). Properties of different artificial antigens immunologically related to tobacco mosaic virus. Biochem. Biophys. Acta 97: 503–509.

Anderer, F. A., and Schlumberger, H. D. (1966). Cross-reactions of antisera against the terminal amino acid and dipeptide of tobacco mosaic virus. Biochim. Biophys. Acta 115: 222–224.

Anderson, T. F., and Stanley, W. M. (1941). A study by means of the electron microscope of the reaction between tobacco mosaic virus and its antiserum. J. Biol. Chem. 139: 339–344.

Barber, P., and Rittenberg, M. B. (1969). Anti-trinitrophenyl (TNP) antibody detection by neutralization of TNP-coliphage T4. Immunochemistry 6: 163–174.

Becker, M. J., Conway-Jacobs, A., Wilchek, M., Haimovich, J. and Sela, M. (1970). Detection of anti-p-azobenzenearsonate antibodies with chemically modified bacteriophage. Immunochemistry 7: 741–743.

Benjamini, E., Shimizu, M., Young, J. D., and Leung, C. Y. (1968a). Immunochemical studies on the tobacco mosaic virus protein. VII. The binding of octanoylated peptides of the tobacco mosaic virus protein with antibodies to the whole protein. Biochemistry 7: 1261–1264.

Benjamini, E., Shimizu, M., Young, J. D., and Leung, C. Y. (1968b). Immunochemical studies on the tobacco mosaic virus protein. VI. Characterization of antibody populations following immunization with tobacco mosaic virus protein. Biochemistry 7: 1253–1260.

Benjamini, E., Shimizu, M., Young, J. D., and Leung, C. Y. (1969). Immunochemical studies on tobacco mosaic virus protein. IX. Investigations on binding and antigenic specificity of antibodies to an antigenic area of tobacco mosaic virus protein. Biochemistry 8: 2242–2246.

Benjamini, E., Young, J. D., Peterson, W. J., Leung, C. Y., and Shimizu, M. (1965). Immunochemical studies on the tobacco mosaic virus protein. II. The specific binding of a tryptic peptide of the protein with antibodies to the whole protein. Biochemistry 4: 2081–2085.

Benjamini, E., Young, J. D., Shimizu, M., and Leung, C. Y. (1964). Immunochemical studies on the tobacco mosaic virus protein. I. The immunological relationship of the tryptic peptides of tobacco mosaic virus protein to the whole protein. Biochemistry 3: 1115–1120.

Bowman, B. V., and Patnode, R. A. (1964). Neutralization of bacteriophage ϕX174 by specific antiserum. J. Immunol. 92: 507–514.

Burnet, F. M., Keogh, E. V., and Lush, D. (1937). The immunological reactions of the filterable viruses. Aust. J. Exp. Biol. Med. Sci. *15:* 227–368.

Carter, B. G., Yo, S. L., and Sehon, H. (1968). The use of bacteriophage neutralization technique for the detection of antihapten antibody. Can. J. Biochem. *46:* 261–265.

Caspar, D. L. (1963). Assembly and stability of the mosaic virus particle. Adv. Protein Chem. *18:* 37–121.

Davenport, F. M., Minuse, E., Hennessy, A. V., and Francis, T., Jr. (1969). Interpretations of influenza antibody patterns of man. Bull. W.H.O. *41:* 453–460.

Dayhoff, M. O. (1969). Virus coat proteins. In *Atlas of Protein Sequence and Structure*, Vol. 4, National Biomedical Research Foundation (Silver Spring, Md., xxvi + 109 text pp. + 252 data pp.).

Dudley, M. A., Henkens, R. W., and Rowlands, D. T., Jr. (1970). Kinetics of neutralization of bacteriophage f2 by rabbit γG-antibodies. Proc. Natl. Acad. Sci. *65:* 88–95.

Dulbecco, R., Vogt, M., and Strickland, A. G. R. (1956). A study of the basic aspects of neutralization of two animal viruses, Western equine encephalitis virus and poliomyelitis virus. Virology *2:* 162–205.

Fazekas de St. Groth, S. (1961). Methods in immunochemistry of viruses. 2. Evaluation of parameters from equilibrium measurements. Aust. J. Exp. Biol. Med. Sci. *39:* 563–582.

Fazekas de St. Groth, S. (1962). The neutralization of viruses. Adv. Virus Res. *9:* 1–125.

Fazekas de St. Groth, S. (1967a). Cross recognition and cross reactivity. Symp. Quant. Biol. *32:* 525–535.

Fazekas de St. Groth, S. (1967b). Reply to E. Haber in Discussion. Symp. Quant. Biol. *32:* 535–536.

Fazekas de St. Groth, S. (1969). The antigenic subunits of influenza viruses. II. The spectrum of cross reactions. J. Immunol. *103:* 1107–1115.

Fazekas de St. Groth, S., and Reid, A. F. (1958). The neutralization of animal viruses. II. A critical comparison of hypotheses. J. Immunol. *80:* 225–235.

Fazekas de St. Groth, S., Watson, G. S., and Reid, A. F. (1958). The neutralization of animal viruses. I. A model of virus-antibody interaction. J. Immunol. *80:* 215–224.

Fazekas de St. Groth, S., and Webster, R. G. (1961). Methods in immunochemistry of viruses. I. Equilibrium filtration. Aust. J. Exp. Biol. Med. Sci. *39:* 549–562.

Fazekas de St. Groth, S., and Webster, R. G. (1963a). The neutralization of animal viruses. III. Equilibrium conditions in the influenza virus-antibody system. J. Immunol. *90:* 140–150.

Fazekas de St. Groth, S., and Webster, R. G. (1963b). The neutralization of animal viruses. IV. Parameters of the influenza virus-antibody system. J. Immunol. *90:* 151–164.

Fazekas de St. Groth, S., and Webster, R. G. (1966a). Disquisitions on original antigenic sin. I. Evidence in man. J. Exp. Med. *124:* 331–345.

Fazekas de St. Groth, S., and Webster, R. G. (1966b). Disquisitions on original antigenic sin. II. Proof in lower creatures. J. Exp. Med. *124:* 347–361.

Fazekas de St. Groth, S., Webster, R. G., and Davenport, F. M. (1969). The antigenic subunits of influenza viruses. I. The homologous antibody response. J. Immunol. *103:* 1099–1106.

Fraenkel-Conrat, H. (1965). Structure and function of virus proteins and of viral nucleic acid. In *The Proteins* Ed. 2, Vol. 3, Neurath, H. ed., Academic Press (New York, 585 pp.), pp. 99–151.

Francis, T. (1953). Influenza: the newe acquayantance. Ann. Intern. Med. *39:* 203–221.

Francis, T., Jr., Davenport, F. M., and Hennessy, A. V. (1953). A serological recapitulation of human infection with different strains of influenza virus. Trans. Assoc. Am. Physicians 66: 231–239.

Franklin, R. E., Caspar, D. L. D., and Klug, A. (1959). The structure of viruses as determined by X-ray diffraction. In Plant Pathology, Problems and Progress, 1908–1958, Holton, C. S. et al., eds. University of Wisconsin Press (Madison, 492 pp.), pp. 461–477.

Fritz, R. B., Lassiter, S., and Day, E. D. (1967). The effect of iodination on anti-fibrinogen antibodies with respect to precipitating and adsorption activities. Immunochemistry 4: 283–293.

Goodman, J. W., and Donch, J. J. (1964). Neutralization of bacteriophage by intact and degraded rabbit antibody. J. Immunol. 93: 96–100.

Goodman, J. W., and Donch, J. J. (1965). Phage-neutralizing activity in light polypeptide chains of rabbit antibody. Immunochemistry 2: 351–357.

Greenbury, C. L., Moore, D. H., and Nunn, L. A. C. (1965). The reaction with red cells of 7S rabbit antibody, its subunits, and their recombinants. Immunology 8: 420–431.

Haber, E. (1967). Discussion following F. de St. Groth's paper. Symp. Quant. Biol. 32: 535.

Haber, E., Richards, F. F., Spragg, J., Austen, K. F., Vallotton, M., and Page, L. B. (1967). Modifications in the heterogeneity of the antibody response. Symp. Quant. Biol. 32: 299–310.

Haimovich, J., Hurwitz, E., Novick, N., and Sela, M. (1970). Use of protein-bacteriophage conjugates for detection and quantitation of proteins. Biochim. Biophys. Acta 207: 125–129.

Haimovich, J., Novik, N., and Sela, M. (1969). Inhibition of the inactivation of modified phage. Isr. J. Med. Sci. 5: 438 incl.

Haimovich, J., and Sela, M. (1966). Inactivation of poly-DL-alanyl bacteriophage T4 with antisera specific toward poly-DL-alanine. J. Immunol. 97: 338–343.

Haimovich, J., and Sela, M. (1969a). Inactivation of bacteriophage T4, of poly-D-alanyl bacteriophage and of penicilloyl bacteriophage by immunospecifically isolated IgM and IgG antibodies. J. immunol. 103: 45–55.

Haimovich, J., and Sela, M. (1969b). Protein-bacteriophage conjugates: application in detection of antibodies and antigens. Science 164: 1279–1280.

Haimovich, J., Sela, M., Dewdney, J. M., and Batchelor, F. R. (1967). Anti-penicilloyl antibodies:' detection with penicilloylated bacteriophage and isolation with a specific immunoadsorbent. Nature 214: 1369–1370.

Haimovich, J., Tarrab, R., Sulica, A., and Sela, M. (1970). Antibodies of different specificities in normal rabbit sera. J. Immunol. 104: 1033–1034.

Harris, J. I., and Knight, C. A. (1955). Studies on the action of carboxypeptidase on tobacco mosaic virus. J. Biol. Chem. 214: 215–230.

Hornick, C. L., and Karush, F. (1969). The interaction of hapten-coupled bacteriophage ϕX174 with antihapten antibody. In Topics in Basic Immunology, Sela, M., and Prywes, M., eds. Academic Press (New York, 180 pp.), pp. 29–36.

Jerne, N. K., and Avegno, P. (1956). The development of the phage-inactivating properties of serum during the course of specific immunization of an animal: reversible and irreversible inactivation. J. Immunol. 76: 200–208.

Kabat, E. A. (1970). Discussion following Professor Morgan's paper. Ann. N. Y. Acad. Sci. 169: 131–133.

Klinman, N. R., and Karush, F. (1967). Equine antihapten antibody. V. The nonprecipitability of bivalent antibody. Immunochemistry 4: 387–405.

Klinman, N. R., Long, C. A., and Karush, F. (1967). The role of antibody bivalence in the neutralization of bacteriophage. J. Immunol. *99:* 1128–1133.

Krueger, R. G. (1970). Effect of antigenic stimulation on the specificity of antibody produced by rabbits immunized with bacteriophage MS-2. J. Immunol. *104:* 1117–1123.

Krummel, W. M., and Uhr, J. W. (1969). A mathematical and experimental study of the kinetics of neutralization of bacteriophage φX174 by antibodies. J. Immunol. *102:* 772–785.

Lafferty, K. J. (1960). The neutralization of animal viruses. Ph.D. Dissertation, Australian National University, Canberra.

Lafferty, K. J. (1963). The interaction between virus and antibody. II. Mechanism of the reaction. Virology *21:* 76–90.

Mäkelä, O. (1966). Assay of anti-hapten antibody with the aid of hapten-coupled bacteriophage. Immunology *10:* 81–86.

Mamet-Bratley, M. D. (1966). Evidence concerning homogeneity of the combining sites of purified antibody. Immunochemistry *3:* 155–162.

Pappenheimer, A. M., Jr., Lundgren, H. P., and Williams, J. W. (1940). Studies on the molecular weight of diphtheria toxin, antitoxin, and their reaction products. J. Exp. Med. *71:* 247–262.

Pappenheimer, A. M., Jr., and Robinson, E. S. (1937). A quantitative study of the Ramon diphtheria flocculation reaction. J. Immunol. *32:* 291–300.

Porter, E. F., and Pappenheimer, A. M., Jr. (1939). Antigen-antibody reactions between layers adsorbed on built-up stearate films. J. Exp. Med. *69:* 755–765.

Rappaport, I. (1959). The reversibility of the reaction between rabbit antibody and tobacco mosaic virus. J. Immunol. *82:* 526–534.

Rohrmann, G. F., and Krueger, R. G. (1970). Precipitation and neutralization of bacteriophage MS-2 by rabbit antibodies. J. Immunol. *104:* 353–358.

Rowlands, D. T., Jr. (1967). Precipitation and neutralization of bacteriophage f2 by rabbit antibodies. J. Immunol. *98:* 958–964.

Stanley, W. M. (1935). The crystallization of tobacco mosaic virus. Science *81:* 644–645.

Stemke, G. W., and Lennox, E. S. (1967). Bacteriophage neutralizing activity of fragments derived from rabbit immunoglobulins by papain digestion. J. immunol. *98:* 94–101.

Taussig, M. J. (1970). Bacteriophage linked assays for antibodies to protein antigens. Immunology *18:* 323–330.

Webster, R. G. (1966). Original antigenic sin in ferrets: the response to sequential infections with influenza viruses. J. Immunol. *97:* 177–183.

Webster, R. G., and Laver, W. G. (1966). Influenza virus subunit vaccines: immunogenicity and lack of toxicity for rabbits of ether- and detergent-disrupted virus. J. Immunol. *96:* 596–605.

Webster, R. G., and Laver, W. G. (1967). Preparation and properties of antibody directed specifically against the neuraminidase of influenza virus. J. Immunol. *99:* 49–55.

Young, J. D., Benjamini, E., Stewart, J. M., and Leung, C. Y. (1967). Immunochemical studies on tobacco mosaic virus protein. V. The solid-phase synthesis of peptides of an antigenically active decapeptide of tobacco mosaic virus protein and the reaction of these peptides with antibodies to the whole protein. Biochemistry *6:* 1455–1460.

8

ANTIBODY REACTIONS WITH MULTIVALENT ANTIGENS
II. Precipitation Reactions

1. Introduction

Svante Arrhenius (1859–1927) coined the term "immunochemistry" in 1904 during a lectureship at the University of California at Berkeley. Better known for his theory of electrolytic dissociation in 1887 and as Nobel Prize winner in 1903, the Swedish chemist published his Berkeley lectures under the title *Immunochemistry* (Arrhenius, 1907) with the following prefatory remarks:

> "I have given to these lectures the title "Immuno-chemistry," and wish with this word to indicate that the chemical reactions of substances that are produced by the injection of foreign substances into the blood of animals, *i.e.* by immunisation, are under discussion in these pages. From this it follows also—that the substances with which these products react, as proteins and ferments, are to be here considered with respect to their chemical properties."

During the formative years of biochemistry considerable interest was displayed in the precipitates that formed in natural fluids such as milk, plasma, and fruit juices. For one thing such precipitates generally represented substances of increased purity that would lend themselves more easily to analysis, and it was natural that casein, fibrin, and pectin would become the initial targets for investigation. For another, the soluble material (serum) remaining after precipitation (in the case of milk and plasma) was enriched enough in albumins that it also became readily subject to analysis.

One of the ways of purifying albumins still further was to inject the serum of milk or blood from one animal into one of another species and later to combine the serum of the immune animal with that of the original. In this way milk serum albumins (now known as lactalbumin) or blood serum albumins could also be made to precipitate. By cross-immunizations it was found that "nearly the whole quantity of the albuminous substances [in the original serum], but only a very small fraction of those [in the immune serum], enter into the precipitate" (Arrhenius, 1907). It was clear to Arrhenius and other physical chemists of the era, however, that something was different about immune precipitation. The antibody apparently was not acting as a catalyst, in the way rennet did in the formation of casein, but rather as a participant in a bimolecular reaction. The nature of the precipitation reaction, however, was so peculiar that a rational mechanism and a mathematical model were not easily derived from it. The most startling feature was the complete solubility of the precipitate in a solution of excess antigen. Although complex formations had been met in inorganic chemistry in which one of the reactants would, in excess, solubilize what it had precipitated in more dilute solution, the phenomenon had not been met before in biochemistry.

Arrhenius tabulated the data of his colleague, Hamburger, to indicate the manner in which peak precipitation would occur and derived an equation that expressed the whole process. A rabbit antiserum had been prepared against sheep serum and then tested against sheep, goat, and bullock sera for precipitation. Varying volumes of the test antigens were added to constant volumes (0.4 cc) of rabbit antiserum in a funnel-shaped vessel which extended into a calibrated capillary tube of 0.04-cc volume, divided into units of 0.0004 cc. By vigorous hand centrifugation for 1.5–2 hr, the precipitates would pack into the capillary tubes where their volume could be measured. The data in Table 8-1 are given in terms of 0.0004-cc volume units of precipitate for various volumes (in cc) of added test antigen. The calculated values were obtained from equations that were remarkable in concept for that era.

A bimolecular reaction was assumed in which the soluble reactants were in equilibrium with the insoluble product according to the law of mass action. At equilibrium between the two phases the solubility product law was then utilized, expressing the product of the concentration of reactants as, K, an equilibrium constant. A was given as multiples of the number of equivalents of 2% sheep serum that would form an optimum precipitate with rabbit antiserum, and B was given as multiples of the number of equivalents of undiluted rabbit serum that would form 100 units of precipitate at optimum. In these experiments 1 ml of diluted sheep serum was found to contain 40 equivalents and 1 ml of undiluted rabbit antiserum, 300 equivalents; i.e., 2.5 ml of 2% sheep serum were equivalent to 0.33 ml of rabbit antiserum, and the two together would form a full capillary of 100

TABLE 8-1

Precipitation of Sheep, Goat, and Bullock Sera with Rabbit Anti-Sheep Serum

Volume of Antigen		Volume Units of Precipitate Formed (P)*					
		Sheep		Goat		Bullock	
Amount	Equivalent†	Observed	Calculated	Observed	Calculated	Observed	Calculated
cc							
0.002	0.08	1	0.5	1	0.4	1	0.5
0.04	1.6	2	1.3	2	1.2	2	1.3
0.1	4	3	3.5	4	3.4	4	3.4
0.15	6	6	5.3	5	5.2	5	5.2
0.2	8	7	7.2	6	7	7	6.7
0.6	24	21	21.5	16	21	16	19
1	40	35	34	26	32	20	24
1.5	60	39	48	30	43	22	26
2	80	60	57	35	48	25	26
3	120	67	66	40	51	28	25
5	200	64	65	50	47	22	21
7	280	58	58	52	40	10	17
10	400	49	46	34	27	7	11
12	480			27	18	5	7
15	600	10	19	9	5	3	1
18	720	5	3	8	0	2	0
20	800	2	0	4	0	1	0

* One volume unit of precipitate equals 0.0004 cc.

† Number of equivalents of 2% sheep serum that would optimally precipitate undiluted rabbit antiserum. Amount of antiserum was fixed at 0.4 cc, enough to precipitate 120 equivalents from 3 cc of 2% sheep serum at optimum.

(From Arrhenius, 1907.)

precipitin units. The precipitate, P, that was formed was assumed to be homogeneous and to contain equivalent precipitin units of both antigen and antibody such that the amounts of A and B left in solution would be $(A - P)$ and $(B - P)$. The total volume V would be the same for each and the concentrations would therefore be $(A - P)/V$ and $(B - P)/V$. Thus,

$$\left(\frac{A - P}{V}\right)\left(\frac{B - P}{V}\right) = K \tag{8.1}$$

or

$$(A - P)(B - P) = K \cdot V^2 \tag{8.2}$$

Since B was kept at 0.4 cc or 120 precipitin units the final equation was

$$(A - P)(120 - P) - K \cdot V^2 \qquad (8.3)$$

Values for K were obtained by plotting the observed values $(A - P)$ $(120 - P)$, against V^2. In the case of sheep serum, $K = 250$; goat serum, $K = 200$; bullock serum, $K = 85$. The calculated values for P in Table 8-1 were obtained by assuming these K values.

Remarkable as the concept is upon which this first precipitin equation was based, it is for the most part erroneous (wherein lies an example of the danger of curve fitting to observed data). Discussion of its flaws will be instructive in understanding the precipitin reaction for what it is.

The first flaw is the assumption that the formed precipitate is homogeneous. It is not homogeneous, but rather a mixture of several components varying in the ratio of antigen to antibody and in total aggregated size. The nature of some of these antigen-antibody complexes will be discussed in a subsequent section and their inhomogeneity will then become apparent.

The second flaw is the assumption that the number of equivalents worked out between rabbit antiserum and its homologous antigen, sheep serum, should hold for cross-reacting antigens. The same number of equivalents A were assigned to a given volume of goat or bullock serum as to sheep serum, and the number of equivalents in 0.4 ml of rabbit serum was assumed to be 120 regardless of the antigen against which it was used. Equivalence zones should have been worked out for each system.

The third flaw is the assumption that the precipitation reaction is volume-independent and requires only considerations of concentration to be valid. Actually, volumes are critical in obtaining quantitative precipitin data and must be kept constant to obtain the most meaningful and reproducible curves.

The fourth flaw is the assumption that the precipitation reaction is practically over by the time the first precipitate is observed. The attainment of a reproducible amount of precipitate takes several hours and, because it is temperature-dependent, requires application of constant temperature.

The fifth flaw is the assumption that the amount of precipitate formed is directly proportional to the amount of antigen precipitated. A variant of the first flaw, this draws attention to the necessity of analyzing the formed precipitate for its antigen and antibody content before applying the data to antigenic analysis.

The sixth flaw is the assumption that the volume of precipitate obtained after packing in a centrifuge is a precise measure of the amount of precipitate present. In protein work such a measure is one of the least precise.

The seventh and perhaps the most serious flaw is the assumption that the law of mass action can be simply applied to the precipitation reaction—to the simple interactions of free haptens and antibodies, yes, but not to the complex interactions that lead up to precipitation.

In spite of the invalid assumptions that made this first mathematical expression of the precipitin reaction erroneous, two conclusions were drawn that were valid, basic, and extremely important: that antibodies are bound to the precipitates they help form and that an equivalence zone exists where antigen and antibody form the optimum amount of precipitate.

The most appealing observations made during the early years of immunochemistry were, perhaps, those of von Dungern (1903). In retrospect they appear to have a contemporary flavor and in them is contained the prototype of the modern experiment. Rabbit antisera were prepared against octopus, crab, and mollusc plasmas and shown to react with hemocyanins to form blue-colored precipitates. (Hemocyanins are blue proteins that form the major part of many invertebrate plasma proteins. They contain no heme but do have copper-peptide prosthetic groups.) By manipulations of reactant concentrations that formed the precipitates von Dungern was able to demonstrate that, in either direction from apparent optimum, hemocyanin precipitates would change in composition. He further showed that the hemocyanins, while in the form of specific precipitates, would become colorless when exposed to CO_2 and would regain their color when exposed to air (O_2). These experiments, while not particularly quantitative, demonstrated the value of having a direct measure of antigen with which to follow the process of precipitation.

2. Quantitative precipitation of pneumococcal polysaccharides

The more than 75 types and subtypes of pneumococci (Heidelberger, 1956) receive their specificities from capsules which, under optimal conditions of growth, cover a maximum number of organisms. Loss of virulence on the part of the organisms is associated with capsular loss and also with the loss of immunological specificity.

Heidelberger and Avery (1923) demonstrated the polysaccharide nature of the solubilized specific substance from Type II pneumococcus capsules, and in a second paper (1924) reported that the polysaccharides from Types II and III organisms were chemically different. S-III was soon shown to be an aldobiuronic acid (Heidelberger and Goebel, 1927) that was nitrogen-free and that was freely soluble in salt form. That this early form of S-III was partially degraded by heat, as shown by Heidelberger, Kendall, and Scherp (1936), did not detract from its usefulness as a purified and nitrogen-free antigen in the study of the precipitation reaction with anti-S-III. The structure of S-III was confirmed by Reeves and Goebel (1941) as that of an aldobiuronic acid and was shown to have a β-D-configuration.

Repeating Unit of S-III Polyaldobiuronic Acid

The usefulness of the S-III polysaccharide in the quantitative study of the precipitin reaction is readily apparent. As shown by Heidelberger and Kendall (1929) the difference in the original nitrogen content of the antibody solution and that remaining after precipitation and centrifugation of the specific precipitate produced an accurate measure of the amount of precipitated antibody in absolute weight units since the antigen contained no nitrogen. Increased precision was obtained by using specifically purified antibody as the starting material and thereby decreasing the amount of original nitrogen (by eliminating nitrogen-containing nonspecific protein).

With the advent of more precise micromethods for determining precipitated antibody nitrogen, thus making direct nitrogen analyses of washed precipitates possible, the precipitin reaction could be investigated in depth.

Heidelberger's review (1939) sums up the application of the quantitative technique in the study of antigen-antibody reactions. When small amounts of S-III were added to a large amount of horse anti-S-III, 240 mg of antibody were precipitated per mg of S-III. When increasing amounts of S-III were added to separate portions of antibody, increasing amounts of precipitate were obtained with no discontinuity and with no antigen detectable in the soluble phase at a dilution of $1:1 \times 10^7$. Antibody was still present in the separated soluble phase since additional precipitate would form when S-III was added to it. This whole region was called the *antibody excess zone*. The *equivalence zone* was reached at the point where neither S-III nor anti-S-III was demonstrable, except perhaps in very small amount, in the soluble phase. As S-III continued to be added a point was eventually reached where antibody nitrogen in the precipitate remained at the maximum but where S-III began to appear in the supernatant fluid. This was the end of the equivalence zone and the beginning of the *first zone of antigen excess*. With a much larger excess of S-III added to antibody an *inhibition zone or second zone of antigen excess* was finally reached in which, as S-III continued to be added, less and less precipitate formed until its appearance was finally prevented. A graphical precipitin curve, recording these events, is shown in Figure 8-1.

When the reaction was confined to the antibody excess region where the amount of added S-III was completely precipitated, it was observed that as the amount of added S-III was increased, the amount of antibody nitrogen that was precipitated with the added S-III did not increase proportionately, i.e., that the ratio of antibody nitrogen to S-III in the formed precipitate did not remain constant (Heidelber-

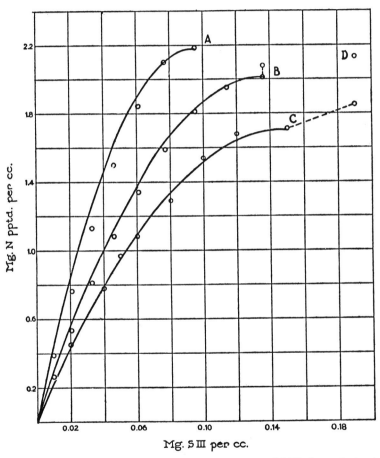

FIG. 8-1. Precipitation titration of anti-S-III by additions of S-III. *Curve C*, standard method at 37°C; *curves A* and *B*, serial additions of S-III in small amounts at 0°C and 37°C, respectively. The higher values obtained with *B* than with *C* demonstrate the Danysz (1902) phenomenon. The higher values obtained with *A* than with *B* demonstrate the temperature effect. (Heidelberger and Kendall, 1935a.)

ger and Kendall, 1935a).

An empirical relationship was worked out, nevertheless, since it was observed that plotting the ratio of antibody nitrogen to added S-III against added S-III resulted in a linear relationship (keeping in mind that added S-III was also precipitated S-III). Thus,

$$\frac{\text{pptd Ab N}}{\text{added S-III}} = a - b \text{ (added S-III)} \tag{8.4}$$

$$\frac{\text{pptd Ab N}}{\text{pptd S-III}} = a - b \text{ (added S-III)} \tag{8.5}$$

where conditions are confined to antibody excess regions and all added antigen is also precipitated antigen (Fig. 8-2).

The constants can be evaluated by considering the ratio R for the two components at equivalence (usually the mid-point):

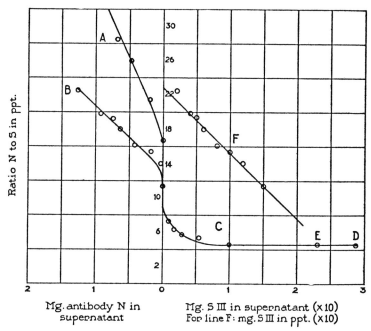

FIG. 8-2. Precipitation titration of anti-S-III by additions of S-III. The *line F* is the pertinent one for the text discussion. Note that the abscissa for F is milligrams of S-III in precipitate, which is also milligrams of added S-III since the titration was carried out in antibody excess. *Curves A* and *B* also represent antibody excess; *curve C*, antigen excess. *Curve A* to *point E* is for antibody B-62 at 0°C. *Curve B* to *point D* is for antibody B-61 at 37°C. *Point D* should read 3.68. (From Heidelberger and Kendall, 1935b.)

$$R = \left(\frac{\text{pptd Ab N}}{\text{pptd S-III}}\right)_{\text{equiv}} \tag{8.6}$$

First, it will be noted that the intercept a on the ordinate is double the value obtained within the equivalence zone, i.e., $a = 2R$. Thus,

$$\lim_{\substack{\text{added S-III} \\ \to 0}} \frac{\text{pptd Ab N}}{[\text{pptd S-III}]} = a = 2R \tag{8.7}$$

and

$$\lim_{\substack{\text{added S-III} \\ \to \text{equiv}}} \frac{\text{pptd Ab N}}{[\text{pptd S-III}]} = R \tag{8.8}$$

Therefore, at equivalence,

$$R = 2R - b \, (\text{added S-III})_{\text{equiv}} \tag{8.9}$$

and

$$b = R/(\text{added S-III})_{\text{equiv}} \tag{8.10}$$

Since

$$(\text{added S-III})_{\text{equiv}} = (\text{pptd S-III})_{\text{equiv}} \tag{8.11}$$

and

$$(\text{pptd S-III})_{\text{equiv}} = (\text{pptd Ab N})_{\text{equiv}}/R \tag{8.12}$$

letting

$$A = (\text{pptd Ab N})_{\text{equiv}}$$
$$b = R^2/A$$

The completed formula can then be written as

$$\frac{\text{pptd Ab N}}{\text{added S-III}} = 2R - \frac{R^2}{A}(\text{added S-III}) \tag{8.13}$$

$$\frac{N}{S} = 2R - \frac{R^2}{A} S \tag{8.14}$$

It was of interest to evaluate the precipitin reactions of antibodies obtained from rabbit anti-S-III to see if the empirical relationships would still hold. As an extension of the study it was also of interest to note any changes in precipitin response as the rabbits were immunized by repeated injections (Heidelberger and Kendall, 1937). An initial course of 15 injections were administered over a period of 4–5 weeks to two rabbits, 3–4 injections per week, with dosages increasing from 1 ml to 3 ml containing 0.05 mg of bacterial N/ml. The first bleeding occurred 4 days after the last injection in the first course; the second, after a week's rest, a course of 12 injections, and another week's rest; the third bleeding, similar to the second; and the fourth, likewise.

The first observation was that the data for precipitation of rabbit anti-S-III with S-III were linear when plotted in the same manner as horse anti-S-III. The second observation was that the value R increased during immunization. The third was that the value R was different for each rabbit at a given stage of immunization as it had been for individual horse antibody preparations (Table 8-2).

When it is recalled that R equals the ratio of antibody nitrogen to S-III at the mid-point of equivalence it can easily be understood that there is no set stoichiometric formula expressing equivalence such that all antisera could be equated at that point. This is not surprising in view of what has already been said about heterogeneity, but it has complicated theoretical treatment of the reaction almost beyond experimental verification. Two general assumptions of Heidelberger and Kendall (1935b) and of Marrack (1938) still stand in spite of controversy over a number of other points: (a) Multivalency of antigen and antibody were assumed (and there is no longer any doubt about this assumption); (b) the behavior of the antibody mixture was taken as that of a single substance on the average. (The precision of the equation could not be expected without this being true.)

Before precipitation occurred a number of bimolecular reactions were assumed to take place with the rate of formation of reaction

TABLE 8-2
Precipitation Equation of S-III with Various Antisera

Species	Antiserum No.	Equation
Horse	BVA	$N/S = 27.2 - 45.6S$
	B36	$N/S = 24.8 - 82.7S$
	B61	$N/S = 22.8 - 76.0S$
Rabbit	3.51—1st bleeding	$N/S = 12.7 - 40.3S$
	2nd	$N/S = 14.5 - 52.6S$
	3rd	$N/S = 16.1 - 64.8S$
	4th	$N/S = 16.7 - 69.7S$
	3.50—1st bleeding	$N/S = 14.9 - 46.2S$
	2nd	$N/S = 15.6 - 60.8S$
	3rd	$N/S = 16.8 - 70.6S$

(From Heidelberger and Kendall, 1937.)

products being proportional to the concentration of reacting substances. This seemed to be the only way of explaining why discrete steps in composition were not found in going from one end of the antibody excess region to the other. *The composition of the precipitate would depend more on the proportions in which the components were mixed than upon the antibody concentration at equilibrium or at the end of the reaction.* There were many objections to this idea, most of them following Marrack (1938), in questioning the apparent irreversibility that would be necessary to "fix" the compositions of soluble reaction products before they formed aggregates.

Heidelberger's answer to this objection was to perform another experiment (Heidelberger, Treffers, and Mayer, 1940). It had already been established that the general form of the precipitin equation would hold for rabbit anti-egg albumin (anti-EA) in its reaction with EA. On the other hand, it was also known that a sample of Pappenheimer's horse anti-EA was "incomplete," that it would bind but not precipitate EA. The experiment that could be performed with the horse and rabbit anti-EA antisera was to find out how long it would take for horse anti-EA (H) to form a soluble complex with EA, then to dissociate reversibly, and finally to make EA available for precipitation with added rabbit anti-EA (R). It was found that if R were added to H-EA as little as 18 sec after H and EA were mixed, only 0.02 mg of nitrogen precipitated out of a total of 0.18 mg in 1 day. Not until after 2–3 weeks did the reverse reaction of H-EA dissociation complete itself and make EA available for precipitation with R. When 3:1 R and H were mixed and then added to EA, 0.12 mg out of 0.18 mg of total available nitrogen was precipitated, showing that the velocities of initial reactions of R and H were comparable. When R was added immediately before H, complex formation of R-EA was complete and precipitation maximal. *Thus, it was demonstrated that the concentration of initial reactants and the rate of formation of soluble reaction products did indeed affect the nature of the precipitate and that equilibrium processes involved in precipitation were much slower.**

---

* It is enlightening to compare the results obtained by Heidelberger, Treffers, and Mayer (1940) with those recent ones of Klinman, Rockey, Frauenberger, and Karush (1966). The latter group followed the development of anti-Lac-human serum albumin (HSA) in a single horse with respect to distribution of antibody activity among six different immunoglobulins, and found that early serum, high in precipitable IgG, precipitated Lac-HSA. However, as IgT became the major component in later serum, no precipitation of Lac-HSA occurred. When IgG in the late serum was separated and tested, it was capable of precipitating the conjugated Lac-protein. Changes in the precipitability of serum in the horse were thus easily attributed to the relative competition between mixtures of precipitable bivalent IgG and nonprecipitable *bivalent* IgT, a conclusion drawn likewise by Heidelberger, Treffers, and Mayer (1940) for a very similar system.

This does not prove conclusively that Heidelberger and Kendall (1935b) were right in their theory, but it does mean that the objections to their theory were certainly not the right ones. Heidelberger (1939), himself, felt that

> "... this oversimplification of the quantitative theory as it now stands ... at least permits many calculations and predictions to be made with accuracy and a certain degree of utility ... The theory was offered, in the realization of many weaknesses, as a temporary expedient which might be useful until antibody possessed of uniform reactivity could be isolated."

The *empirical precipitation equation* has suffered unduly because of the unrest concerning its meaning. Although it can be derived from the Heidelberger-Kendall theory, *it does not depend upon that theory for its validity*. Unlike the Arrhenius equation, no assumptions were necessary to formulate this one, and no attempt was made to cover all regions with one formula.

Other empirical formulas were found on occasion to provide better linearity. One of these was worked out for a protein-antiprotein system in which the test antigen was coupled to a colored dye (Heidelberger and Kendall, 1935c). Total precipitated nitrogen was determined directly, antigen nitrogen was determined by its known ratio to the colorimetric amount of antigen present, and antibody nitrogen was obtained by difference. The equation was

$$N = 3RD - 2\sqrt{\frac{R^3 D^3}{A}} \qquad (8.15)$$

where

R = ratio of N to D at equivalence, i.e., $A{:}D$
N = antibody nitrogen
D = dye-antigen nitrogen
A = maximum precipitable antibody nitrogen

A more familiar form and one used for demonstrating linearity is

$$\frac{N}{D} = 3R - 2\sqrt{\frac{R^3}{A}}\sqrt{D} \qquad (8.16)$$

where N/D is plotted against the square root of added antigen nitrogen or $\sqrt{D}$. This was the form used by Kabat and Berg (1953) to describe the precipitin reactions of human anti-dextran antibodies with a number of native and clinical dextrans (Table 8-3).

An example of the power inherent in the intelligent use of the quan-

TABLE 8-3
Empirical Precipitin Equations for Dextran-Anti-Dextran Systems

Dextran	Antiserum	Equation
Native (B742)*	1-D-2	$N/D = 0.87 - 0.06D^{1/2}$
	20-D-2	$N/D = 0.92 - 0.05D^{1/2}$
	30-D-2	$N/D = 0.79 - 0.04D^{1/2}$
	49-D-2	$N/D = 0.63 - 0.03D^{1/2}$
Clinical	1-D-2	$N/D = 12.1 - 3.1D^{1/2}$
(N150N)†	20-D-2	$N/D = 12.8 - 2.8D^{1/2}$
	30-D-2	$N/D = 11.9 - 2.5D^{1/2}$
	49-D-2	$N/D = 11.7 - 3.0D^{1/2}$

* The ratio of 1,6 to non-1,6 links in dextran was 1.9.
† The ratio of 1,6 to non-1,6 links in dextran was 32–49.
(From Kabat and Berg, 1953.)

titative precipitin reaction is found in a procedure for antibody purification that was predicted on the basis of the reaction. Heidelberger, Kendall, and Teorell (1936) had noted the following:

1.24 mg of horse anti-S-III Ab N pptd by 0.1 mg of S-III in 0.15 M NaCl

1.01 mg of horse anti-S-III Ab N pptd by 0.1 mg of S-III in 1.75 M NaCl

It seemed to Heidelberger and Kendall (1936) that if the reaction were carried out in 0.15 M NaCl and the precipitate were collected and washed, and if then the precipitate were agitated in 1.75 M NaCl, then 0.23 mg of nitrogen should dissociate in the form of antibody. If this indeed were true, then salt dissociation should form the basis of a purification procedure for anti-S-III antibody. The technique was tried and the predicted amount of antibody in 90–98% purity was obtained in a number of trials.

It was this simple procedure that led to the finding that horse, cow, and pig anti-pneumococcal polysaccharide antibodies were IgM whereas those from rabbit, monkey, and man were IgG (Heidelberger and Pedersen, 1937; Kabat and Pedersen, 1938; Tiselius and Kabat, 1938, 1939; and Kabat, 1939).

The immunological specificity of pneumococcal polysaccharides and the cross-reactions displayed among them has been the main subject of study by Heidelberger and his colleagues, and the development of quantitative techniques for antigenic analysis was pursued to make detailed exploration possible. One of the many problems solved by application of quantitative technique concerned an atypical Type III pneumococcus isolated by Sugg, Gaspari, Fleming, and Neill (1928). The work of Cooper, Edwards, and Rosenstein (1929) had

shown that the atypical strain cross-reacted with anit-S-III but failed
to remove all anti-S-III activity. The new form was then called Type
VIII, and Goebel (1935) confirmed the nature of its difference from
Type III. Though its polysaccharide contained the same aldobiuronic
acid as S-III, there was a glucose in addition. It was not until 1957 that
Jones and Perry tentatively worked out the fine structure of S-VIII
as containing a repeating unit of

[-4- β-D-glucuronic-(1 → 4)- β-D-glucose-(1 → 4)-
α-D-glucose-(1 → 4)- α-D-galactose-(1 →)]

In a cross-reaction study Heidelberger, Kabat, and Shrivastava (1937)
showed that although a horse anti-S-III reagent contained 30% cross-
reacting antibody that would react with S-VIII, a rabbit anti-S-III contained little or no cross-reacting antibody even though it would react
in very high titer with S-III. The subtle differences in structures between the two cellobiuronic acids were enough to make it not always
possible to protect individuals against both pneumococcal types by
immunization with only one. In spite of this both types of antisera in
high dilution were found to precipitate the soluble sodium salts of
oxidized cotton cellulose (Heidelberger and Hobby, 1942), indicating
that the latter contained cellobiuronic acid residues.

As reagents for identifying specific polysaccharide groupings from
a number of other sources, the anti-pneumococcal polysaccharides
have been extremely invaluable. The hydrolyzed polysaccharide from
the slime of *Sphaerotilus natans* was found to form precipitates, e.g.,
with anti-S-III and anti-S-VIII, showing the presence of the cellobiuronic acid, β-D-glucuronopyranosyl-(1 → 4)-D-glucose (Heidelberger, Gaudy, and Wolfe, 1964). Chemical modification of S-III by
complete acetylation, which esterified the carboxyl groups, was found
to destroy its binding capacity for anti-S-III, but when progressive
deacetylation was carried out reactivity was regained until, with all
acetyl groups removed, the material reacted with anti S-III as well
as it had before acetylation. It was of interest, however, that esteri-
fication of 35% of the carboxyl groups and conversion to the amide
gave a product 86–90% as reactive as the native material. It was
understandable from these results why anti-S-III reacted so well
with oxidized cotton cellulose—the latter contained 16–21%
carboxylic acid groups.

The cyclic process of investigations involving the pneumococcal
polysaccharide systems still continues—cyclic in the sense that as
new structures are found, they eventually become identified and
purified, and in turn help to characterize the very antiserum reagents
that led to their identification. These lead back to methods for

preparing pneumococcal polysaccharides in a less degraded and more complete state and permit more extended and detailed cross-reaction studies among the various types. The end result is new knowledge about the structures and specific groupings of poly-saccharides in general. Sometimes this can lead to the elucidation of a repeating unit as in the case of S-VI, in which O-α-D-galacto-pyranosyl-(1 → 3)-O-D-glucopyranosyl-(1 → 3)-O-α-L-rhamnopyrano-syl-(1 → 3)-D (or L)-ribitol was obtained (Rebers and Heidelberger, 1961). It was found that the adjacent units in the undegraded poly-saccharide were joined together by phosphate diester linkages in head-to-tail fashion and that type specificity came in three parts (Heidelberger and Rebers, 1960): linear chains of (1 → 3)-linked L-rhamnose, (1 → 3)-linked D-glucose, and (1 → 2)-linked D-galactose. The cross-reaction of anti-S-VI with polysaccharide prepared from group A hemolytic streptococci (known to contain L-rhamnose) sug-gested that the group A sugar might also contain (1 → 3)-linked rham-nose residues, and this was confirmed by chemical studies (Hey-mann, Manniello, and Barkulis, 1963).

The quantitative precipitin reaction need not be confined to poly-saccharides and proteins but can be extended to the agglutination of bacteria and other particulate materials. Heidelberger and Kabat (1937) demonstrated this in the case of horse anti-S-I in its precipita-tion of Type I pneumococcus. Several controls were of course neces-sary. (One serious problem was to control for the amount of S-I that tended to leach out from the organism and form precipitates in-dependent of the bacteria.) A technique was finally worked out, using purified antibody, that provided reproducible data and, most important, that gave rise to linearity when the precipitin equation was used. In the region of antibody excess the bacteria were found to agglutinate easily and to resuspend uniformly. A temperature differ-ence was found such that the equations were, in 0.15 M NaCl,

$$N/S = 8.0 - 26.9S \text{ at } 37°C$$

and

$$N/S = 5.7 - 11.6S \text{ at } 0°C$$

The increased value of R (4.0 vs. 2.85) at the higher temperature (in-creased amount of antibody bound per cell) was explained as a me-chanical difference in which more surface S-I was present at 37°C than at 0°C. In terms of the amount of S-I present in the bacteria (which would have precipitated anti-S-I if in the freely soluble form), less than a maximum number of bacteria were precipitated per equivalent amount of antibody. This was quite reasonably taken to indicate that not all S-I was available in reactive form at the cell surface.

In the same way that the dissociation of specific precipitates was predicted to and did take place in strong salt, dissociation of specific agglutinates was similarly found to occur (Heidelberger and Kabat, 1938).

3. Precipitation and solubilization in antigen-excess regions

Although the most useful regions for quantitative immunochemical determinations have been those expressive of antibody excess and of equivalence, the region of antigen excess has provided an area for some of the more revealing studies on the nature of antigen-antibody interaction. Marrack's (1938) description of what probably happens is still more or less acceptable today:

> "... no precipitation will occur in the post-zone (antigen excess) owing to the formation of small aggregates ... protected by the excess of antigen. With smaller quantities of antigen continuously larger aggregates will be formed, possibly arranged as a lattice with incomplete packing of the antibody molecules. These may settle, leaving the supernatant fluid cloudy, owing to the presence in it of large aggregates. At optimum proportions a continuous lattice will be formed."

Marrack regarded the optimum proportion to be that ratio of antibody to antigen which is capable of forming a stable lattice, and by this view, but for different reasons, was in accord with Taylor (1931) and with Burnet (1931). A stable lattice

> "... will be determined partly by a question of size. In the instance in which the antigen, serum globulin, is of approximately the same size as the antibody the ratio is 1 to 4. This would be given by a lattice ... with each antigen molecule surrounded by 16 antibody molecules and each antibody molecule by 4 antigen molecules."

How a stable lattice is achieved with bivalent antibody and multivalent antigen is still unknown since the number of possibilities is large; however, the essential correctness of Marrack's framework theory for the final product is supported by much evidence.

In the area of antigen excess the problem is made simpler since complex formation itself is simpler. Early work with systems in antigen excess was hampered, however, by the lack of physical instrumentation with which to exploit the soluble phases. Immunochemistry had been essentially an exploitation of precipitating systems since separations, so necessary to analysis, could easily be achieved. With the advent of ultracentrifugation and electrophoresis, however, the soluble phases could be explored in depth. Heidelberger and Pedersen (1937) demonstrated that several species of complexes apparently could exist in solution, and latter work confirmed this. One of the most basic and detailed confirmatory studies was that of Singer and Campbell (1951, 1952).

Crystalline bovine serum albumin (BSA) was used as antigen, and rabbit IgG anti-BSA as antibody. In order to determine the relative amounts of BSA and anti-BSA in any given complex, the BSA was iodinated with an average of 5 atoms of iodine per antibody molecule. Thus, analysis of a given complex for total nitrogen and iodine would provide data for calculating BSA and anti-BSA. Before proceeding with analyses of complexes it was necessary to determine the effect of iodination upon BSA-anti-BSA interaction, there being essentially none for the particular antibody in the study. The procedure that was used in the main study included the following steps:

(1) IgG purified by precipitation with one-third saturated ammonium sulfate.

(2) Specific BSA-anti-BSA precipitates formed in equivalence zone with BSA-5I and washed with cold saline.

(3) Washed (BSA-5I)-anti-BSA redissolved in antigen excess.

(4) Solution of the complex brought to half saturated ammonium sulfate to form a precipitate, with unbound albumin remaining in solution. (This is the basis of the Farr technique that was developed in 1958.)

(5) Precipitate suspended in buffered saline *where it completely redissolves.*

(6) Solution analyzed for iodine and nitrogen to give total antigen and antibody content.

(7) Solutions of greater antigen excess prepared by adding known amounts of BSA-5I to solution from Step 6.

(8) Ultracentrifugation carried out in phosphate, pH 7.6, $\mu = 0.1$, and 21°C

(9) Electrophoresis carried out in Veronal, pH 8.5, $\mu = 0.1$.

Several species of antigen-antibody complexes as well as free antigen were separated by sedimentation in the ultracentrifugal field but as antigen excess increased the faster sedimenting complexes disappeared considerably until in high antigen excess only one prominent peak was obtained—the *a* complex. Electrophoretic resolution was poor, but a separate fast-moving peak was obtained agreeing in composition with the *a* complex. The question at the time was concerned with the ratio of antigen to antibody in the a complex and the valency of the antibody. From certain assumptions the composition of the a complex was taken as $(Ag)_2Ab$ and that of another, the b complex, as $(Ag)_3(Ab)_2$. As the complexes became faster sedimenting (i.e., as their molecular weight increased) their relative antigen content continually decreased until precipitation finally occurred.

The question now is no longer one of valency since that has been answered from a completely independent series of experiments. The composition of the complexes as determined by Singer and Campbell (1952) can be taken as completely valid. *The question now concerns the rôle of equilibrium processes in determining the composition of the final precipitate including that at optimal proportions.* Singer and Campbell (1953) observed that the various components in antigen excess must be in a very rapidly adjusted equilibrium. Otherwise, no resolution into separate peaks in the ultracentrifuge would have resulted. Reequilibration due to ultracentrifugal or electrophoretic fields, however, may have prevented determination of the exact distribution of the various species in the original equilibrium mixture, as Singer and Campbell pointed out.

The modern view of the nature of soluble complexes that go on to form turbid aggregates and finally stable precipitates would hold that since the forward reaction between antibody and antigen (hapten) is generally so much more rapid than the reverse reaction, build-up of soluble complexes would be expected. Aggregation, although less rapid than dissociation of soluble complexes, would therefore begin to take place. The dissociation of aggregates *into soluble complexes* would be less rapid than their formation so that eventually aggregate build-up would occur. Finally, binding and precipitation of aggregates would take place. In such a complex series of steps, an overall equilibrium would not be expected until precipitation had ceased, but even then readjustments in composition of the various precipitated components would be expected to occur before the most stable form of precipitate was reached and thermodynamic equilibrium was thereby established. It is clear that until intensive physicochemical measurements are made through the intelligent application of phase rule and phase diagrams, the nature of precipitate composition must remain in obscurity (Day, 1966).

By 1955 Singer and Campbell had evaluated a number of homogeneous solutions of antigen-antibody complexes. Through use of the electrophoretic technique by which free antigen could be measured, there was no longer a need for the iodinated antigens; both BSA and egg albumin (EA), because of their greater mobility and distinct separation from the complexes, could be easily determined. The difference between added BSA (or EA) and free BSA (or EA) gave the value for bound antigen. Assuming that all antibody was complexed, the ratio r of bound antigen molecules to bound antibody molecules could be determined.

The data were plotted in two ways: r vs. percentage of total antigen that was free, in the 1955 papers (Singer and Campbell, 1955a, b); and $1/r$ vs. $1/[Ag]$, in Singer (1957, 1965). $[Ag]$ was the concentration of free antigen divided by the concentration of total antigen; $1/[Ag]$ was therefore a reciprocal of the percentage. In the first plot, extrapolation to 100% free antigen (i.e., infinite antigen excess) gave r as 2, the valence of antibody. In the second plot (Fig. 8-3) extrapolation to the point where $1/[Ag]$ equated unity, i.e., where all antigen was again free, gave a value for $1/r$ of 0.5 and again a value of 2 for the valence of antibody. (In the 1955 plot the curve was also completed in the other direction to 0% free antigen, but an error in extrapolation was made since the ratio r of bound antigen to bound antibody was assumed to be 0 at 0% free antigen. At the point where there is no longer free antigen, the equivalence zone is entered, the ratio of bound antigen to bound antibody becomes that at the edge of the equivalence zone, and a value considerably greater than zero is obtained.)

4. The Goldberg equation

Goldberg (1952) developed a theory and an equation to unify the

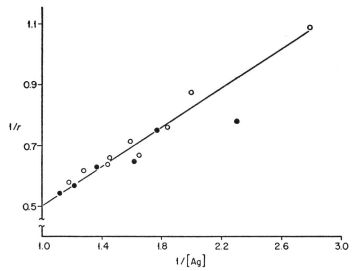

FIG. 8-3. Soluble complexes of bovine serum albumin (○) and egg albumin (●) with their respective antibodies in antigen excess. The parameter r is the number of moles of antigen bound per mole of antibody; $[Ag]$ is the concentration of free antigen divided by the concentration of total antigen in the solution. (From Singer, 1957.)

precipitation reaction from far antibody excess to far antigen excess. The derivation is considerably complex and there is not space here to set it down. Essentially, however, it is a distribution formula which takes into account at any point in composition the number of every kind of antigen-antibody combination as well as free antigen and/or free antibody. It requires knowledge of valence of antigen, the extent of the reaction, and composition of the total mixture.

m_{ik} = number of aggregates composed of i bivalent antibody and k f-valent antigen

fG = number of antigen sites (valence) per antigen times number of antigen molecules in system

$2A$ = number of antibody sites in whole system

fk = number of antigen sites in an aggregate

q = number of free antibody sites in an aggregate

p = fraction of antigen sites in system (fG) that have reacted (also called extent of reaction)

$r = fG/2A$ = ratio of antigen sites to antibody sites in system.

The distribution is written in simplified form without including univalent antibody (which is now unnecessary) and is the form used by Singer and Campbell (1953):

$$m_{ik} = fG \frac{(fk - k)!}{(fk - 2k + 2 - q)k!\, q!}$$

(8.17)

$$\cdot r^{k-1} p^{k+i-1}(1 - p)^{fk-k-i+1}(1 - pr)^{i-k+1}$$

The Heidelberger-Kendall precipitin equation (cf. Paragraph 2) was rewritten in terms of molarity and used the concept that $2R$ (where the ratio of antibody to antigen was at infinite antibody excess) was the effective antigen valence. Just as in infinite antigen excess antibody would be bound by antigen according to its valence (as shown by Singer and Campbell) so in infinite antibody excess antigen would be bound by antibody according to antigen valence, antibody reacting as if univalent. Therefore, since

$$2R = f$$

and

$$R^2/A = f^2/4A$$

it follows from the Heidelberger-Kendall equation that

$$A/G = f - f^2G/4A$$

(8.18)

The data from a number of papers in the literature that had been taken from experiments by Heidelberger and Kendall (1935d), Kabat and Heidelberger (1937), and Pappenheimer (1940) were converted to a mole to mole basis for antibody and antigen, and compared with calculated data from the Goldberg equation. (It can be seen that R, the ratio of bound antibody to bound antigen, is given by i/k, the number of aggregated bivalent antibodies over the number of aggregated f-valent antigens.) Two sets of data could be obtained from the Goldberg equation: maximal and critical ratios, i.e., those for the maximum extent of reaction (p_{max}) and those below which precipitation does not occur (p_c). The data for EA-anti-EA (a Heidelberger-Kendall experiment) that were considered by Goldberg (typical of several such experiments in the paper) are shown in Table 8-4. The agreement between the experimentally determined values, R, and the theoretical values, i/k, is remarkable. One must remember, however, that remarkable agreement between observed and calculated values were also obtained by Arrhenius (1907) even though his theoretical concept proved to be erroneous. Remarkable disagreement may disprove a theory, but remarkable agreement does not by the same token prove it.

It is natural that such a sweeping theory of the precipitation reaction, based on the distribution equation, should have its champions and its critics. All would agree, no doubt, that it does give a semiquantitative expression of the over-all precipitation reaction and the soluble aggregate formation, in spite of its drawbacks and shortcomings, and that it gives credence to Marrack's (1938) framework theory. Criticism centers mainly on the inability of the theory, based as it is upon homogeneous equilibria, to describe adequately and accurately phenomena that are based upon a two-phase system (minimally). In the antigen excess region *where a single phase system of*

TABLE 8-4

Theoretical and Experimental Values of Precipitate Ratios for EA-Rabbit Anti-EA

Experimental		Theoretical	
A/G	K	$(i/k)_{max}$	$(\bar{i}/k)_c$
21	3.9	4.0	
13	3.5	4.0	
7.6	3.3	4.0	3.5
4.8	2.9	4.0	2.8
3.8	2.7	3.7	2.5
2.9	2.4	2.6	2.2
2.6	2.3	2.3	2.0
2.3	2.1	2.1	1.9

(From Goldberg, 1952.)

homogeneous complexes in equilibrium can be established, the Goldberg equation has proved to be a powerful tool. Out of it has come an equation for calculating the intrinsic equilibrium constant between antigen and antibody that has proven extremely reliable (Singer, 1965, p. 307):

$$K_i = \frac{pM_A}{2C_A(1-p)\left(1 - p\,\dfrac{fC_GM_A}{2C_AM_G}\right)} \qquad (8.19)$$

where

K_i = intrinsic equilibrium constant in M^{-1}
p = fraction of antigen sites that have reacted
C_G = concentration of antigen in grams/liter
C_A = concentration of antibody in grams/liter
M_A = molecular weight of antibody
M_G = molecular weight of antigen
f = valency of antigen
2 = valency of antibody

5. Consequences of monogamous bivalent binding in precipitin reaction

From Chapter 5 we can obtain the equation that expresses the axiom of all immunochemistry—that at all times the number of bound antibody sites equals the number of bound antigen sites:

$$jbnA = lqsP \qquad (8.20)$$

where

A = number of antibody molecules
P = number of antigen molecules
n = antibody valence
s = antigen valence
b = fraction of antibody molecules bound
q = fraction of antigen molecules bound
j = fraction of antibody sites bound in bound antibody
l = fraction of antigen sites bound in bound antigen.

Monogamous bivalent binding means that at all times from equivalence to far antibody excess the fraction of antibody sites bound in bound antibody molecules

$$j = 1$$
$$n = 2$$

At far antibody excess also

$$q = 1$$
$$l = 1$$

Therefore,

$$2bA = sP_0 \tag{8.21}$$

and

$$\frac{b_0 A_0}{P_0} = \frac{s}{2} \tag{8.22}$$

But we have already defined bA/P as f in Scatchard derivations and

$$f_0 = \frac{s}{2} \tag{8.23}$$

Thus, we see that the so-called effective antigenic valence, traditionally designated f, is f_0, and that the true antigenic valence is $2f_0$. At equivalence

$$b = 1$$
$$j = 1$$
$$n = 2$$
$$q = 1$$

and

$$2A_e = lsP_e \tag{8.24}$$

The traditional designation of A_e/P_e from the Heidelberger-Kendall equation is R. Thus,

$$R = ls/2 \tag{8.25}$$

Under the conditions of the linear Heidelberger plot we know that $2R = f_0$, and that, therefore,

$$f_0 = ls$$
$$s/2 = ls$$
$$l = 1/2.$$

In other words, assuming monogamous bivalent binding, the condition for an ideal Heidelberger linear equation is that half the antigenic determinants be covered at equivalence and half empty. For highly multivalent antigens it is much more likely that many fewer than half the determinants are covered at equivalence; thus, the Heidelberger plot must deviate and curve upward. The value l will range from its low value at equivalence to one at far antibody excess while the value b will range from one at equivalence to a low value at far antibody excess. How these two quantities vary essentially describes the shape of the precipitin curve in antibody excess regions.

It is interesting to note the parameters influencing the affinity constant at $l = 1/2$:

$$j = 1$$
$$n = 2$$
$$q = 1$$

$$K_{12} = \frac{lqsP}{(nA - bnA)(sP - slP)} \tag{8.27}$$

$$= \frac{l}{(2A - 2bA)(1 - l)} \tag{8.28}$$

$$= \frac{l}{2A(1 - b)(1 - l)} \tag{8.29}$$

When

$$l = 1/2$$
$$K_{12} = \frac{1}{2A(1 - b)} = \frac{1}{2aA} \tag{8.30}$$

If one could establish with reasonable certainty that point in the precipitin reaction, near equivalence, at which half the antigenic determinants were covered, and had a means of measuring free antibody molecules at that point, e.g., ^{125}I-antibody in supernatant fluids, one would have an automatic measure of the equilibrium constant.

The molar ratio of antibody to phage particles in Figure 7-16c (p. 294), taken from Rowlands (1967), shows the typical curve upward to a much higher f_0 than twice the R value at equivalence. Monogamous bivalent binding was assumed in that discussion and it was calculated that $s = 2f_0$ 180, the approximate subunit valence of the phage particle. The curvilinear Heidelberger plot obtained by Rowlands was very similar to the one obtained by Rappaport (1957) for TMV virus.

In the case of soluble macromolecular proteins it is a matter of chance whether linearity or a curvilinear plot is obtained. Fritz, Lassiter, and Day (1967a) obtained precipitin curves with ^{125}I-labeled porcine fibrinogen and ^{131}I-labeled rabbit γG anti-fibrinogen (Fig. 8-4), and found that linear Heidelberger plots of the precipitin data could be constructed (Fig. 8-5). The fibrinogen in that assay was purified through a mild salting-out procedure. Fibrinogen,

purified after an initial cold ethanol precipitation as fraction I, contained a much more open structure and, as might be expected,
exhibited a much higher valency. At equivalence the same number
of molecules were involved in precipitation in both fibrinogens, but
since the value l was considerably lower in the latter at equivalence
the consequence was a curvilinear plot from the precipitin reactions
with four different antibody preparations (Figs. 8-6 and 8-7).

The iodination of the antibody γG in each of the four antibody
preparations with varying amounts of iodine reagent caused a decrease in the effective antigenic valences, f_0, with increasing ratios
of iodine atoms per mole γG (Fig. 8-8) but did not lower the values of
f at equivalence (Fritz, Lassiter, and Day, 1967b). Heterogeneity of
antibody populations was thereby displayed since, if a single form of
antibody were the only one progressively destroyed, there would have
been no change in f_0 at infinite antibody excess and the curves would
have extrapolated to the same point. The slopes would have changed
instead in the same way as obtained by dilution to weaker antibody
titers.

The effect of iodination upon the precipitibility could have been
directed against the secondary effects leading to aggregation rather
than upon primary binding. To test for this possibility, the antibodies
were also adsorbed with fibrin as a natural immunoadsorbent, and the
same sensitivity to iodination was displayed in the primary binding

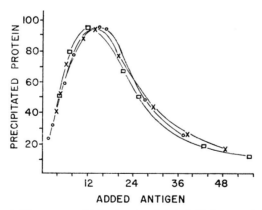

Fig. 8-4. Precipitin curves obtained using labeled fibrinogen, labeled antibody,
and paired labeling on both fibrinogen and antibody: (O) labeled antigen; (□)
labeled antibody; (×) paired labeling. Antigen was DFN, globulin was anti-DFN
(#68), and data were corrected for variations in antibody concentrations. Each precipitin tube contained 1 mg γ-globulin dissolved in a 0.5-ml volume. Units of both ordinate
and abscissa are in terms of micrograms of protein. (From Fritz, Lassiter, and Day,
1967a.)

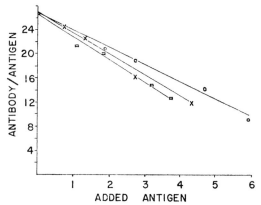

FIG. 8-5. Plots of data obtained from antibody excess regions of precipitin curves in Figure 8-4: (○) labeled fibrinogen; (□) labeled antibody; (×) paired label. Antigen was DFN, globulin was anti-DFN (#68). Molar ratios based on molecular weights of 160,000 for γ-globulin and 330,000 for porcine fibrinogen. Units of abscissa are 10^{-5} μmoles of protein. (From Fritz, Lassiter, and Day, 1967a.)

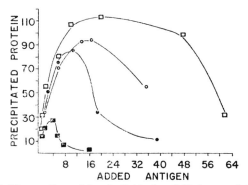

FIG. 8-6. Precipitin reactions of four individual anti-fibrinogen globulins with LFN: (○) globulin 68; (●) globulin 78; (□) globulin 98; (■) globulin 108. Units of both ordinate and abscissa are in terms of micrograms of protein. (From Fritz, Lassiter, and Day, 1967a.)

leading to adsorption (Fig. 8-9). The individuality of each antibody γG was preserved, #38 exhibiting extreme sensitivity to low iodine/antibody ratios and #98 exhibiting considerably less sensitivity.

The biphasic nature of the adsorption curves was interpreted as additional evidence of antibody heterogeneity, one population particularly sensitive and the other not so much. The proportions of each population in the individual antisera obviously varied and antiserum #38 seemed particularly rich in the iodine-sensitive type.

Interestingly enough, as the values of f_0 decreased in the precipitin reaction while the values of f_e remained relatively constant with in-

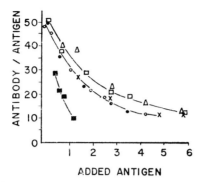

FIG. 8-7. Plots of data from antibody excess regions of precipitin curves obtained using four individual antifibrinogen globulins: (O) globulin 68; (●) globulin 78; (□) globulin 98; (■) globulin 108; (×) globulin 68 + normal pig serum; (△) globulin 98 + normal pig serum. Units of abscissa are 10^{-5} μmoles of protein. (From Fritz, Lassiter, and Day, 1967a.)

creasing iodination the effect was to approach the conditions for a linear Heidelberger plot (Table 8-5). In order to obtain estimates of the values for f_0 from the curvilinear Heidelberger plots, the relation $\log f$ vs. P was used (Fig. 8-10).

6. Further effects of radioiodination on antibody activity

The popularity of iodination of antibody results from its chemical simplicity of reaction, the ease of incorporation of radioactivity into the antibody molecule through the use of radioiodine, and the selectivity of tyrosine as its main (though by no means sole) target of attack. The difficulty of ascribing loss of antibody activity to iodination of a tyrosine within the active site can be readily understood when it is remembered that rabbit IgG contains 56 tyrosine residues per molecule (molecular weight of 160,000), and that, therefore, a total of 112 atoms of iodine could be incorporated before exhaustion of all tyrosine residues. It is true that surface tyrosines would be most amenable to attack and with them those that are near active site centers, but the heavy chain tyrosines that are most closely associated with combining site activity may escape iodination that heavily attacks light chain tyrosines.

In addition to the 56 tyrosines there are also 16 histidines, 14 methionines, and 20 tryptophans that can react with iodine, and long before all tyrosines become exhausted many of these other residues will become involved.

The data of Koshland, Englberger, and Gaddone (1965) answer one question negatively once and for all: Is tyrosine a universally essential amino acid for site activity? They prepared two different antihapten

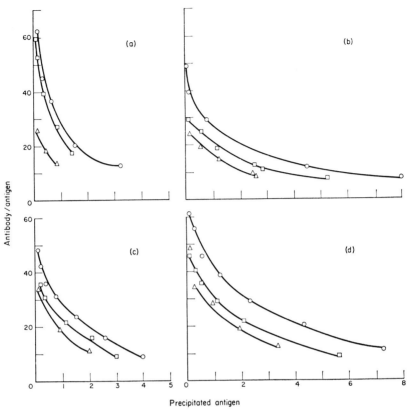

FIG. 8-8. Molar antibody/antigen ratios in antibody excess of four individual antibody globulins iodinated at various levels as a function of precipitated fibrinogen. Molecular weight of globulin assumed to be 160,00 and that of porcine fibrinogen to be 330,000. Units of abscissa are 10^{-5} μmoles. (*a*) Globulin 38 iodinated at 0.6 (O), 1.5 (□), and 3.8 (△) iodine atoms/globulin molecule. (*b*) Globulin 68 iodinated at 1.0 (O), 8.1 (□), and 13.0 (△) iodine atoms/globulin molecule. (*c*) Globulin 78 iodinated at 1.0 (O), 5.7 (□), and 10.7 (△) iodine atoms/globulin molecule. (*d*) Globulin 98 iodinated at 1.5 (O), 9.2 (□), and 16.4 (△) iodine atoms/globulin molecule. (From Fritz, Lassiter, and Day, 1967b.)

antibodies, one against *p*-azophenyltrimethylammonium ion (Apz) and the other against *p*-azophenylarsonate (Rpz). Anti-Apz antibody with an average of *140 iodine atoms* per molecule still retained 15% of its binding sites and 30% of its binding affinity even after treatment with 10 M urea for 3 hr to expose all available tyrosine groups. In contrast to this, anti-Rpz had lost all its activity by the time *60 iodine atoms* had been added (Fig. 8-11). Equilibrium dialysis measurements were made of the binding capacity of anti-Apz, and the familiar Scatchard plots of binding capacity against hapten concentration

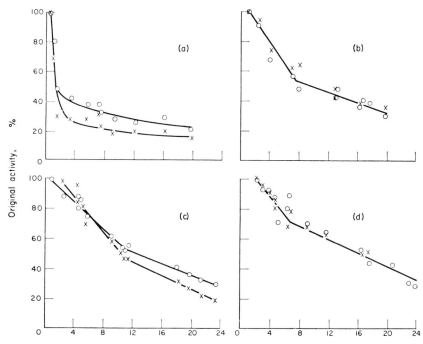

FIG. 8-9. Precipitin (×) and adsorption (○) activities of four individual anti-fibrinogen globulin preparations at various levels of iodination. Precipitin activity is taken as the percentage of globulin precipitated at equivalence and adsorption activity is the percentage of radiolabeled globulin adsorbed to an excess of insoluble fibrin after correction for nonspecific uptake. (a) Globulin 38, (b) globulin 68, (c) globulin 78, and (d) globulin 98. (From Fritz, Lassiter, and Day, 1967b.)

gave the typical Karush-type curves (Fig. 8-12).

The data of Johnson, Day, and Pressman (1960) on the effect of iodination on antibody activity are not so simply interpretable, the reason being that precipitation and other complicated systems were used as the basis of measurement: precipitation of egg albumin and BSA, hemolysis of red cells, *in vitro* binding of radioiodinated antibody to red cells, and *in vivo* binding of radioiodinated antibody to rat kidney and liver were used. Only one thing was clear: that levels of iodination over an average of *two* iodine atoms per molecule resulted in progressive loss of precipitating activity with 50% loss occurring in most instances if only an average of eight were introduced and essentially 100% loss at a level of 30 atoms per molecule (Fig. 8-13). The application of the results to trace labeling with radioactive iodine was apparent, indicating that certain precipitating and absorption systems could be followed equally well with classical or radioactive methods of measurement as long as no more than two atoms of iodine

TABLE 8-5

Effect of Iodination of Anti-Fibrinogen Globulins on Molar Antibody/Antigen Ratios at Equivalence and Infinite Antibody Excess

Antiserum Globulin	Iodine Atoms/ Molecule γG	f_e	f_0	l
38	1.5	10.3	62	0.17
	3.8	11.6	31	0.37
	9.5	8.5	22	0.39
68	1.5	12.4	48	0.27
	8.1	7.9	29	0.27
	13.0	8.9	22	0.40
	16.1	9.8	18	0.54
78	1.0	11.7	38	0.31
	5.7	11.3	34	0.30
	10.4	11.2	27	0.30
	10.7	11.0	27	0.41
98	1.5	15.7	57	0.28
	9.2	14.6	41	0.36
	11.6	14.6	38	0.38
	17.5	13.9	34	0.39

f_0 = moles Ab/moles Ag at infinite Ab excess, obtained by extrapolation of log (Ab/Ag) vs. Ag to Ag = 0; f_e = moles Ab/moles Ag at mid-point of equivalence; l = fraction of total antigen sites that are occupied at equivalence, monogamous bivalent binding of antibody assumed.

(Data from Fritz, Lassiter, and Day, 1967b.)

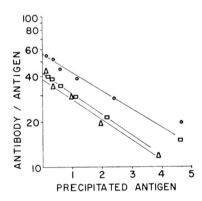

FIG. 8-10. Logarithm of molar antibody/antigen ratios (i.e., f) in antibody excess of anti-fibrinogen globulin 98 as a function of precipitated fibrinogen (i.e., P). Levels of iodination: 1.5 (O), 9.2 (□), and 16.4 (△) iodine atoms/molecule γG. (From Fritz. Lassiter, and Day, 1967b.)

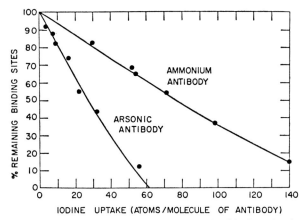

FIG. 8-11. Effect of iodination on the number of effective binding sites in ammonium and arsonic antibodies. (Koshland, Englberger, and Gaddone, 1965.)

were introduced per antibody molecule.

Since primary binding of Apz by anti-Apz antibodies was so insensitive to iodination in assays of Koshland *et al.*, it followed that a precipitin reaction involving Apz haptenic determinants in a carrier protein should also be iodine insensitive with respect to antibody. Fritz, Lassiter, and Day (1968) raised antibodies against Apz coupled to porcine fibinogen and tested them for precipitin reactivity with Apz-bovine γG. The results showed that the precipitins from two of three rabbits were indeed quite iodine insensitive. A third, however, was particularly iodine sensitive, and when checked by equilibrium dialysis, was found to decrease in activity with increasing ratios of iodine per molecule of γG. The report of Grossberg, Radzimski, and Pressman (1962) conflicted, with respect to anti-Apz iodine sensitivity, with that of Koshland, Englberger, and Gaddone (1965). The conflict can now be seen to reflect differences in rabbit responses to the ammonium hapten—most often raising antibodies insensitive to iodination, occasionally raising a different population.

Overall one would judge that the study of the precipitin reaction as a means of probing primary binding phenomena leaves much to be desired. Yet it needs to be understood for itself since it does stand at the focus of so much immunochemical information.

7. Fluorescence polarization in the measurement of binding in multivalent systems

The risk one takes in measuring macromolecule interaction by ultracentrifugal, electrophoretic, and viscosimetric techniques is

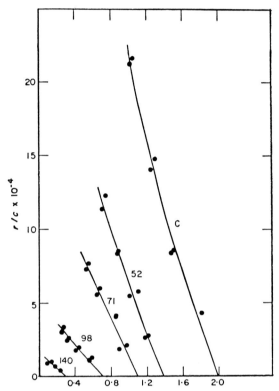

FIG. 8-12. Scatchard plot, r/c vs. r showing the effect of iodination on the binding activity of ammonium antibody. The parameter r is the number of hapten molecules bound per molecule of antibody. The parameter c is the concentration of free hapten at equilibrium. *Curve C* represents untreated antibody. The *numbers* beside the remaining curves represent the atoms of iodine substituted per molecule of antibody. Percentage of remaining antibody activity after iodination can be calculated by dividing $r \times 100$ (at $r/c = 0$) by 2.0. (From Koshland, Englberger, and Gaddone, 1965.)

that conformational structures important to the interaction may be distorted by such hydrodynamic changes. Dandliker and his colleagues (reviewed by Dandliker and de Saussare, 1970) chose the technique of fluorescence polarization to circumvent this problem. By so doing they also opened the door to what may become the most central unambiguous technique for the study of multivalent-antigen-multivalent-antibody interaction. In essence if one has a ligand that is labeled with a fluorescent compound and interacts the ligand with a receptor (antibody, enzyme, etc.) the complex that is formed will fluoresce polarized light to a much greater extent that the unbound form. The "frozen assembly of isotropic molecules" will always give rise to much greater intensity of polarized light than a "randomly oriented assembly of molecules free to rotate and non-isotropic."

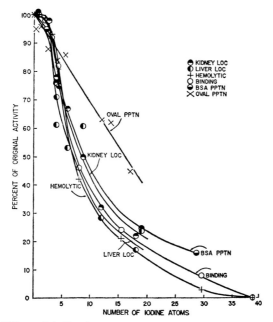

FIG. 8-13. Effect of iodination on antibody activity. Ordinate is percentage of original activity which remains after iodination. Abscissa is the average number of iodine atoms per 160,000 molecular-weight unit of rabbit IgG. The antifibrinogen antibodies shown in Figure 8-8 retained 20% activity even in the most sensitive cases. (From Johnson, Day, and Pressman, 1960.)

It holds that the molar concentrations of the free and bound forms of fluorescent ligand, F_f and F_b, are related to the molar fluorescence intensity, Q and polarization p by the equation

$$\frac{F_b}{F_f} = \frac{Q_f}{Q_b}\frac{(p - p_f)}{(p_b - p)} = \frac{Q_f - Q}{Q - Q_b} \qquad (8.31)$$

The law of mass action applies and, for nonuniform binding sites, the Sips distribution of binding energies closely approximates reality; therefore, one can easily derive the Sips form of the Law in terms of fluorescence intensities of the free and bound forms:

$$\log F_f \log = (1/a)\left(\frac{F_b}{F_{max} - F_b}\right) - \log K_0 \qquad (8.32)$$

The addition of nonfluorescent competing ligand N_b changes the equation to

$$\log F_f = (1/a)\log\left(\frac{F_b}{F_{max} - F_b - N_b}\right) - \log K_0 \qquad (8.33)$$

One recognizes in these Dandliker equations a rearrangement of the Sips equation

$$\log \frac{r}{n-r} = a \log c + a \log K_0 \tag{8.34}$$

$$\log c = (1/a) \log \left(\frac{r}{n-r}\right) - \log K_0 \tag{8.35}$$

By means of fluorescence polarization Dandliker, Schapiro, Meduski, Alonso, Feigen, and Hamrick (1964) found, for example, that when the fluorescent dye, fluorescein, reacted with anti-fluorescein the equilibrium constant ($K_0 = 5.4 \times 10^6$ M^{-1}) was nearly two orders of magnitude lower than the equilibrium constant for fluorescein-ovalbumin conjugate in its interaction with anti-fluorescein ($K_0 = 2.11 \times 10^8$ M^{-1}). A summary of equilibrium and heterogeneity constants for a number of fluorescent ligands (Table 8–6) and their corresponding antibodies and Fab fragments reveals the range of the fluorescence polarization technique that has already been explored.

That the kinetics of macromolecular antigen-antibody interaction can also be followed by fluorescence polarization was shown by Dandliker and Levison (1968). The work of Levison, Kierszenbaum, and Dandliker (1970) on the effect of chaotropic ions on antigen-antibody interaction (cf. Chapter 4) also involved the same technique. For the rate equation

$$\left(\frac{dp}{dt}\right)_0 = \frac{Q_b}{Q_f}(p_b - p_f)k(A)_0{}^{N_1}(P){}^{N_2-1} \tag{8.34}$$

where

$$p = \text{polarization}$$
$$t = \text{time}$$
$$Q = \text{fluorescence intensity}$$
$$k = \text{empirical rate constant}$$
$$A = \text{molar antibody concentration}$$
$$P = \text{molar antigen concentration}$$
$$N_1 = \text{order of reaction with respect to } A$$
$$N_2 = \text{order of reaction with respect to } P$$

To obtain forward and reverse reaction rate constants (k_1 and k_2, respectively) an integrated equation is obtained in which log ($p_e - p$) vs. t is linear (p_e, equilibrium value; p, instantaneous value):

$$\log (p_e - p) = \log (p_e - p_f) - \left(\frac{k_1(A)^{N_1} + k_2}{2.3}\right)t \tag{8.35}$$

TABLE 8-6

Affinity and Heterogeneity Constants Obtained by the Method of Fluorescence Polarization

Ligand	Antibody	K_0	a
		M^{-1}	
Fluorescein-ovalbumin (FO)	anti-FO	2.1×10^8	0.84
Fluorescein-ovalbumin	anti-O	1.8×10^8	0.65
Fluorescein-ovalbumin	anti-FO Fab	2.6×10^8	1.0
Dansylated-bovine serum albumin	anti-BSA	2.0×10^8	0.61
Bovine serum albumin (BSA)*	anti-BSA	3.4×10^8	0.83
Fluorescein hapten	anti-FO	8.0×10^6	0.54
Fluorescein hapten	anti-FO Fab	8.0×10^7	0.62
Fluorescent penicilloyl hapten	anti-P-RSA	9.0×10^6	0.71
Fluorescent penicilloyl hapten	anti-P-hemocyanin	4.7×10^7	0.73

* Determined as competitor of dansylated-BSA by Equation 8.33.
(From Dandliker and de Saussure, 1970.)

The slope changes with varying antibody concentration and the plot of slope vs. A (as long as N_1 is first-order, i.e., one) is also linear so that

$$\frac{d \log (p_e - p)}{dA} = -k_1 \tag{8.36}$$

when $N_1 = 1$. The intercept is k_2, the slope is k_1. Within the range of antibody concentrations in which N_1 could be designated either as first order or pseudo-first order, Dandliker and Levison (1968) found that fluorescein-ovalbumin interacted with antiovalbumin at the rate of $k_1 = 2 \times 10^5$ M^{-1} sec^{-1} and dissociated at the rate of $k_2 = 1 \times 10^{-3}$ sec^{-1}. The overall equilibrium constant was very close to that obtained previously by strict equilibrium measurements: $K_{12} = k_1/k_2 = 2 \times 10^8$ M^{-1}.

Dandliker and de Saussure (1970) have stated that "to extend the usefulness of fluorescence polarization into many interesting areas where it is desired to quantify antigens, it would be necessary to label the antibody." Since fluorescent-labeled antibodies and Fab are so readily available, as they pointed out, the studies need only to be made. One should imagine that for such work with univalent fluorescent Fab the following equations would then apply:

$$\log \left(\frac{f}{n - f} \right) = a \log d + a \log K_0 \tag{8.37}$$

$$\log d = (1/a) \log \left(\frac{f}{n - f} \right) - \log K_0 \tag{8.38}$$

$$\log F_f = (1/a) \log \left(\frac{F_b}{F_{max} - F_b} \right) - \log K_0 \qquad (8.39)$$

where equation (8.37) is the parallel Sipsian form described in Chapter 5 and where F_b and F_f are bound and free forms of fluorescent Fab. It can be seen that equation (8.39) is identical to that of equation (8.32). The rate equations also apply except that now equation (8.35) becomes

$$\log (p_e - p) = \log (p_e - p_f) - \left(\frac{k_1(P)^{N_2} + k_2}{2.3} \right) t \qquad (8.40)$$

First order or pseudo-first order must now be established for the ligand or antigen concentration P rather than for antibody concentration A.

8. Fluorescence quenching

By following the molar fluorescence of fluorescein-conalbumin conjugate in its interaction with varying concentrations of anti-fluorescein-conalbumin, Tengerdy (1966) was able to establish the points at which maximum fluorescence was obtained, an index of bound ligand. From these data it was possible to obtain Scatchard plots (Fig. 8-14) showing the heterogeneous binding that occurred at different antibody levels. An association constant of 4.7×10^7 M^{-1} was obtained.

9. Primary binding vs. precipitin reactions

It must be obvious by now that the principal means of studying antigen-antibody interaction is essentially a partitioning technique by which free and bound forms of either added antibody or added antigen can somehow be measured. Equilibrium dialysis partitions free hapten from the bound form; equilibrium filtration partitions free antibody from the bound; ultracentrifugal techniques sediment the complexes faster than the unbound antigen or antibody; precipitin reactions separate insoluble aggregated complexes from soluble components; solid-phase column or bulk adsorption of antibodies by immunoadsorbents separate specific from nonspecific entitites. Of the above reactions only one is a dependent secondary process subsequent to primary binding, and that one is the precipitin reaction.

Another technique of measuring primary binding is the preferential salting-out of complexes by half-saturated ammonium sulfate, leaving unbound antigen in solution (γG precipitates at this concentration). Singer and Campbell (1951, 1952) introduced the technique to sepa-

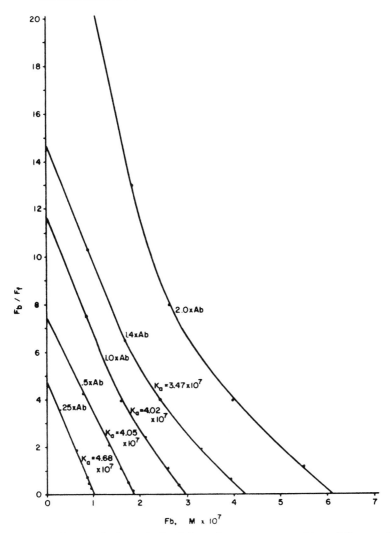

FIG. 8-14. Scatchard plots obtained from fluorescence quenching of fluorescein-conalbumin by anti-fluorescein-conalbumin. $1.0 \times Ab$ = 0.146 mg/ml. (From Tengerdy, 1966.)

rate BSA-anti-BSA complexes from BSA (cf. Paragraph 3) and Farr (1958) showed how it could be used as a quantitative measure by the partitioning of radioactive antigen between the soluble free and insoluble bound phases. Minden, Reid, and Farr (1966), Farr and Minden (1968), and Minden, Anthony, and Farr (1969) have since extended the technique and presented comparative data on its superior quantitative performance over six other primary binding techniques.

The procedure is limited, of course, to antigens not precipitable by half-saturated ammonium sulfate (HSAS), but this includes a great many. A particularly interesting study was that of Wold, Young, Tan, and Farr (1968) on the formation of antibody deoxyribonucleic acid (DNA) complexes that would precipitate from HSAS, leaving free DNA in solution.

The radioimmunoassay technique has been particularly important in the detection and evaluation of small peptidal hormones such as angiotensin (Sundsfjord, 1970), thyrotropin (Freychet, Rosselin, and Dolais, 1968), human growth hormone (Hunter and Greenwood, 1962), and gastrin (Yip and Jordon, 1970). In the last mentioned, for example, rabbit-anti-porcine-gastrin-BSA antiserum of very high titer permitted the precipitation and measurement of less than $10\mu\mu g$ of natural gastrin in the presence of known microamounts of radio-iodinated synthetic gastrin. Midgley, Niswender, and Rebar (1969) and Midgley, Rebar, and Niswender (1969) have critically reviewed the radioimmunoassay techniques and discussed in particular the minimum criteria for specificity and freedom from interference by unwanted   substances.

Steensgaard and Hill (1970) made a particularly intriguing study of ^{131}I-labeled human serum albumin (^{131}I-HSA) and anti-HSA antibodies at various regions of antigen excess from low to high, and employed a rate-zonal centrifugation procedure that placed complexes at various places in a weak isokinetic gradient according to sedimentation properties (Fig. 8-15).

Not only soluble macromolecules but insoluble particulate materials of uniform density can be investigated if isopycnic-zonal procedures are employed. Viruses and subcellular particulate fractions, for example, will float at particular densities in density gradients. Fritz and Beard (1969) in one study showed how BAI-anti-BAI virus complexes would distribute in linear fashion according to complex density and antibody-virus ratio (Fig. 8-16). In the Fritz-Beard assay the increased density contribution of the bound γG to the complex caused the virus to move to denser isopycnic flotation densities. If radioiodinated antibody is used in trace amounts to tag particulate matter it does not affect the final isopycnic flotation density of the particles and can be used under those conditions as an indicator of specificity or cross-reactivity (Day, 1968; Day and Lassiter, 1969).

10. Derivation of equilibrium and heterogeneity constants from precipitin curves

Steiner and Eisen (1965) tested a series of anti-dinitrophenyl

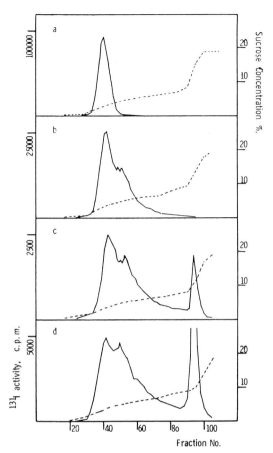

FIG. 8-15. Rate-zoning of HSA-anti-HSA complexes in a B-XIV rotor with an isokinetic gradient: (a) Nonreacted ^{131}I-HSA, 4.4S; (b) ^{131}I-HSA purified monomer in far antigen excess with anti-HSA; Singer complexes Ag_2Ab and Ag_3Ab_2 appear as 9S and 11S; (c) in moderate antigen excess a 30S component also appears; (d) near equivalence in antigen excess the 30S component predominates. (From Steensgaard and Hill, 1970.)

(DNP) antibodies, graded according to binding affinity, for their ability as precipitins to react with DNP-HSA. According to equilibrium dialysis and fluorescence quenching methods the equilibrium constants ranged from less than 10^6 M^{-1} for sera obtained at 10 days after immunization to more than 10^7 M^{-1} for sera obtained 8 weeks after immunization. The precipitin and Heidelberger plots obtained with four such antisera are shown in Figure 8-17. It can be seen that the "effective antigenic valence," f, increased with time (as did the system described in Table 8-2) and that this effect was a

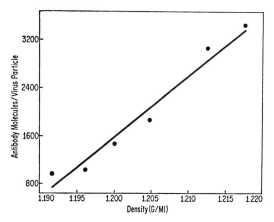

FIG. 8-16. Equilibrium density of BAI-anti-BAI virus complexes in a potassium tartrate gradient after centrifugation for 2 hr at 131,000 × G in an SW-50 rotor. Density of virus alone was 1.176 gm/ml; density of ^{125}I-γG was 1.381 gm/ml but the unbound ^{125}I-γG remained at or near the origin of 1.120 gm/ml while the bound ^{125}I-antibody moved with the virus. (From Fritz and Beard, 1969.)

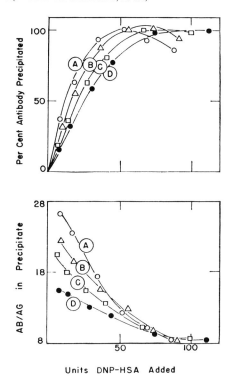

FIG. 8-17. Precipitin reactions of DNP-HSA with rabbit antisera obtained after a single injection of 2 mg of DNP-BγG in complete Freund's adjuvant. Units DNP-HSA

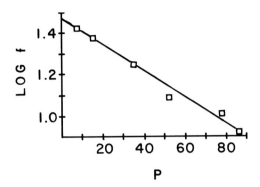

FIG. 8-18. Precipitin data of Steiner and Eisen (Fig. 8-17) transformed into Fritz-Lassiter-Day form. The intercept, 1.47, corresponds to an f_0 of 29.5 mg Ab/mg Ag or 15.7 moles Ab/mole Ag. The antigenic valence s is 31 if monogamous bivalent binding is assumed.

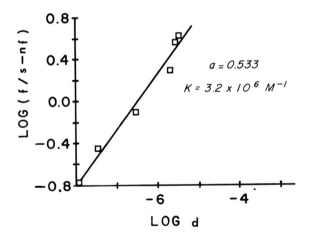

FIG. 8-19. Precipitin data of Steiner and Eisen (Fig. 8-17) transformed into Sipsian form using antigenic valence as obtained in Figure 8-18.

are expressed as milligrams of antigen added, normalized with respect to the maximum antibody precipitated. (*Upper*) Percentage of antibody precipitated vs. DNP-HSA added. (*Lower*) Weight ratio antibody:DNP-HSA in precipitate vs. DNP-HSA added. (*A*) Pooled sera 8 weeks, (*B*) 5 weeks, (*C*) 3 weeks, and (*D*) 10 days after immunization. (From Steiner and Eisen, 1965.)

function, in this case at least, of increasing affinity. When the data from the four plots of Figure 8-17 are transformed into terms of f (moles bound antibody/mole added antigen) and d (moles free antibody), Scatchard and Langmuir plots can be constructed.

Given a knowledge of antigenic valence, Sipsian plots can also be drawn to calculate association and heterogeneity constants. The data of the A plot in Figure 8-17 are shown graphically as $log\ f$ vs. P in Figure 8-18 where f is mg antibody bound/mg total antigen P in the system (i.e., bA/P). An intercept of 1.47 is obtained corresponding to 29.5 mg antibody per mg antigen. In molar terms this becomes 15.7 moles Ab/mole Ag. The antigenic valence s then becomes 31.4 by these calculations (assuming monogamous bivalent binding). The Sips plot (Fig. 8-19) was obtained from

$$\log \frac{f}{s - nf} = a \log d + a \log K_0$$

$$\log \frac{f}{31 - 2f} = a \log d + a \log K_0$$

A heterogeneity constant of 0.533 and an association constant of 3.2×10^6 M^{-1} were obtained. The problem of converting precipitin to equilibrium data rests in the fact that equilibria do not discriminate between what is soluble nonprecipitable complex and what is contained in the precipitate itself whereas most precipitin reactions pertain only to the latter. If soluble complex formation is suspect then transformation of data is not valid.

REFERENCES

Arrhenius, S. (1907). The precipitins and their antibodies. In *Immunochemistry*, Macmillan (New York, 309 pp.), pp. 263–299.

Burnet, F. M. (1931). The interactions of staphylococcus toxin anatoxin and antitoxin. J. Pathol. Bacteriol. *34:* 471–492.

Cooper, G., Edwards, M., and Rosenstein, C. (1929). The separation of types among the pneumococci hitherto called group therapeutic antiserums for those types. J. Exp. Med. *49:* 461–474.

Dandliker, W. B., and de Saussure, V. A. (1970). Fluorescence polarization in immunochemistry. Immunochemistry *7:* 799–828.

Dandliker, W. B., and Levison, S. A. (1968). Investigation of antigen-antibody kinetics by fluorescence polarization. Immunochemistry *5:* 171–183.

Dandliker, W. B., Schapiro, H. C., Meduski, J. W., Alonso, R., Feigen, G. A., and Hamrick, J. R., Jr. (1964). Application of fluorescence polarization to the antigen-antibody reaction. Immunochemistry *1:* 165–191.

Danysz, J. (1902). Contribution a l'étude des propriétés et de la nature des mélanges. Des toxines avec leurs antitoxines. Ann. Inst. Pasteur *16:* 331–345.

Day, E. D. (1966). *Foundations of Immunochemistry*, The Williams & Wilkins Co. (Baltimore, 209 pp.), pp. 132–145.

Day, E. D. (1968). Myelin as a locus for radioantibody adsorption in vivo in brain and brain tumors. Cancer Res. *28:* 1335–1343.

Day, E. D., and Lassiter, S. (1969). Multi-compartment distribution analysis of anti-brain radioantibodies in density gradients. J. Immunol. *103:* 550–555.

Farr, R. S. (1958). A quantitative immunochemical measure of the primary interaction between I*BSA and antibody. J. Infect. Dis. *103:* 239–262.

Farr, R. S., and Minden, P. (1968). The measurement of antibodies. Ann. N. Y. Acad. Sci. *154:* 107–114.

Freychet, P., Rosselin, G., and Dolais, J. (1968). Radioimmunological study of cross-reactions presented by human thyrotropin. In *Protein Polypeptide Hormones, Proceedings of the International Symposium, 1968*, Margoulies, M., ed., Excerpta Medica Foundation (Amsterdam, 1969), pp. 348–350.

Fritz, R. B., and Beard, J. W. (1969). Density of BAI strain A avian leukosis virus-antibody complexes relative to antigen-antibody ratio. J. Immunol. *102:* 1326–1329.

Fritz, R. B., Lassiter, S., and Day, E. D. (1967a). A quantitative precipitin study of porcine fibrinogen employing paired labels. J. Immunol. *98:* 1213–1217.

Fritz, R. B., Lassiter, S., and Day, E. D. (1967b). The effect of iodination on anti-fibrinogen antibodies with respect to precipitating and adsorption activities. Immunochemistry *4:* 283–293.

Fritz, R. B., Lassiter, S., and Day, E. D. (1968). The effect of iodination on the precipitin reaction. The anti-*p*-azophenyltrimethylammonium (anti-Ap) hapten system. Immunochemistry *5:* 557–565.

Goebel, W. F. (1935). Chemo-immunological studies on the soluble specific substance of pneumococcus. II. The chemical basis for the immunological relationship between the capsular polysaccharides of types III and VIII pneumococcus. J. Biol. Chem. *110:* 391–398.

Goldberg, R. J. (1952). A theory of antibody-antigen reactions. I. Theory for reactions of multivalent antigen with bivalent and univalent antibody. J. Am. Chem. Soc. *74:* 5715–5725.

Grossberg, A. L., Radzimiski, G., and Pressman, D. (1962). Effect of iodination on the active site of several antihapten antibodies. Biochemistry *1:* 391–401.

Heidelberger, M. (1939). Quantitative absolute methods in the study of antigen-antibody reactions. Bacteriol. Rev. *3:* 49–95.

Heidelberger, M. (1956). Chemical constitution and immunological specificity. Annu. Rev. Biochem. *25:* 641–658.

Heidelberger, M., and Avery, O. T. (1923). The soluble specific substance of pneumococcus. I. J. Exp. Med. *38:* 73–79.

Heidelberger, M., and Avery, O. T. (1924). The soluble specific substance of pneumococcus. II. J. Exp. Med. *40:* 301–316.

Heidelberger, M., Gaudy, E., and Wolfe, R. S. (1964). Immunochemical identification of the aldobiuronic acid of the slime of Sphaerotilus natans. Proc. Natl. Acad. Sci. *51:* 568–569.

Heidelberger, M., and Goebel, W. F. (1927). The soluble specific substance of pneumococcus. V. On the chemical nature of the aldobiuronic acid from the specific polysaccharide of Type III pneumococcus. J. Biol. Chem. *74:* 613–618.

Heidelberger, M., and Hobby, G. L. (1942). Oxidized cotton, immunologically specific polysaccharide. Proc. Natl. Acad. Sci. *28:* 516–518.

Heidelberger, M., and Kabat, E. A. (1937). Chemical studies on bacterial agglutination. III. A reaction mechanism and a quantitative theory. J. Exp. Med. *65:* 885–902.

Heidelberger, M., and Kabat, E. A. (1938). Studies on antibody purification. II. The

REACTIONS OF ANTIBODIES

dissociation of antibody from pneumococcus specific precipitates and specifically agglutinated pneumococci. J. Exp. Med. 67: 181–199.

Heidelberger, M., Kabat, E. A., and Shrivastava, D. L. (1937). A quantitative study of the cross reaction of Types III and VIII pneumococci in horse and rabbit antisera. J. Exp. Med. 65: 487–496.

Heidelberger, M., and Kendall, F. E. (1929). A quantitative study of the precipitin reaction between Type III pneumococcus polysaccharide and purified homologous antibody. J. Exp. Med. 50: 809–823.

Heidelberger, M., and Kendall, F. E. (1935a). The precipitin reaction between Type III pneumococcus polysaccharide and homologous antibody. II. Conditions for quantitative precipitation of antibody in horse sera. J. Exp. Med. 61: 559–562.

Heidelberger, M., and Kendall, F. E. (1935b). The precipitin reaction between Type III pneumococcus polysaccharide and homologous antibody. III. A quantitative study and a theory of the reaction mechanism. J. Exp. Med. 61: 563–591.

Heidelberger, M., and Kendall, F. E. (1935c). A quantitative theory of the precipitin reaction. II. A study of an azoprotein-antibody system. J. Exp. Med. 62: 467–483.

Heidelberger, M., and Kendall, F. E. (1935d). A quantitative theory of the precipitin reaction. III. The reaction between crystalline egg albumin and its homologous antibody. J. Exp. Med. 62: 697–720.

Heidelberger, M., and Kendall, F. E. (1936). Quantitative studies on antibody purification. I. The dissociation of precipitates formed by pneumococcus specific polysaccharides and homologous antibodies. J. Exp. Med. 64: 161–172.

Heidelberger, M., and Kendall, F. E. (1937). A quantitative theory of the precipitin reaction. IV. The reaction of pneumococcus specific polysaccharides with homologous rabbit antisera. J. Exp. Med. 65: 647–660.

Heidelberger, M., Kendall, F. E., and Scherp, H. W. (1936). The specific polysaccharides of types I, II, and III pneumococcus. A revision of methods and data. J. Exp. Med. 64: 559–572.

Heidelberger, M., Kendall, F. E., and Teorell, T. (1936). Quantitative studies on the precipitin reaction. Effect of salts on the reaction. J. Exp. Med. 63: 819–826.

Heidelberger, M., and Pedersen, K. O. (1937). The molecular weight of antibodies. J. Exp. Med. 65: 393–414.

Heidelberger, M., and Rebers, P. A. (1960). Immunochemistry of the pneumococcal types II, V, and VI. I. The relation of type VI to type II and other correlations between chemical constitution and precipitation in antisera to type VI. J. Bacteriol. 80: 145–153.

Heidelberger, M., Treffers, H. P., and Mayer, M. (1940). A quantitative theory of the precipitin reaction. VII. The egg albumin-antibody reaction in antisera from the rabbit and horse. J. Exp. Med. 71: 271–282.

Heymann, H., Manniello, J. M., and Barkulis, S. S. (1963). Structure of streptococcal cell walls. I. Methylation study of C-polysaccharide. J. Biol. Chem. 238: 502–509.

Hunter, W. M., and Greenwood, F. C. (1962). Preparation of iodine-131 labelled human growth hormone of high specific activity. Nature 194: 495–496.

Johnson, A., Day, E. D., and Pressman, D. (1960). The effect of iodination on antibody activity. J. Immunol. 84: 213–220.

Jones, J. K. N., and Perry, M. B. (1957). The structure of the type VIII pneumococcus specific polysaccharide. J. Am. Chem. Soc. 79: 2787–2793.

Kabat, E. A. (1939). The molecular weight of antibodies. J. Exp. Med. 69: 103–118.

Kabat, E. A. (1961). Kabat and Mayer's Experimental Immunochemistry, Ed. 2, Charles C Thomas (Springfield, Ill., 905 pp.).

Kabat, E. A., and Berg, D. (1953). Dextran—an antigen in man. J. Immunol. 70: 514–532.

Kabat, E. A., and Heidelberger, M. (1937). A quantitative theory of the precipitin reaction. V. The reaction between crystalline horse serum albumin and antibody formed in the rabbit. J. Exp. Med. 66: 229–250.

Kabat, E. A., and Pedersen, K. O. (1938). The molecular weights of antibodies, anti-Types I and III. Science 87: 372–373.

Klinman, N. R., Rockey, J. H., Frauenberger, G., and Karush, F. (1966). Equine anti-hapten antibody. III. The comparative properties of γG- and γA-antibodies. J. Immunol. 96: 587–595.

Koshland, M. E., Englberger, F. M., and Gaddone, S. M. (1965). Evidence against the universality of a tyrosyl residue at antibody combining sites. Immunochemistry 2: 115–125.

Levison, S. A., Kierszenbaum, F., and Dandliker, W. B. (1970). Salt effects on antigen-antibody kinetics. Biochemistry 9: 322–331.

Marrack, J. R. (1938). The Chemistry of Antigens and Antibodies, His Majesty's Stationery Office (London, 194 pp.), pp. 169–175.

Midgley, A. R., Jr., Niswender, G. D., and Rebar, R. W. (1969). Principles for the assessment of the reliability of radioimmunoassay methods (precision, accuracy, sensitivity, specificity). Acta Endocrinol. Suppl. No. 142, 163–184.

Midgley, A. R., Jr., Rebar, R. W., and Niswender, G. D. (1969). Radioimmunoassays employing double antibody techniques. Acta Endocrinol. Suppl. No. 142, 247–256.

Minden, P., Anthony, B. F., and Farr, R. S. (1969). A comparison of seven procedures to detect the primary binding of antigen by antibody. J. Immunol. 102: 832–841.

Minden, P., Reid, R. T., and Farr, R. S. (1966). A comparison of some commonly used methods for detecting antibodies to bovine albumin in human serum. J. Immunol. 96: 180–187.

Pappenheimer, A. M. (1940). Anti-egg albumin antibody in the horse. J. Exp. Med. 71: 263–269.

Rappaport, I. (1957). The antibody-antigen reaction. An hypothesis to account for the presence of uncombined antigenic sites in the presence of excess antibody. J. Immunol. 78: 246–255.

Rebers, P. A., and Heidelberger, M. (1961). The specific polysaccharide of type VI pneumococcus. II. The repeating unit. J. Am. Chem. Soc. 83: 3056–3059.

Reeves, R. A., and Goebel, W. F. (1941). Chemoimmunological studies on the soluble specific substance of pneumococcus. V. The structure of the type III polysaccharide. J. Biol. Chem. 139: 511–519.

Rowlands, D. T., Jr. (1967). Precipitation and neutralization of bacteriophage f2 by rabbit antibodies. J. Immunol. 98: 958–964.

Singer, S. J. (1957). Physical-chemical studies on the nature of antigen-antibody reactions. J. Cell. Comp. Physiol. 50: Suppl. 1, 51–78.

Singer, S. J. (1965). Structures and function of antigen and antibody proteins. In The Proteins, Ed. 2, Vol. III, Neurath, H., ed., Academic Press (New York, pp. 269–357), p. 291.

Singer, S. J., and Campbell, D. H. (1951). The valence of precipitating rabbit antibody. J. Am. Chem. Soc. 73: 3543–3544.

Singer, S. J., and Campbell, D. H. (1952). Physical chemical studies of soluble antigen-antibody complexes. I. The valence of precipitating rabbit antibody. J. Am. Chem. Soc. 74: 1794–1802.

Singer, S. J., and Campbell, D. H. (1953). Physical chemical studies of soluble antigen-antibody complexes. II. Equilibrium properties. J. Am. Chem. Soc. 75: 5577–5578.

Singer, S. J., and Campbell, D. H. (1955a). Physical chemical studies of soluble antigen-antibody complexes. III. Thermodynamics of the reaction between bovine serum albumin and its rabbit antibodies. J. Am. Chem. Soc. 77: 3499–3504.

Singer, S. J., and Campbell, D. H. (1955b). Physical chemical studies of soluble antigen-antibody complexes. V. Thermodynamics of the reaction between oval-bumin and its rabbit antibodies. J. Am. Chem. Soc. 77: 4851–4855.

Steensgaard, J., and Hill, R. J. (1970). Separation and analysis of soluble immune complexes by rate zonal ultracentrifugation. Anal. Biochem. 34: 485–493.

Steiner, L. A., and Eisen, H. N. (1965). The nature of antigen-antibody interactions. In Immunological Diseases, Samter, M., and Alexander, H. L., eds., Little Brown & Co. (Boston, 966 pp.). 122–130.

Sugg, J. Y., Gaspari, E. L., Fleming, W. L., and Neill, J. M. (1928). Studies on immunological relationships among the pneumococci. I. A. virulent strain of pneumococcus which is immunologically related to, but not identical with typical strains of type III pneumococci. J. Exp. Med. 47: 917–931.

Sundsfjord, J. A. (1970). Radioimmunoassay of angiotensin II in plasma. Acta Endocrinol. 64: 181–192.

Taylor, G. L. (1931). The results of some quantitative experiments on the serum precipitation reaction. J. Hyg. 31: 56–83.

Tengerdy, R. P. (1966). Equilibrium and kinetic studies of the reaction between conalbumin and anticonalbumin. Immunochemistry 3: 463–477.

Tiselius, A., and Kabat, E. A. (1938). Electrophoresis of immune serum. Science 87: 416–417.

Tiselius, A., and Kabat, E. A. (1939). An electrophoretic study of immune sera and purified antibody preparations. J. Exp. Med. 69: 119–131.

von Dungern, E. (1903). Bindungsverhältnisse bei der Präzipitinreaktion. Zentrralbl. Bakteriol. Orig. 34: 355–380.

Wold, R. T., Young, F. E., Tan, E. M., and Farr, R. S. (1968). Deoxyribonucleic acid antibody: a method to detect its primary interaction with deoxyribonucleic acid. Science 161: 806–807.

Yip, B. S. S. C., and Jordon, R. H., Jr. (1970). Radioimmunoassay of gastrin using antiserum to porcine gastrin. Proc. Soc. Exp. Biol. Med. 134: 380–385.

9

THE ACTIVE CENTERS OF
MULTIVALENT ANTIGENS

1. Serum albumins

Lapresle (1955) and, shortly thereafter, Porter (1957) began studies on the fragments of these most popular of all native antigens in order to determine the nature, variety, and position of the antigenic determinants, and, in particular, those determinants that distinguish between specificity and cross-reactivity. Lapresle, Kaminski, and Tanner (1959) obtained enzymatic split products of human serum albumin (HSA) which possessed different distributions of specific determinants and Lapresle and Webb (1964) found one fragment of 11,000 molecular weight which would inhibit but not precipitate with bivalent antibody; Lapresle and Webb (1965) then isolated another fragment, Fl, of 6600 molecular weight that contained no tyrosine or tryptophan, but did likewise inhibit whole anti-HSA antibody. The fragment, when coupled to p-aminobenzylcellulose (PAB-cellulose), acted as an immunoadsorbent and it would also induce antibody formation; however, anti-Fl would not precipitate human serum albumin (Lapresle and Goldstein, 1969). When F1 or HSA were conjugated to red blood cells anti-F1 would agglutinate the cells; when HSA was polymerized with gluteraldehyde, anti-F1 would precipitate the polymer; when F1 was conjugated to red cells by bis-diazotization or tanning processes, anti-F1 would not react. It was apparent, therefore, that the formation of precipitates between bovine serum albumin (BSA)-anti-BSA involved heterogeneous determinants one of which, F1, was present as a single active antigenic center. Homogenous antibody that was directed only against F1 would not form complexes greater than HSA-Ab-HSA and would not precipitate.

In this demonstration we find the main difference between multivalent antigens that have repeating determinants—cell-wall polysaccharides, dextrans, viruses, synthetic polymers, symmetric multichain macromolecules such as γG, etc.—and those multivalent antigens which are univalent with respect to each specificity.

2. Homogeneous antibodies among myeloma proteins that react with multivalent antigens

Metzger (1967) recognized the problem of univalent specificity determinants in searching for proteins that would interact with homogeneous myeloma immunoglobulins:

> " ... the very fact that an antibody is homogeneous may make its detection more difficult than the detection of heterogeneous antibodies. Many immunologic assays are highly dependent on the number of antigen-antibody cross-links that can form. A heterogeneous population of antibodies amplifies the valency of an antigen, thereby favoring such multiple interactions. Unless the antigen has repeating determinants, it can only be monovalent with respect to a homogeneous antibody. If the latter itself is only divalent (γG), the reaction may be much more difficult to observe than if the antibody is polymeric (γM). Even in the presence of repeating antigenic determinants, γM antibodies may show one thousand times as much activity as γG."

The Waldenstrom macroglobulin γM proteins were often found to possess reactivity for γG and would precipitate γG antigens in the classical manner of precipitins. Yet it was difficult to establish a valence for their interaction (Stone and Metzger, 1967). γM$_{LAY}$, for example, was found to be specific for the Fc portion of human γG, and confined its binding properties to its Fab portions. It had a defined and limited valence and had all the other characteristics of an antibody. The valence qeustion arose because the 18S protein, although composed of 10 Fab binding sites, would bind only 5 γG molecules; likewise, its 7S bivalent subunit would bind only one γG. Nearly 90% of the Fab fragments, however, were active, and, allowing for some loss in activity from fragmentation, all could be considered so. It later was established by means of the preparation of tryptic Fab$_{\mu}$ fragments (Stone and Metzger, 1968), a much gentler procedure, that indeed all Fab$_t$ units of γM$_{LAY}$ would bind with γG-Fc as established at high γG: Fab molar ratios. A Scatchard plot of ultracentrifugal data for the interaction of Fab$_{\mu\,LAY}$ with γG$_{WAR}$ revealed complete homogeneous binding (Fig. 9-1). The ultracentrifugal patterns determined that no more than one Fab would bind with γG at even high Fab: γG molar ratios (Fig. 9-2). A heterogeneity constant of 1.0 and an association constant of 6.2×10^4 M^{-1} described the homogeneous binding of the antibody. Of interest in the context of this chapter was the finding that each γG molecule or Fc fragment contained only one determinant site for Fab attachment. Steric hindrance appeared

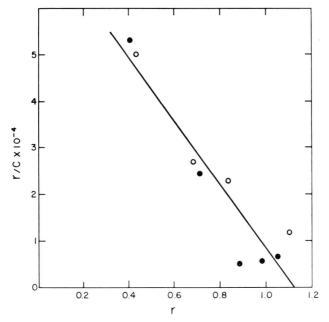

FIG. 9-1. Scatchard plot of ultracentrifugal data for the interaction of $Fab\mu_{Lay}$ with γG_{War}. Data plotted so as to give valence of the γG antigen: r = moles of $Fab\mu$ bound per mole γG; c = unbound $Fab\mu$ concentration. Solvent: 0.01 μ of PO_4-0.05 M NaCl, pH 6.0. Temperature: 20–25°C. (●) $Fab\mu$ unreduced; (○) $Fab\mu$ reduced. Line drawn by method of least squares. (From Stone and Metzger, 1968.)

to prevent the approach of more than one γG or Fc to each pair of binding sites in γM or γM_s; but monogamous bivalent binding was discounted because of the one-to-one binding relationship between Fab_μ and Fc_γ.

The determinant in γG was found not only in human but also in primate sources. The chimpanzee and baboon, of the same hominoid infraorder as man, and the rhesus monkey and crab-eating macaque, of cercopithecoid infraorder, all contained γG that reacted with γM_{LAY} as easily as human γG (Fig. 9-3). All ceboids and lemuriforms reacted either poorly or not at all. Two lorsiforms—the potto and the bushbaby—had globulins that would precipitate γM_{LAY} completely but would only compete as inhibitors for human γG to the extent of 20%.

Another interesting feature of the primate study was the comparative ease with which rabbit anti-human γG antibodies could be used to distinguish among the minor structural features of other primate globulins. The heterogeneous nature of the rabbit antisera with antibodies against a number of antigenic active centers (specificities)

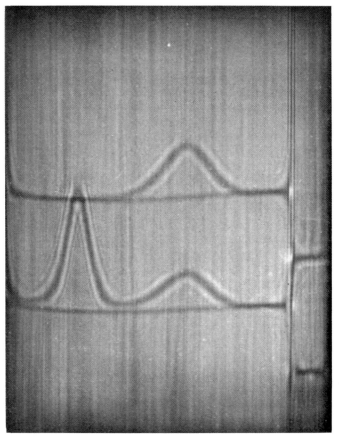

Fɪɢ. 9-2. Photograph of schlieren patterns obtained by sedimenting 1.38×10^{-4} M Fabμ (reduced) fragments in the presence (*lower cell*) and absence (*upper cell*) of 3.60×10^{-5} M human γG (γG $_{War}$). Solvent: 0.01 μ of PO$_4$-0.05 M NaCl, pH 6.0. Temperature: 22.3°C. Bar angle 60°. Picture taken 75 min after speed (56,000 rpm) reached. Area measurements indicated 30% binding. (From Stone and Metzger, 1968.)

made the selectivity possible. Directed as it was against a single anti-genic center that was univalent per γG molecule, the γM$_{LAY}$ anti-body reagent displayed singular stoichiometry and limited cross-reactivity. And the cross-reactivity was not due to mixed determi-nants but to a true energetic difference typical of cross-reacting haptenic analogs.

3. Conformational determinants

In their discussion of antigenic determinants Sela, Schechter, Schechter, and Borek (1967) distinguished clearly between *sequential*

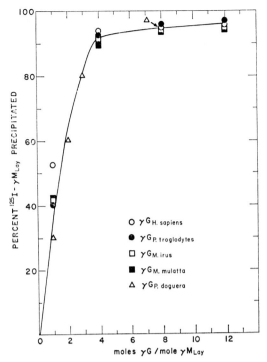

FIG. 9-3. Precipitation of γM_{Lay} by DEAE-purified γG from the higher anthropoids—man, chimpanzee, crab-eating macaque, rhesus monkey, and baboon. Two prosimians, the potto and the bushbaby (not shown) all precipitated as effectively. (From Stone and Metzger, 1969.)

and *conformational* determinants. An amino acid sequence in random coil form would be expected to raise antibodies that would react with peptides of identical or similar sequence. A conformational determinant that depended upon the steric conformation of an antigenic macromolecule would not necessarily react with peptides either derived from that area of the molecule or from similar sequential alignments. It was their opinion that most native proteins as antigens raised antibodies mostly against conformational rather than sequential determinants. They considered many of the antibodies in Lapresle's work to be directed against conformational structures of HSA, pointing out that large but not small peptides would inhibit most of the anti-HSA antibodies. It would not be unlikely that the γG determinant seen by γM_{LAY} was also conformational particularly since there was only one in a structure, Fc, that was dimeric in a sequential sense.

Bovine pancreatic ribonuclease depends for its native conformation upon the positions of its four disulfide bonds and upon hydrogen bonding. The disulfide bridges between residues 26–84, 40–95, 58–110, and 65–72 form a stabilized structure that in turn helps form a groove in the molecular surface, bounded by residues 7–11, 41–45, and 119–123. It is in the groove that the active site for cleavage of intranucleotide bonds of mammalian RNA is believed to reside. The sequential pattern of the single chain enzyme (Table 9-1) is considerably less revealing of the actual enzyme than the three-dimensional conformational model built up from X-ray crystallographic data, but the underlined residues in the sequence illustrate how far away the active site amino acids may be sequentially but how close three-dimensionally.

Brown, Delaney, Levine, and Van Vunakis (1959) prepared antibodies against the bovine ribonuclease (RNAase) enzyme and also against a modified form, RNase oxidized with performic acid, to produce a random coil devoid of disulfide bridges. They found that antibodies to native RNAase did not react with the random coil and that antibodies to the random coil did not react with the native RNase. The difference between conformational and sequential determinants was readily demonstrated by this one experiment and confirmed by Brown (1962) who showed that heterogeneous rabbit

TABLE 9-1

Bovine and Rat Ribonuclease Sequences Aligned for Maximum Homology

Species	Sequence						Residue Positions
Bovine	KE	TAAA*K*	*FERQ*H	MDSST	SAASS	SNYCN	(1–27)
Rat	GESRE	SSAD*K*	*FKRQ*H	MDTEG	PSKSS	PTYCN	(1–30)
Bovine	QMMKS	RNLTK	DRC*KP*	*VNT*FV	HESLA	DVQAV	(28–57)
Rat	QMMKR	QGMTK	GSC*KP*	*VNT*FV	HEPLE	DVQAI	(31–60)
Bovine	CSQKN	VACKN	GQTNC	YQSYS	TMSIT	DCRET	(58–87)
Rat	CSQGQ	VTCKN	GRDNC	HKSSS	TLRIT	DCRLK	(61–90)
Bovine	GSSKY	PNCAY	KTTQA	MKHII	VACEN	GPYVP	(88–117)
Rat	GSSKY	PNCTY	NTTNS	EKHII	IACDG	NPYVP	(91–120)
Bovine	V*HFDA*	SV					(118–124)
Rat	V*HFDA*	SV					(121–127)

Active site residues (bovine numbering): 7–11, 41–45, 119–123, in italics. Disulfide bridges (bovine numbering): 26 to 84, 40 to 95, 58 to 110, 65 to 72. (From Dayhoff, 1969, pp. D130-D131.)

Bovine sequence is that of Smyth, Stein, and Moore (1963); rat sequence, Beintema and Gruber (1967). See Dayhoff for these references and for additional information.

antibodies to the performic acid-oxidized RNase were specificially inhibited by sequential peptides 38–61, 40–61, and 105–124 from two different areas of the enzyme. Peptide 38–61 was most inhibitory. Mills and Haber (1963), after reducing RNase in 8 M urea, reoxidized the protein to form a mixture of molecules with disulfide bridges between the "wrong" pairs of cysteine residues, a "urox"-RNase. This newly conformed structure also reacted very poorly with antibodies to the native enzyme.

Wondering if all disulfide bridges were essential for RNase activity, Neumann, Steinberg, Brown, Goldberger, and Sela (1967) treated the enzyme in the absence of urea with phosphorothioate, a compound that selectively opened two of the four disulfide bridges. Both the native biological and the native immunological activities were preserved, but when the enzyme was further treated by the same mild reagent to open all bridges, enzyme activity was lost and cross-reactivity with antibodies against the native enzyme was drastically diminished.

Parallel to the studies on the active antigenic centers of native ribonuclease, which still remain to be pinpointed, has developed the very important immunochemical discipline concerned with antibodies to biologically active molecules (Cinader, 1967). Ribonuclease has been one of the central functional compounds in that study. Very early Branster and Cinader (1961) began an investigation of the mechanism by which anti-RNase affected RNase activity.

The inhibitory capacity of rabbit anti-RNase antiserum was established (Fig. 9-4) and the increase in this capacity with continued immunization over a period of a year was observed. During the intervening years it became suspected that not all antibodies were inhibitory, however, and finally Suzuki, Pelichova, and Cinader (1969) and Pelichova, Suzuki, and Cinader (1970) were able to separate chromatographically two populations of anti-RNase antibodies, one inhibitory of RNase and the other hyperactivating (Fig. 9-5). The two types of antibodies were partially competitive for each other and quite likely directed at least partially toward the same active antigenic center. There was no way to distinguish the possible presence of a third population in the activating antibody—one that would block inhibitory antibody binding but otherwise have no effect upon biological activity.

The overall neutralizing curve produced by a typical anti-RNase antiserum that contained both inhibiting and activating antibodies was viewed as dependent upon three factors: total antibody concentration with respect to antigen which would determine whether the system was in antigen or antibody excess; relative concentrations

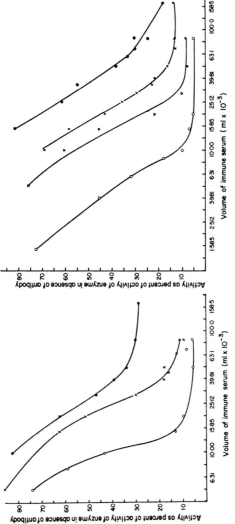

FIG. 9-4. Inhibition of bovine pancreatic RNase activity for RNA substrate by rabbit antibody. Increase in inhibitory activity with time. (*Left*) Rabbit serum #570, 5 days after first course of immunization (●); 110 days later, and 5 days after boosting (×); 356 days later and 5 days after boosting (○). (*Right*) Rabbit serum #619, 5 days (●), 33 days (×), and 252 days (○) after first course of immunization. (From Branster and Cinader, 1961.)

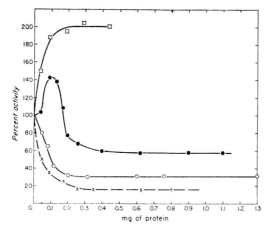

FIG. 9-5. Effect of two chromatographically separated rabbit anti-RNase antibody populations upon RNase activity. Activating (□); inhibiting (×); 1:1 mixture (●); 1:9 mixture of activating and inhibiting antibody (○). (From Pelichova, Suzuki, and Cinader, 1970.)

of the two (or three) types of antibodies; and binding affinity of each type with RNase determinants. Competition would depend upon concentration and upon the degree of reversibility of the antigen-antibody bonds. Ordinarily the enhancing capacity of activating antibody would be observed in zones of high antigen excess and would be reduced by the presence of inhibiting antibody. The product of affinity and free equilibrium concentration of reactants can thus be seen to be most critical in the final shape of the neutralization curve.

The idea of an activating antibody—actually a hyperactivation antibody—suggests that some native enzymes can be made better enzymes (at least more active) through the aegis of antibody binding. Does this mean that tertiary structures can be remodeled by antibody to assume conformations more amenable to substrate binding and catalysis? Pollock, who was the first to observe an activating enzyme (Pollock, 1963, 1964) in his work with penicillinases, thought that this might be the case. By preparing mutationally altered analogs of wild-type bacterial penicillinases Pollock, Fleming, and Petrie (1967) were able to test the effect of activating antibody upon a series of inactive mutein enzymes whose one-step structural-gene alterations were minimal (Fig. 9-6). It is not yet clear whether the clear-cut enzyme activation produced in the mutant penicillinases was due to specific conformational changes induced by complementation with antibody or stabilization of weakened tertiary structure. Either way the conformational nature of the antigenic determinants was proved.

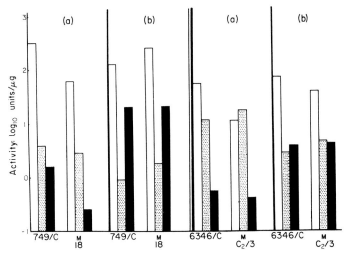

Fig. 9-6. Activation of mutant penicillinases with antibody. Wild-type penicillinases: 749/c and 6346/c. Mutant penicillinases: M18 from 749/c and $MC_2/3$ from 6346/c. (a) No antiserum, (b) specific anti-749/c antiserum added. *White bars* = benzylpenicillin substrate; *speckled bars* = benzylcephalosporin C substrate; *black bars* = methicillin substrate. Note almost identical activities of wild and mutant penicillinases in the presence of activating antibody. (From Pollock, Fleming, and Petrie, 1967.)

4. Two models of antigens with mixed conformational determinants and sequential determinants—lysozyme and sperm whale myoglobin

Crystalline egg-white lysozyme in solution will hydrolyze *Micrococcus lysodeikticus*, and tri-N-acetyl-ᴅ-glucosamine (tri-NAG) will inhibit the enzyme competitively. Antibodies against crystalline egg-white lysozyme will inhibit the enzyme by specific binding such that there is correlation between inhibition and degree of binding. However, as shown in Figure 9-7, when tri-NAG is first bound to the enzyme site the binding of antibody is diminished from 100% to only 60% (Von Fellenberg and Levine, 1967). Using 75% binding as the end point, antibody binding is cut to 30%, only 40% of its original capacity (Fig. 9-8). By this experiment two possibilities were open: (a) antibodies might be directed against amino acids in the active enzyme site, and (b) antibodies might be directed against native conformational determinants that are shifted in the presence of tri-NAG.

The investigators, having apprised themselves that the lysozyme-tri-NAG complex did produce conformational changes, if however small, whereas NAG did not produce such changes, then went on to show that antibody binding was unaffected by the presence of NAG.

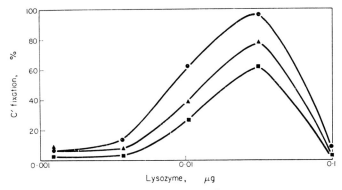

FIG. 9-7. Diminished binding of anti-lysozyme (1/13,000 dilution) with lysozyme in the presence of enzyme bound tri-NAG. No tri-NAG (●), 100 μg (▲), 300 μg (■). Binding was measured by the secondary technique of microcomplement fixation. (From Von Fellenberg and Levine, 1967.)

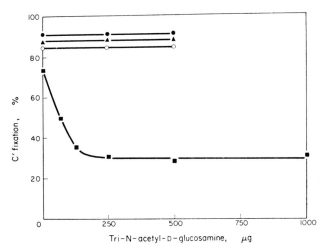

FIG. 9-8. Diminished binding of anti-lysozyme (0.03 μg lysozyme-anti-lysozyme, diluted 1/13,000) resulting from tri-NAG binding to lysozyme (■). Effect is specific. Controls: pepsinogen-anti-pepsinogen (●), ribonuclease-anti-ribonuclease (○), β-lactoglobulin-anti-β-lactoglobulin (▲). (From Von Fellenberg and Levine, 1967.)

They were, therefore, inclined to pinpoint the antigenic determinant as a conformational one at the left side of the well known cleft of the enzyme active center—the region that X-ray analysis had shown would tilt when closed (see Dayhoff, 1969, her figure 7-6). The cleft begins at a point between residues 37 and 114, proceeds to a region between residues 52 and 90, and terminates near residue 101 (see Table 9-2). It runs more or less vertically, almost bisecting the structure and involves, among others, the glutamic acid and aspartic

TABLE 9-2

Amino Acid Sequence of Chicken Egg-White Lysozyme Aligned for Maximum Homology with Sequence of Related Bovine Lactalbumin

Protein	Sequence						Residue Number
Lyso-zyme	KVFGR	CELAA	AMKRH	GLDNY	RGYSL	GNWVC	(1–30)
Lactal-bumin	EQLTK	CEVFR	ELK--	DLKGY	GGVSL	PEWVC	(1–28)
Lyso-zyme	AAKFE	SNFNT	QATNR	NTDGS	TDYGI	LQINS	(31–60)
Lactal-bumin	TTFHT	SGYBT	ZAIVZ	B-BZS	TBYGL	FZIBB	(29–57)
Lyso-zyme	RWW*CN*	*DGRTP*	*GSRNL*	*CNIPC*	*SALLS*	SDITA	(61–90)
Lactal-bumin	KIWCK	BBZBP	HSSBI	CNSIC	DKFLB	BBLTB	(58–87)
Lyso-zyme	SVNCA	KKIVS	DGDGM	NAWVA	WRNRC	KGTDV	(91–120)
Lactal-bumin	BMICV	KKIL–	DKVGI	NYWLA	HKALC	SEKLD	(88–116)
Lyso-zyme	QAWIR	GC–RL					(121–129)
Lactal-bumin	Q–WL–	–CEKL					(117–123)

Canfield and Liu (1965) sequence for lysozyme. Disulfide bonds are 6:127, 30:115, 64:80, and 76:94. Loop peptide 64–83 with disulfide bridge 64:80 is italicized. Glutamic and aspartic acids at 35 and 52 participate in stabilizing activated complex. Brew, Vanaman, and Hill (1967) sequence for lactalbumin. Protein contains 4 disulfide bonds.

(From Dayhoff, 1969, pp. D132-D133.)

acid residues 35 and 52 which participate in stabilizing the activated complex. A hexameric-NAG would stretch from one end of the cleft to the other.

Arnon (1968), realizing that rabbit anti-lysozyme antibodies actually were considerably heterogeneous with respect to lysozymal determinants, began fractionating the antibodies with respect to their different specificities. A loop peptide (Arnon and Sela, 1969) was eventually isolated which contained the residues 64–83 joined by cysteines 64:80 into a native cyclic structure. The peptide was, in essence, an isolated conformational determinant. Anti-loop antibodies which could be isolated either as a fraction from lysozyme-cellulose immunoadsorbents or as a specific entity from loop-cellulose immunoadsorbents, were shown to be able to distinguish between the intact loop and the open chain peptide derivative. They reacted with the former but not the latter. Arnon, Maron, Sela, and Anfinsen (1971) then went on to synthesize the conformationally dependent loop, conjugated it with poly (DL-alanyl)-poly(L-lysine), raised antibodies against it, and demonstrated specificity of the antibodies for the native conformational structure.

Gerwing and Thompson (1968) worked with an unlooped structure, the T-11 peptide, which stretched from asparagine residue #74 to the lysine residue #96, thus overlapping the sequence of Arnon but not containing the conformational structure. The peptide exhibited haptenic activity. Investigating further, Thompson and Levy (1970) prepared a synthetic decapeptide, NLCNIPCSAL, representative of residues 74–83, and showed that it was even more potent haptenically the larger T-11 peptide. That it terminated at the same place as the loop peptide of Arnon and Sela was aimed at suggesting the sequential nature of the loop peptide rather than its conformational structure. Thus, it was possible that this active antigenic center could select and raise both conformational-dependent and sequential-specific antibodies.

Young and Leung (1969, 1970) employed cyanogen bromide cleavage to obtain both N-terminal and C-terminal peptides 1–12 and 106–129. Both were immunologically active sequential determinants. On the other hand, Bonavida, Miller, and Sercarz (1969), by showing that CNBr-treated lysozyme would inhibit up to 70% binding of antilysozyme with native lysozyme, interpreted their findings as suggesting considerable retention of native conformation in the CNBr cleavage products. Habeeb and Atassi (1969) modified lysozyme by substituting 2-nitrophenyl sulfonyl chloride at the six tryptophan residues. The effect was to eliminate enzyme activity by hitting tryptophan in the active site as well as to induce conformational changes. Cross-reactivity with antibody against native enzyme was nil; immunogenicity was poor. Using carbamylation to modify lysozyme Strosberg and Kanarek (1970) determined that α-amino group substitution had little or no effect upon interaction with anti-native-enzyme antibodies whereas substitution upon the ϵ-amino groups of lysine altered the antigenic properties. With their particular antisera it was also found that CNBr cleavage products were much reduced in activity as were carboxymethylated derivatives that were modified at their methionine residues.

The overall view of lysozyme immunochemistry confirms the multiplicity of determinants originally suggested by Arnon (1968) and the presence among them of both conformational and sequential varieties. The need for homogeneous antibodies directed toward individual determinants is obvious to pursue the study of the immunochemical nature of the enzyme much further. Particularly nagging is the persistent question of antibody activity against the substrate-binding sites originally raised by Von Fellenberg and Levine (1967).

Simultaneously in the same publication the two research teams, Perutz, Rossmann, Cullis, Muirhead, Will, and North (1960) and Kendrew, Dickerson, Strandberg, Hart, Davies, Phillips, and Shore (1960), announced the three-dimensional structures of hemoglobin and myoglobin, respectively, down to a resolution as low as 2 Ångstroms. This was an important achievement whose total effect has not yet been felt even after a decade. Hemoglobins and myoglobins diverged from a common globin ancestor perhaps one billion years ago with over 300 changes occurring between them per chain in the ensuing interval, remarkable for a chain only 141–153 residues long (Dayhoff, 1969). Even more remarkable has been the preservation of the general shape of the folded molecule with insertions and deletions occurring principally at the ends of the α-helical regions.

Immunochemical interest in sperm whale myoglobin (sequence, Table 9-3; conformation, Fig. 9-9) was sparked by the work of Crumpton (1965). The removal of ferrihaem from metmyoglobin was known to produce a conformational change that led to the formation of apomyoglobin. When antibodies, prepared against apomyoglobin, were reacted with metmyoglobin, the release of ferrihaem was induced. The antibodies had caused a conformational change in globin structure. When antibodies, prepared against metmyoglobin, were reacted with apomyoglobin, the precipitate which they formed took up ferrihaem and metmyoglobin was produced in the complex. These antibodies had also caused a conformational change in globin structure. The detection of the antibodies against myoglobin

TABLE 9-3
Amino Acid Sequence of Sperm Whale Myoglobin

Sequence						Residue Positions
VLSEG	EWQLV	LHVWA	KVEAD	VAGHG	QDILI	(1–30)
RLFKS	HPETL	EKFDR	FKHLK	TEAEM	KASED	(31–60)
LKKHG	VTVLT	ALGAI	LKKKG	HHEAE	LKPLA	(61–90)
QSHAT	KHKIP	IKYLE	FISEA	IIHVL	HSRHP	(91–120)
GNFGA	DAQGA	MNKAL	ELFRK	DIAAK	YKELG	(121–150)
YQG						(151–153)

Edmundson (1965) sequence. α-Helices: 3–18, 20–35, 36–39, 51–56, 58–77, 86–94, 100–118, 125–148.

(From Dayhoff, 1969, p. D64.)

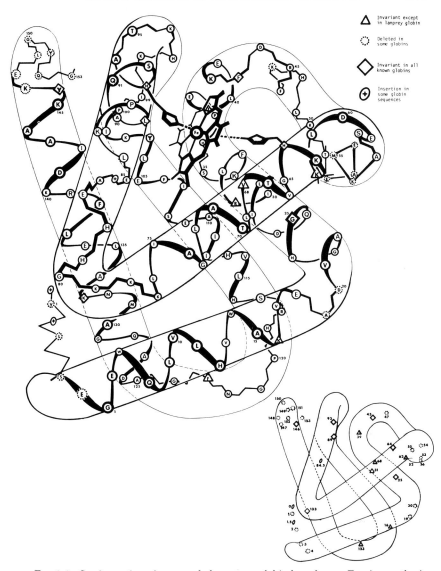

FIG. 9-9. Conformation of sperm whale metmyoglobin based upon Fourier synthesis at 2 Å of Kendrew *et al.* (1960), the two-dimensional representation of Dickerson (1964), and the sequence numbering of Edmundson (1965). Amino acid -carbon atoms without side chains shown. (From Dayhoff, 1969, p. 20.)

conformational determinants stood in contrast to other types of antibodies which Crumpton and Wilkinson (1965) found against sequential determinants. These latter types could be inhibited by chymotryptic peptides whereas the former could not. One of these was C-terminal and cross-reactive with a synthetic heptapeptide of the C-terminal sequence, KELGYQG (Crumpton, Law, and Strong, 1970). Interestingly enough the immunodominant amino acid was leucine, residue 149. Hexa-, penta-, and tetrapeptides were tested and the impression was gained that lysine, residue 147, was also important but not essential. It could be replaced with phenylalanine or p-methoxyphenylalanine without affecting reactivity with antibody.

Givas, Centeno, Manning, and Sehon (1968) also worked with the same nonhelical C-terminal heptapeptide, KELGYQG, using it to displace rabbit anti-myoglobin antibodies from an immunoadsorbent of myoglobin-DX840-31 and Sephadex-G-25 mixture. The antibodies, specifically eluted with the heptapeptide, showed greater restriction of electrophoretic heterogeneity than antibodies nonspecifically eluted with glycine-HCl buffer at pH 2.5, and much greater restriction than whole rabbit serum (Fig. 9-10). Moreover, the antibody eluted with the heptapeptide failed to give a precipitate with whole myoglobin, thus demonstrating the univalency of the determinant.

A series of immunochemical studies from Atassi's laboratory were concerned with the location of region and specific site of determi-

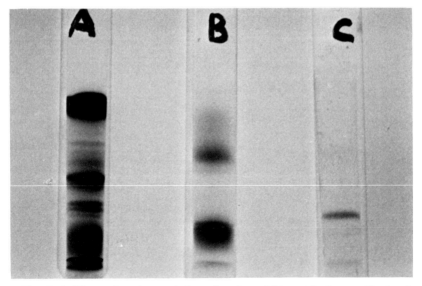

Fig. 9-10. Electrophoretic restriction of antimyoglobin antibody, specific for C-terminal heptapeptide, *disc C*, as compared with anti-myoglobin antibodies nonspecifically eluted with glycine-HCl buffer at pH 2, *disc B*, and with whole serum, *disc A*. (From Givas, Centeno, Manning, and Sehon, 1968.)

nants involved in antigenicity (Atassi and Saplin, 1968; Atassi and Caruso, 1968; Atassi, 1968, 1969; and Atassi and Thomas, 1969). By residue modification studies it could be concluded that methionine residues at positions 55 and 131 were not involved and that tyrosine 103 also was not important. Tyrosines 146 and/or 151 were present in the regions of a sequential antigenic reactive site and one or more of the arginines (31, 45, 118, and 139) seemed to be involved in the conformational determinant of metmyoglobin. The model of sperm whale myoglobin will continue to invite the interest of immunochemists for years to come. For one thing there is the promise of Givas, Centeno, Manning, and Sehon (1968): " . . . it is planned to establish the degree of homogeneity of the combining sites of purified [anti-myoglobin] antibodies in terms of their binding constants."

5. Some additional known native antigens

The sequences of bovine chymotrypsinogen and bovine trypsin are aligned for maximum homology in Table 9-4. Trypsin is formed by the

TABLE 9-4

Amino Acid Sequences of Bovine Chymotrypsinogen A and Trypsinogen Aligned for Maximum Homology

Protein	Sequence						Position of Residues
Chymotrypsinogen A	CGVPA	IQVPL	SGLSR	IVNGE	EAVPG	SWPWQ	1–30
Trypsinogen	-----	----V	DDDDK	IVGYY	TCGAN	TVPYQ	1–21
Chymotrypsinogen A	VSLQD	K---T	GFHFC	GGSLI	NENWV	VTAAH	31–57
Trypsinogen	VSLN-	----S	GYHFC	GGSLI	NSQWV	VSAAH	22–46
Chymotrypsinogen A	CGVTT	SD-VV	VAGEF	DQGSS	SEKIQ	KLKIA	58–86
Trypsinogen	CYKSG	IQ--V	RLGQD	NINVV	EGNQQ	FISAS	47–74
Chymotrypsinogen A	KVFKN	SKYNS	LTINN	--DIT	LLKLS	TAASF	87–114
Trypsinogen	KSIVH	PSYNS	NTLNN	--DIM	LIKLK	SAASL	75–102
Chymotrypsinogen A	SQTVS	AVCLP	SASDD	FAAGT	TCVTT	GWGLT	115–144
Trypsinogen	NSRVA	SISLP	TSCA-	-SAGT	QCLIS	GWGNT	103–130
Chymotrypsinogen A	RYTNA	NTPDR	LQQAS	LPLLS	NTNCK	K--YN	145–172
Trypsinogen	KSSGT	SYPDV	LKCLK	APILS	NSSCK	S--AY	131–158
Chymotrypsinogen A	GTKIK	DAMIC	AG-AS	GV-SS	CMGDS	GGPLV	173–200
Trypsinogen	PGQIT	SNMFC	AGYLE	GGKDS	CQGDS	GGPVV	159–188
Chymotrypsinogen A	CKKNG	AWTLV	GIVSW	GSS-T	CSTST	-PGVY	201–228
Trypsinogen	CSGK-	---LQ	GIVSW	GS--G	CAQKN	KPGVY	189–212
Chymotrypsinogen	ARVTA	LVNWV	QQTLA	AN			229–245
Trypsinogen	TKVCN	YVSWI	KQTIA	SN			213–229

Trypsinogen sequence revised from original by Walsh and Neurath (1964). Chymotrypsinogen revised, Brown and Hartley (1966). The 42-residue peptide of α-chymotrypsin contains peptides 131–141, 190–207, and 217–229 linked by disulfide bonds 136:201 and 191:220 (Sanders, Walsh, and Arnon, 1970).

removal of a short peptide from the N-terminal end. Chymotrypsin is a family formed by the splitting between different residues and the formation of chains held together by disulfide bridges; e.g., α-chymotrypsin A contains chain A (residues 1–13), chain B (16–146), and chain C (149–245). A and B are linked at 1:122, B and C at 136:201.

Arnon and Schechter (1966) prepared antibodies against trypsin, obtained precipitin reactions without enzymatic degradation of the reagent immunoglobulins, and inhibited proteolytic activity. As in many anti-enzyme inhibition reactions this one was also directly related to the size of the substrate. The bulk of the antibodies interacted with regions other than the catalytic sites and inhibited catalysis by steric hindrance. When Arnon and Schechter reacted the antitrypsin antibodies with chymotrypsin there was no precipitate formation, yet there was inhibition of catalytic activity. Following this phenomenon one step further, Sanders, Walsh, and Arnon (1970) prepared anti-chymotrypsin antibodies as well and could show the reverse. Using ^{125}I-labeled enzymes they could show by a modified Farr procedure the degree of specificity and cross-reactivity in each antiserum (Table 9-5).

Because of the similarity in cross-reactivity between the two antisera the question was raised whether this might be a result of a common antigenic determinant in the two enzymes. Peptic digests of chymotrypsin were therefore made, incubated with purified antitrypsin antibodies, salted out in 40% ammonium sulfate, and eluted at an acid pH by a procedure that would at the same time physically separate released antibody from the peptide. The cross-reacting peptide that was isolated with the antibody and that was therefore common to both enzymes—denoted the "42-residue peptide"—was found to be over 50% homologous with trypsin as compared with a 40% overall homology between the two whole proteins. The peptide represented residues 131–141.190–207.217–229 in chymotrypsin and residues of the same numbering in trypsin. Based upon a conformational structure (Fig. 9-11) the 42-residue peptide can be seen

TABLE 9-5
*Amount of ^{125}I-labeled Enzyme Bound to Antibody**

	^{125}I-Chymotrypsin	^{125}I-Trypsin	Cross-reaction
	$\mu moles$	$\mu moles$	%
Antitrypsin	0.28	1.36	20.2
Antichymotrypsin	0.70	0.14	19.6

* Enzyme, 4 μg, + γG, 2 μg, incubated 1 hr, 37°C, cooled to 4°, precipitated in 40% ammonium sulfate, washed, counted.
(From Sanders, Walsh, and Arnon, 1970.)

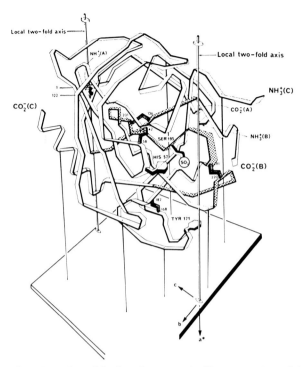

Fig. 9-11. Drawing of model of α-chymotrypsin X-ray structure determined by Matthews *et al.* (1967). Shaded area denotes 42-residue peptide isolated by binding with antitrypsin antibodies. See Table 9-4 for sequences. (From Sanders, Walsh, and Arnon, 1970.)

in its original native position. Two separate cross-reacting determinants were found in the peptide since by CNBr-cleavage two separate immunologically active peptides could be obtained. One fragment was homologous to the corresponding tryptic region in 10/12 residues; the other had a sequence of four identical residues. Besides the importance of the information itself, the technique used by these investigators showed the way to a direct method for separating in one step the active antigenic centers of a molecule from those that do not bind.

The zymogen-enzyme difference in trypsin is so slight that complete cross-reactivity is most often obtained with antisera against either form with either form (Arnon and Neurath, 1970). The antisera here, too, do not appear to be involved directly in catalytic sites since chemical modifications that would affect site reactivity did not affect antigenic properties and vice versa. Moreover, as Barrett and Epperson (1967) revealed, activation of either trypsinogen or chymotrypsinogen could take place even in the presence of antisera.

The newly formed enzymes, however, could not be detected until after dissociation with 0.001 M HCl.

Staphylococcal nuclease is an interesting antigen since it lacks disulfide structure, has a relatively low α-helix content, and maintains a high degree of flexibility in solution. Yet general antibody reactivity for the native enzyme "is at least an order of magnitude greater than its capacity for nuclease fragments" (Omenn, Ontjes, and Anfinsen, 1970a, b). The 149-residue-long sequence of *Staphylococcus aureus* V8 nuclease is completely known (Taniuchi, Anfinsen, and Sodja, 1967; Taniuchi, Cusumano, Anfinsen, and Cone, 1968) and both the N-terminal 18–33 and the C-terminal 127–149 peptides have been observed as antigenically active. The group raised the interesting idea that because of its high flexibility in solution the enzyme might be "especially susceptible to antibody recognition of both conformational and linear determinants."

Evidence that purine determinants were involved in the appearance of anti-DNA antibodies in lupus erythematosus serum was given by Stollar and Levine (1963). It was noted that denatured but not native deoxyribonucleic acid (DNA) would react with the antibodies and that the reaction was inhibited by purine derivatives. Using synthesized polyfunctional antigens containing uracil and 5-acetyluracil residues, Tanenbaum and Beiser (1963) obtained rabbit antibodies that would also cross-react much more strongly with denatured DNA than with the so-called native product. Extending the work still further, Erlanger and Beiser (1964) found that antibodies to nucleosides and nucleotides (conjugated to BSA) would react with thermally denatured DNA but not ribonucleic acid (RNA). Plescia, Braun, and Palczuk (1964) conferred antigenic properties upon thermally denatured calf thymus DNA and T4 phage DNA by complexing them with methylated BSA and found specific differences in immunological reactivity between the two DNA products with little cross-reactivity. Sela, Ungar-Waron, and Schechter (1964) synthesized multichain polypeptides containing uridine-5'-carboxylic acid residues, produced anti-uridine antibodies in rabbits against the material, and found that the antibodies reacted with both thermally denatured RNA and DNA, as well as polyuridylic acid, but not polyadenylic acid, native *Escherichia coli* RNA, or double-stranded calf thymus DNA. Ungar-Waron, Hurwitz, Jaton, and Sela (1967) conjugated nucleoside 5'-carboxylic acids to multichain polypeptides and made antibodies to uridine, deoxyuridine, thymidine, cytidine, and adenosine. All reacted with heat denatured DNA and two with heat treated RNA, but none reacted with native DNA.

Some patient sera were eventually found that would react with native DNA, with denatured DNA, and with both forms without evidence of specificity for one form or the other (Stollar and Sandberg, 1966; Tan, Schur, Carr, and Kunkel, 1966; Arana, and Seligmann, 1967). Thus, it must have come as some surprise to all concerned when Tan and Natali (1970) made their comparative study of antibodies to native and denatured DNA. Whereas rabbit antibodies against heat denatured DNA, as expected, did not cross-react with native DNA, one systemic lupus erythematosus serum in their hands, while not cross-reacting very much at all with denatured DNA, reacted very well indeed with native DNA!

Within the immunoglobulins themselves we have already noted certain allotypic antiserum reactions that required multichain and conformational structures for their full expression. Hirose and Osler (1967) noted that rabbits immunized with heavy chains of human γG developed antibodies of two types: one type against native conformational determinants present in intact γG, the other against new determinants that emerged in intact γG only by heat denaturation or urea treatment. Apparently the turbid solutions of polymerized heavy chains were representative of the latter. Yagi, Rutishauser, and Pressman (1968) discovered a most intriguing conformational effect—reminiscent of ferrihaem release from metmyoglobin but in reverse—by the treatment of light-chain-anti-light-chain complexes with Fd fragment. The light chain-Fd recombinant caused the release of some of the antibody—a conformational change resulting in the loss of some light chain determinants. Antibody against the conformational determinants of human light chain-Fd recombinant were found by Rivat, Rivat, and Ropartz (1969) not to bind to the separate chains; in addition, an antibody that would not react with either Fc or Fab was found, an anti-$(\gamma L)_2$, that would react only with conformational determinants of the intact γG or whole recombinants.

The chemical modification of immunoglobulins brought about by iodination has already been discussed. Not much conformational change has ever been noted with iodination but direct effects have been conferred instead upon individual residues in and around the binding site. Polyalanylation (Fuchs and Sela, 1965) neither has much effect upon binding affinity, nor does it bring about conformational changes (Karush and Sela, 1967). Alanine enrichment to the extent of 200–800 residues/mole, using N-carboxy-DL-alanine anhydride, increases solubility but leaves most of the original charged groups at the exterior of the globulin molecule. In equine γT there is loss in binding activity by polyalanylation but only after dissociation, attributable to a conformational change in heavy-light chain combining regions (Genco, Karush, and Tenenhouse, 1968). Some modifications are reversible such as that produced by complete maleylation of amino groups of antihapten antibodies. Anti-Rp and anti-Xp activity can be destroyed by the effect (but not anti-Ap or anti-Fp) and completely restored upon removal of the groups (Freedman, Grossberg, and Pressman, 1968). Arginine likewise can be modified with a 2,3-butanedione reagent (after protectively acetylating lysines) to the extent of 70% with loss only in anti-Xp, anti-Rp, and anti-succinamate activity, but not in anti-Ap or anti-3-azopyridine activity (Grossberg and Pressman, 1968). Chemical modifications which do not affect the globular $(Fab)_2$ combining regions may yet have an effect on other parts of immunoglobulin molecules to interfere with sequential and conformational determinants that ordinarily are detected by antiimmunoglobulin antibody reagents. Other biological properties of the immunoglobulins may also be affected such as transport, complement binding, and opsonic activities. For example, with regard to the last-mentioned Messner, Parker, and Williams (1970) were able to show that antibody reactivity with staphylococcal antigens was not appreciably affected by acetylation, carbamylation, or amidination, yet the opsonic activity was decreased with increasing modification and was already completely destroyed by the time 50% substitution was reached.

Another interesting series of compounds of immunochemical interest that have biological functions and that are affected by antibody binding are the toxins and the venoms. Some of the simpler ones have been sequenced such as the 26-residue-long melitten peptide of the honeybee, the 14- and 19-residue-long neurotoxins I and II of the scorpion, and the partially sequenced peptides of three strains of botulinus toxin from *Clostridium botulinum*. Others, such as staphylococcal enterotoxins B and C, are in the process of evaluation—with the help of combined chemical modification and immunochemical approaches. Enterotoxin C, a 34,100 molecular weight protein, induces vomiting in monkeys but when its 21 tyrosyl residues are completely acetylated its biological function is lost along with its ability to combine with antibody against the native protein (Borja and Bergdoll, 1969). Acetylation of only 5 tyrosyl groups diminishes neither toxic nor immunologic properties. Which type of determinants, conformational or sequential, is involved in the immunological process—measured in this case by precipitin reactions and Heidelberger-type plots—is uncertain, but the location of the active toxic center in the molecule is somehow intimately involved. A similar association of toxic and immunologic properties occurs in enterotoxin B (Chu, Crary, and Bergdoll, 1969) since guanidination does not alter either one whereas acetylation, succinylation, and carbamylation reduce and, at extremes, destroy both. In this case it appears that the reduction of biological and antigenic activities is due to the loss of net positive charge.

Not only tertiary but also quaternary antigenic structures may be important to antibody binding, thus calling for an additional class of antigenic determinants—not only sequential or primary and conformational or tertiary, but also associative or quaternary. An example was predicted for but not yet found in the hemocyanins whose macromolecular organization was approached immunochemically by Weigle (1964) and morphologically through electron microscopy by Fernandez-Moran, van Bruggen, and Ohtsuki (1966). Keyhole limpet hemocyanin (KLH) at pH 8.5 exists in the monomeric dissociated form with a molecular weight of 8×10^5; at pH 6.9 or less it assumes an associated decagonal quaternary form with a molecular weight of 8×10^6. Weigle (1964) prepared rabbit antisera against both the associated and dissociated forms (which at physiological pH *in vivo* probably assumed the same intermediate mixture), and found that each antiserum contained antibodies that reacted to a higher extent with dissociated KLH than with associated $(KLH)_{10}$. Recalculation of his data in molar terms shows that 380 moles of anti-$(KLH)_{10}$ were bound to 10 subunits of dissociated KLH in antibody excess whereas only 165 moles, less than half, were bound to a 10-subunit associated complex; also that 440 moles of anti-KLH were bound to 10 subunits of KLH in contrast to 200 moles antibody bound per mole of 10-unit KLH. The difference in binding could have been attributed to a difference in number of available determinants due to the burial of determinants within the associated structure or due to change in subunit conformation accompanying association. The findings of Rutishauser, Ritterberg, and Campbell (1967) provided an answer. They confirmed Weigle's experiments by showing that the difference in antibody/KLH ratios depended upon degree of subunit association; in addition, the complexes that were made at pH 8.8 between antibody and KLH monomers were found to release antibody into solution as they were dialyzed at pH 6.9 under conditions favoring decamers. Complexes that formed between antibody and decamers at pH 6.9 would release monomeric antigen upon dialysis back to pH 8.8. It might have seemed that such a strength of subunit binding that could reverse binding site affinity and elute antibody into solution might also be involved in producing conformation changes in the subunits themselves. The antibodies that were eluted in this case, however, reacted very well indeed with associated $(KLH)_{10}$ and demonstrated that the difference between the two forms was strictly in the antigenic valence. In essence, the antibodies were of a cross-

380 REACTIONS OF ANTIBODIES

reacting variety, but the possibility of preparing quaternary or subunit specific antibodies still remains open. Meanwhile, Rutishauser *et al.* have pointed to a by-product of their study—"a gentle method of isolating small amounts of specific antibody under physiologic conditions."

6. A synthetic antigen with conformational determinants

Sela, Schechter, Schechter, and Borek (1967) reported to the Cold Spring Harbor Symposium the preparation of two types of synthetic polypeptides: one, a branched polypeptide with YAE tripeptides located at the amino termini of poly-DL-alanyl side chains of a poly-L-lysine backbone [(YAE)–A--K, mol. wt. = 75,000]; the other, a polymer of repeating ordered sequence, L-Tyr-L-Ala-L-Glu or $(YAE)_n$, with a molecular weight of 10^5 that under conditions of physiologic pH and ionic strength took on an α-helical form. Antibodies were raised in rabbits against both the (YAE)–A--K and the $(YAE)_n$ antigens and were tested for specificity with the homologous and for cross-reactivity with the heterologous groups. The antibodies showed remarkable specificity for their specific homologous antigen, very little if any cross-reactivity with the other. This demonstration of sequential and conformational determinant specificity and the difference in quality of antibody binding between the two was clear, unambiguous, and very much to the point. As a footnote to this study, however, one may still point out additional nuances that add to the diversity already in view. As one example, Maurer, Clark, and Liberti (1970) found two distinct populations of antibodies in antisera to synthetic poly-α-amino acids rich in glutamyl residues. Many of those raised against calcium glutamyl polypeptides were dependent upon the presence of calcium ion for their interaction with antigen and thus were an example of antibodies to a conformational structure. The function of calcium was found to be that of changing the conformation of the polymer from one form to another. Another population of antibodies was independent of calcium and directed toward sequential type peptidal determinants.

7. The "evolution" of an antigenic determinant—cytochrome *c* in the human, the monkey, and the kangaroo

Electrons from cytochrome *b* are transferred to cytochrome oxidase in mitochondria by cytochrome *c*, one of the most conserved of all polypeptides in evolution. Between human α-hemoglobin and γ-hemoglobin chains there is only 36% homology, yet between human cytochrome *c* and even one of its most distant relatives in *Candida krusei* there remains 51% homology. Between human and wheat cytochromes c there is 59% homology and between the human and the rhesus monkey there is only one residue difference out of the complete 104-residue polypeptide, threonine at position 58 in the monkey instead of isoleucine. Human and chimpanzee cytochromes c are identical. Even between human cytochrome c and that from the kangaroo there are only 10 amino acids different, 9 between the human and the rabbit (Table 9-6). By raising antibodies in rabbits to monomeric cytochromes c from various species Margoliash, Nisonoff, and Reichlin (1970) were able to study the cross-reactions and specifities among a very large number of vertebrate species, 19 in the present series. The binding reactions between antibody and antigen were determined by a quantitative complement fixation technique and by an inhibition method utilizing ^{125}I-cytochrome c of one species, its homologous antibody, and a series of unlabeled

TABLE 9-6

Amino Acid Sequences of Cytochrome c from Four Different Species

Species	Sequence						Residue Position
Human	GDVEK	GKKIF	*IM*KCS	QCHTV	EKGGK	HKTGP	(1–30)
Rhesus monkey	GDVEK	GKKIF	*IM*KCS	QCHTV	EKGGK	HKTGP	
Kangaroo	GDVEK	GKKIF	VQKCA	QCHTV	EKGGK	HKTGP	
Rabbit	GDVEK	GKKIF	VQKCA	QCHTV	EKGGK	HKTGP	
Human	NLHGL	FGRKT	GQA*P*G	YSYTA	ANKNK	GI*I*WG	(31–60)
Rhesus monkey	NLHGL	FGRKT	GQA*P*G	YSYTA	ANKNK	GITWG	
Kangaroo	NL*NGI*	FGRKT	GQA*P*G	F*T*YTD	ANKNK	GI*I*WG	
Rabbit	NLHGL	FGRKT	GQAVG	FSYTD	ANKNK	GITWG	
Human	EDTLM	EYLEN	PKKYI	PGTKM	IF*V*GI	KKK*EE*	(61–90)
Rhesus monkey	EDTLM	EYLEN	PKKYI	PGTKM	IF*V*GI	KKK*EE*	
Kangaroo	EDTLM	EYLEN	PKKYI	PGTKM	IFAGI	KKK*G*E	
Rabbit	EDTLM	EYLEN	PKKYI	PGTKM	IFAGI	KKKDE	
Human	RADLI	AYLKK	ATNE				(91–104)
Rhesus monkey	RADLI	AYLKK	ATNE				
Kangaroo	RADLI	AYLKK	ATNE				
Rabbit	RADLI	AYLKK	ATNE				

Residues in italics are those that differ from rabbit in which antibodies were made. Human: Matsubara and Smith (1962) revised; monkey: Rothfus and Smith, 1965; kangaroo: Nolan and Margoliash, 1966; rabbit: Needleman and Margoliash, 1966.

(From Dayhoff, 1969, pp. D8-D11; Margoliash and Schejter, 1966; Nolan and Margoliash, 1968.)

competitive cytochromes from the other species. A sample of the
results with one serum is given in Table 9-7 along with the
degree of sequence differences (in this case, horse) from the
homologous cytochrome antigen. There were differences noted
between total binding, a measure of both strong and weak antibodies,
and competitive binding, but a reasonable correlation was established
between strength of immunological reactions and relatedness in
amino acid sequence of the cross-reacting cytochromes. There was no
intention in this first report of drawing sweeping conclusions, yet
there was a wealth of data presented in eight different tables from
which three important conclusions could be drawn: (a) some antisera
do not distinguish between cytochromes c of different amino acid
sequences; (b) the immunological distinction in cytochromes c that
differ by single residues may be minor in some cases, major in others;
(c) a small globular protein such as cytochrome c can serve as a model
for the study of the effects of amino acid substitution upon antigenic
determinants.

Nisonoff, Reichlin, and Margoliash (1970) provided an example of

TABLE 9-7

*Correlation between Binding of Rabbit-Anti-Horse Cytochrome c with Various
Cytochromes c and Amino Acid Differences between Horse Cytochrome c
and Others*

Cytochrome c	Homologous Reaction at Maximum in Complement Fixation*	Label Displaced in Binding Competition†	No. of Variant Residues‡
	%	%	
Horse	100	93	0
Donkey	100	91	1
Cow, sheep, pig	60	70	3
Finback whale	45	55	5
Kangaroo	38	55	7
Rabbit	35	50	6
Macaca mulatta	25		11
Chicken, turkey	19	50	11
Human, chimpanzee	16	53	12
Pekin duck	13	45	14
Tuna	27	40	17
Screw worm fly	0	55	24
Samia cynthia	0	30	29
Saccharomyces cerevisiae (iso-1)	5	6	45

* Measures total binding.
† Measures strength of binding.
‡ Rabbit was the source of antiserum, horse of antigen.
(From Margoliash, Nisonoff, and Reichlin, 1970.)

these three conclusions in the case of the monkey and the human and the kangaroo. As has already been stated the human cytochrome c differs from that of the rhesus monkey at only one residue: isoleucine at position 58 in case of human, threonine in the case of monkey. The cytochrome c of rabbit, like that of monkey, contains threonine while the cytochrome c of kangaroo, like that of human, contains isoleucine. When antibodies are produced in rabbits against monkey cytochrome c, there is absolutely no immunological distinction between reactivity with monkey or human antigen, and none is expected. (By the same token, antibodies produced in kangaroos against human cytrochrome c would not be expected to distinguish between human and monkey.) When antibodies are produced in rabbits against human cytochrome c, however, there are between 30 and 40% of the antibodies that do not cross-react with monkey. They are the ones that are specific for the hydrophobic isoleucine residue (and presumably the region around it), and they react only with one other cytochrome c in the list of 19 (those given in Table 9-7 plus snapping turtle and pigeon), that of the kangaroo.* The isoleucine residue thus proved to be the center of a strong antigenic determinant. The authors cautioned as a result of this finding:

> "The [immunodominant] importance of a single isoleucyl residue and appearance in two species not closely related points up an uncertainty in establishing phylogenetic relations immunochemically."

In many ways the result is not unlike that of Karakawa, Maurer, Walsh, and Krause (1970) who prepared antisera against the synthetic random polypeptide, poly $(\text{L-glu}^{42}\text{-L-lys}^{25}\text{-D-ala}^{30})_n$, and found that some of the antibodies cross-reacted with the mucopeptides of gram-positive cocci. D-Alanine turned out to be the critical amino acid in the synthetic polymer that was responsible for the cross-reaction. The peptide portion of the bacterial polymer of N-acetylglucosamine and N-acetylmuramic acid had been known to be the immunodominant tetrapeptide L-ala-D-glu-L-lys-D-ala. Through the use of antisera to the three polymers poly$(\text{L-glu}^{42}\text{-L-lys}^{28}\text{-D-ala}^{30})_n$, poly$(\text{D-glu}^{16}\text{-L-lys}^{16}\text{-DL-ala}^{68})_n$, and poly$(\text{L-glu}^{42}\text{-L-lys}^{28}\text{-L-ala}^{30})_n$, it was determined that only antisera to polymers containing D-alanine would cross-react with the mucopeptide, and by this technique an important puzzle in the antigenic specificity of the gram-positive moiety was solved. From there it is only a few steps to the solution of the perplexing problem of bacterial mucopeptide toxicity.

---

* One would predict a reaction with rattlesnake cytochrome c also, but this was not included in the series.

384 REACTIONS OF ANTIBODIES

REFERENCES

Arana, R., and Seligmann, M. (1967). Antibodies to native and denatured deoxyribonucleic acid in systemic lupus erythematosus. J. Clin. Invest. 46: 1867–1882.

Arnon, R. (1968). A selective fractionation of anti-lysozyme antibodies of different determinant specificities. Eur. J. Biochem. 5: 583–589.

Arnon, R., Maron, E., Sela, M., and Anfinsen, C. B. (1971). Antibodies reactive with native lysozyme elicited by a completely synthetic antigen. Proc. Natl. Acad. Sci. 68: 1450–1455.

Arnon, R., and Neurath, H. (1970). Immunochemical studies on bovine trypsin and trypsinogen derivatives. Immunochemistry 7: 241–250.

Arnon, R., and Schechter, B. (1966). Immunological studies on specific antibodies against trypsin. Immunochemistry 3: 451–461.

Arnon, R., and Sela, M. (1969). Antibodies to a unique region in lysozyme provoked by a synthetic antigen conjugate. Proc. Natl. Acad. Sci. 62: 163–170.

Atassi, M. Z. (1968). Immunochemistry of sperm whale myoglobin. III. Modification of the three tyrosine residues and their role in the conformation and differentiation of their roles in the antigenic reactivity. Biochemistry 7: 3078–3085.

Atassi, M. Z. (1969). Immunochemistry of sperm whale myoglobin. V. Specific modification of the methionine residues with β-propiolactone. Immunochemistry 6: 801–810.

Atassi, M. Z., and Caruso, D. R. (1968). Immunochemistry of sperm whale myoglobin. II. Modification of the two tryptophan residues and their role in the conformation and antigen-antibody reaction. Biochemistry 7: 699–705.

Atassi, M. Z., and Saplin, B. J. (1968). Immunochemistry of sperm whale myoglobin. I. The specific interaction of some tryptic peptides and of peptides containing all the reactive regions of the antigen. Biochemistry 7: 688–698.

Atassi, M. Z., and Thomas, A. V. (1969). Immunochemistry of sperm whale myoglobin. IV. The role of the arginine residues in the conformation and differentiation of their roles in the antigenic reactivity. Biochemistry 8: 3385–3394.

Barrett, J. T., and Epperson, M. S. (1967). The activation of chymotrypsinogen and trypsinogen in the presence of antisera. Immunochemistry 4: 497–499.

Bonavida, B., Miller, A., and Sercarz, E. E. (1969). Structural basis for immune recognition of lysozymes. I. Effect of cyanogen bromide on hen egg-white lysozyme. Biochemistry 8: 968–979.

Borja, C. R., and Bergdoll, M. S. (1969). Staphylococcal enterotoxin C. II. Some physical, immunological, and toxic properties. Biochemistry 8: 75–79.

Branster, M., and Cinader, B. (1961). The interaction between bovine ribonuclease and antibody: A study of the mechanism of enzyme inhibition by antibody. J. Immunol. 87: 18–38.

Brew, K., Vanaman, T. C., and Hill, R. L. (1967). Comparison of the amino acid sequence of α-lactalbumin and hens egg white lysozyme. J. Biol. Chem. 242: 3747–3749.

Brown, J. R., and Hartley, B. S. (1966). Location of disulphide bridges by diagonal paper electrophoresis. The disulphide bridges of bovine chymotrypsinogen A. Biochem. J. 101: 214–228.

Brown, R. K. (1962). Studies on the antigenic structure of ribonuclease. J. Biol. Chem. 237: 1162–1167.

Brown, R. K., Delaney, R., Levine, L., and Van Vunakis, H. (1959). Studies on the antigenic structure of ribonuclease. I. General role of hydrogen and disulfide bonds. J. Biol. Chem. *234:* 2043–2049.

Canfield, R., and Liu, A. K. (1965). The disulfide bonds of egg white lysozyme (muramidase). J. Biol. Chem. *240:* 1997–2002.

Chu, F. S., Crary, E., and Bergdoll, M. S. (1969). Chemical modification of amino groups in staphylococcal enterotoxin B. Biochemistry *8:* 2890–2896.

Cinader, B. (1967). Editor. Antibodies to Biologically Active Molecules: Proceedings of the 2nd Meeting of the Fed. Eur. Biochem. Soc., Vienna, 21–24 April, 1965, Vol. 1, Pergamon Press (Oxford, 424 pp.).

Crumpton, M. J. (1965). Conformational changes in sperm-whale metmyoglobin due to combination with antibodies to apomyoglobin. Biochem. J. *100:* 223–232.

Crumpton, M. J., Law, H. D., and Strong, R. C. (1970). The C-terminal antigenic site of sperm-whale myoglobin: the immunological activities of synthetic peptides related to the C-terminus of myoglobin. Biochem. J. *116:* 923–925.

Crumpton, M. J., and Wilkinson, J. M. (1965). The immunological activity of some of the chymotryptic peptides of sperm-whale myoglobin. Biochem. J. *94:* 545–556.

Dayhoff, M. O. (1969). Evolution of the globins. In *Atlas of Protein Sequence and Structure*, Vol. 4, National Biomedical Research Foundation (Silver Spring, Md., xxxvi + 109 text pp. + 252 data pp.), pp. 20 and D64, myoglobin; 55 and D130–D131, ribonuclease; D132–D133, lysozyme and lactalbumin; D115, trypsin; D118, chymotrypsin; D8–D11, cytochrome *c*.

Dickerson, R. E. (1964). X-ray analysis and protein structure. In *The Proteins*, Ed. 2, Vol. II, Neurath, H., ed. Academic Press (New York, 788 pp.), pp. 634–778.

Edmundson, A. B. (1965). Amino acid sequences of sperm whale myoglobin. Nature *205:* 883–887.

Erlanger, B., and Beiser, S. (1964). Antibodies specific for ribonucleosides and ribonucleotides and their reaction with DNA. Proc. Natl. Acad. Sci. *52:* 68–74.

Fernandez-Moran, H., Van Bruggen, E. F. J., and Ohtsuki, M. (1966). Macromolecular organization of hemocyanins and apohemocyanins as revealed by electron microscopy. J. Mol. Biol. *16:* 191–207.

Freedman, M. H., Grossberg, A. L., and Pressman, D. (1968). The effects of complete modification of amino groups on the antibody activity of antihapten antibodies. Reversible inactivation with maleic anhydride. Biochemistry *7:* 1941–1950.

Fuchs, S., and Sela, M. (1965). Preparation and characterization of poly-DL-alanyl rabbit γ-globulin. J. Biol. Chem. *240:* 3558–3562.

Genco, R. J., Karush, F., and Tenenhouse, H. S. (1968). Equine antihapten antibody. VI. Subunits of polyalanylated γG(T)-immunoglobulin. Biochemistry *7:* 2462–2468.

Gerwing, J., and Thompson, K. (1968). Studies on the antigenic properties of egg-white lysozyme. I. Isolation and characterization of a tryptic peptide from reduced and alkylated lysozyme exhibiting haptenic activity. Biochemistry *7:* 3888–3892.

Givas, Sr. J., Centeno, E. R., Manning, M., and Sehon, A. H. (1968). Isolation of antibodies to the C-terminal heptapeptide of myoglobin with a synthetic peptide. Immunochemistry *5:* 314–318.

Grossberg, A. L., and Pressman, D. (1968). Modification of arginine in the active sites of antibodies. Biochemistry *7:* 272–279.

Habeeb, A. F. S. A., and Atassi, M. Z. (1969). Enzymic and immunochemical properties of lysozyme. II. Conformation, immunochemistry, and enzymatic activity of a derivative modified at tryptophan. Immunochemistry *6:* 555–566.

Hirose, S.-I., and Osler, A. G. (1967). Interaction of rabbit anti-human H chain sera with denatured human γ-globulin and its subunits. J. Immunol. *98:* 618–627.

Karakawa, W. W., Maurer, P. H., Walsh, P., and Krause, R. M. (1970). The role of

D-alanine in the antigenic specificity of bacterial mucopeptides. J. Immunol. *104:* 230–237.

Karush, F., and Sela, M. (1967). Equine anti-hapten antibody. IV. The effect of poly-alanylation on affinity. Immunochemistry *4:* 259–267, 1967.

Kendrew, J. C., Dickerson, R. E., Strandberg, B. E., Hart, R. G., Davies, D. R., Phillips, D. C., and Shore, V. C. (1960). Structure of myoglobin. A three-dimensional Fourier synthesis at 2 Å resolution. Nature *185:* 422–427.

Lapresle, C. (1955). Étude de la dégradation de la serum de la sérum albumine humaine par un extrait de rate de lipin. II. Mise en évidence de trois groupements spécifiques différents dans le motif antigénique de l'albumine humaine et de trois. Ann. Inst. Pasteur *89:* 654–664.

Lapresle, C., and Goldstein, I. J. (1969). Immunogenicity of a fragment of human serum albumin. J. Immunol. *102:* 733–742.

Lapresle, C., Kaminski, M., and Tanner, C. E. (1959). Immunochemical study of the enzymatic degradation of human serum albumin: an analysis of the antigenic structure of a protein molecule. J. Immunol. *82:* 94–102.

Lapresle, C., and Webb, T. (1964). Données actuelles sur les bases chimiques de la spécificité immunologique des protéines. Bull. Soc. Chim. Biol. *46:* 1701–1710.

Lapresle, C., and Webb, T. (1965). Isolation and study of a fragment of human serum albumin containing one of the antigenic sites of the whole molecule. Biochem. J. *95:* 245–251.

Margoliash, E., Nisonoff, A., and Reichlin, M. (1970). Immunological activity of cytochrome *c*. I. Precipitating antibodies to monomeric vertebrate cytochromes *c*. J. Biol. Chem. *245:* 931–939.

Margoliash, E., and Schejter, A. (1966). Cytochrome *c*. Adv. Protein Chem. *21:* 113–286.

Matsubara, H., and Smith, E. L. (1962). The amino acid sequence of human heart cytochrome *c*. J. Biol. Chem. *237:* PC3575–PC3576.

Matthews, B. W., Sigler, P. B., Henderson, R., and Blow, D. M. (1967). Three-dimensional structure of tosyl-α-chymotrypsin. Nature *214:* 652–656.

Maurer, P. H., Clark, L. G., and Liberti, P. A. (1970). Antigenicity of polypeptides (poly α-amino acids): calcium-dependent and independent antibodies. J. Immunol. *105:* 567–573.

Messner, R. P., Parker, C. W., and Williams, R. C., Jr. (1970). Chemical modification of human and rabbit antistaphylococcal γG antibodies: Effect of acetylation, carbamylation, and amidination on opsonic activity. J. Immunol. *104:* 238–246.

Metzger, H. (1967). Characterization of a human macroglobulin. V. A Waldenstrom macroglobulin with antibody activity. Proc. Natl. Acad. Sci. *57:* 1490–1497.

Mills, J. H., and Haber, E. (1963). The effect on antigenic specificity of changes in the molecular structure of ribonuclease. J. Immunol. *91:* 536–540.

Needleman, S. B., and Margoliash, E. (1966). Rabbit heart cytochrome *c*. J. Biol. Chem. *241:* 853–863.

Neumann, H., Steinberg, I. Z., Brown, J. R., Goldberger, R. F., and Sela, M. (1967). On the non-essentiality of two specific disulphide bonds in ribonuclease for its biological activity. Eur. J. Biochem. *3:* 171–182.

Nisonoff, A., Reichlin, M., and Margoliash, E. (1970). Immunological activity of cytochrome *c*. II. Localization of a major antigenic determinant of human cytochrome *c*. J. Biol. Chem. *245:* 940–946.

Nolan, C., and Margoliash, E. (1966). Primary structure of the cytochrome *c* from the great grey kangaroo, *Macropus canguru*. J. Biol. Chem. *241:* 1049–1059.

Nolan, C., and Margoliash, E. (1968). Comparative aspects of primary structures of proteins. Annu. Rev. Biochem. *37:* 727–790.

Omenn, G. S., Ontjes, D. A., and Anfinsen, C. B. (1970a). Immunochemistry of staphylococcal nuclease. I. Physical, enzymatic, and immunologic studies of chemically modified derivatives. Biochemistry 9: 304–312.

Omenn, G. S., Ontjes, D. A., and Anfinsen, C. B. (1970b). Immunochemistry of staphylococcal nuclease. II. Inhibition and binding studies with sequence fragments. Biochemistry 9: 313–321.

Pelichova, H., Suzuki, T., and Cinader, B. (1970). Enzyme-activation by antibody. II. The distribution of activating antibody in chromatographic fractions of ribonuclease antisera and their competition with inhibiting antibody for enzyme sites. J. Immunol. 104: 195–202.

Perutz, M. F., Rossmann, M. G., Cullis, A. F., Muirhead, H., Will, G., and North, A. C. T. (1960). Structure of haemoglobin. A three-dimensional Fourier synthesis at 5.5-Å resolution, obtained by X-ray analysis. Nature 185: 416–422.

Plescia, O. J., Braun, W., and Palczuk, N. C. (1964). Production of antibodies to denatured deoxyribonucleic acid (DNA). Proc. Natl. Acad. Sci. 52: 279–285.

Pollock, M. R. (1963). Penicillinase-antipenicillinase. Ann. N.Y. Acad. Sci. 103: 989–1005.

Pollock, M. R. (1964). Stimulating and inhibiting antibodies for bacterial penicillinase. Immunology, 7: 707–723.

Pollock, M. R., Fleming, J., and Petrie, S. (1967). The effects of specific antibodies on the biological activities of wild-type bacterial penicillinases and their mutationally altered analogues. In Antibodies to Biologically Active Molecules, Cinader, B., ed., Pergamon Press (Oxford, 424 pp.), pp. 139–152.

Porter, R. R. (1957). The isolation and properties of a fragment of bovine-serum albumin which retains the ability to combine with rabbit antiserum. Biochem. J. 66: 677–686.

Rivat, C., Rivat, L., and Ropartz, C. (1969). Mise en évidence de déterminants antigéniques liés à la conformation moléculaire dans les immunoglobulines γG humaines. Immunochemistry 6: 327–335.

Rothfus, J. A., and Smith, E. L. (1965). Amino acid sequence of rhesus monkey heart cytochrome c. J. Biol. Chem. 240: 4277–4283.

Rutishauser, V. S., Ritterberg, M. B., and Campbell, D. H. (1967). Antibody recovery from immune precipitates of a reversibly dissociable antigen—hemocyanin. Immunochemistry 4: 113–116.

Sanders, M. M., Walsh, K. A., and Arnon, R. (1970). Immunological cross reaction between trypsin and chymotrypsin as a guide to structural homology. Biochemistry 9: 2356–2363.

Sela, M., Schechter, B., Schechter, I., and Borek, F. (1967). Antibodies to sequential and conformational determinants. Symp. Quant. Biol. 32: 537–545.

Sela, M., Ungar-Waron, H., and Schechter, Y. (1964). Uridine-specific antibodies obtained with synthetic antigens. Proc. Natl. Acad. Sci. 52: 285–292.

Stollar, D., and Levine, L. (1963). Antibodies to denatured deoxyribonucleic acid in lupus erythematosus serum. IV. Evidence for purine determinants in DNA. Arch. Biochem. Biophys. 101: 417–422.

Stollar, B. D., and Sandberg, A. L. (1966). Comparisons of antibodies reacting with DNA. I. Systemic lupus erythematosus sera and rabbit antibodies induced by DNA-methylated bovine serum albumin complexes. J. Immunol. 96: 755–763.

Stone, M. J., and Metzger, H. (1967). The valence of a Waldenstrom macroglobulin antibody and further thoughts on the significance of paraprotein antibodies. Symp. Quant. Biol. 32: 83–88.

Stone, M. J., and Metzger, H. (1968). Binding properties of a Waldenstrom macroglobulin antibody. J. Biol. Chem. 243: 5977–5984.

388 REACTIONS OF ANTIBODIES

Stone, M. J., and Metzger, H. (1969). The specificity of a monoclonal macroglobulin (γM) antibody: reactivity with primate γG immunoglobulin. J. Immunol. *102:* 222–228.

Strosberg, A. D., and Kanarek, L. (1970). Immunochemical studies on hen's egg-white lysozyme. Role of lysine, histidine, and methionine residues. Eur. J. Biochem. *14:* 161–168.

Suzuki, T., Pelichova, H., and Cinader, B. (1969). Enzyme activation by antibody. I. Fractionation of immune sera in search for an enzyme activating antibody. J. Immunol. *103:* 1366–1376.

Tan, E. M., and Natali, P. G. (1970). Comparative study of antibodies to native and denatured DNA. J. Immunol. *104:* 902–906.

Tan, E. M., Schur, P. H., Carr, R. I., and Kunkel, H. G. (1966). Deoxyribonucleic acid (DNA) and antibodies to DNA in the serum of patients with systemic lupus erythematosus. J. Clin. Invest. *45:* 1732–1740.

Tanenbaum, S. W., and Beiser, S. M. (1963). Pyrimidine-specific antibodies which react with deoxyribonucleic acid (DNA). Proc. Natl. Acad. Sci. *49:* 662–668.

Taniuchi, H., Anfinsen, C. B., and Sodja, A. (1967). The amino acid sequence of an extracellular nuclease of *Staphylococcus aureus.* III. Complete amino acid sequence. J. Biol. Chem. *242:* 4752–4758.

Taniuchi, H., Cusumano, C. L., Anfinsen, C. B., and Cone, J. L. (1968). Correction of the amino acid sequence of staphylococcal nuclease, strain V8. J. Biol. Chem. *243:* 4775–4777.

Thompson, K. E., and Levy, J. G. (1970). Effect of sequential degradation on the haptenic activity of a tryptic peptide isolated from reduced and alkylated egg-white lysozyme and the haptenic properties of its amino-terminal residue. Biochemistry *9:* 3463–3468.

Ungar-Waron, H., Hurwitz, E., Jaton, J.-C., and Sela, M. (1967). Antibodies elicited with conjugates of nucleosides with synthetic polypeptides. Biochim. Biophys. Acta *138:* 513–531.

Von Fellenberg, R., and Levine, L. (1967). Proximity of the enzyme active center and an antigenic determinant of lysozyme. Immunochemistry *4:* 363–365.

Walsh, K., and Neurath, H. (1964). Trypsinogen and chymotrypsinogen as homologous proteins. Proc. Natl. Acad. Sci. *52:* 884–889.

Weigle, W. O. (1964). Immunochemical properties of hemocyanin. Immunochemistry *1:* 295–302.

Yagi, Y., Rutishauser, V., and Pressman, D. (1968). Release of anti-L-chain antibody from antigen-antibody complexes by Fd fragment. Immunochemistry *5:* 67–74.

Young, J. D., and Leung, C. Y. (1969). Immunological studies on lysozyme and carboxymethylated lysozymes. Fed. Proc. *28:* 326 incl.

Young, J. D., and Leung, C. Y. (1970). Immunochemical studies on lysozyme and carboxymethylated lysozyme. Biochemistry *9:* 2755–2762.

10

AFFINITY AND THE IMMUNE RESPONSES

1. Parameters of immune responses

To discuss the immune response fully and adequately and to evaluate the research in that area with responsible criticism one would need as many pages as are contained in this whole book. A good beginning, however, would be to replace the commonly used phrase—the immune response—with the more descriptive plural form, the immune responses.

One would need to consider age, sex, race, and environment before arriving at an adequate description of any particular normal immune response. And, if "it does not yet seem justified to speak of normal human immunoglobulin levels" (Kalff, 1970), how much less justified it must yet be to speak of normal immune responses.

One would need to consider the region of the body most expressive of any particular immune response. Immunologists of the past have been trained to think in terms of serum levels of immunoglobulins as guides from which to measure the immune response and in terms of γG as the most typical and predominant immunoglobulin. Yet it is perfectly clear that serum levels are not expressive at all of man's immune response to the common cold or to poliomyelitis. Nasal washes contain much higher titers of antibody to rhinovirus that has been sniffed, and the antibody is almost exclusively confined to 11.6–12.6S γA (Cate, Rossen, Douglas, Butler, and Couch, 1967). The feces of poliomyelitic children contain very high titers of poliovirus neutralizing antibody (Steigman and Lipton, 1959; Lipton and Steigman, 1963), and the feces of children, following Sabin oral poliovirus vaccinations, likewise contain high titers of neutralizing antibody (Kawakami, Tatsumi, Tatsumi, and Kono, 1966). That such coproantibodies are principally γA has been shown by Keller and Dwyer (1968). One might have argued in the past that antibodies in the respiratory passages and intestinal tract were transported there by the circulation from remote synthesizing depots, but it is now well enough documented that *de novo* local

389

synthesis of antibody is primarily responsible, and that γA is considerably more prominent than γG along the mucosal surfaces. Although immunoglobulin levels in various regions are not indices of any particular immune responses yet they do reflect the differences in the distributions of immunocytes that synthesize one type of immunoglobulin or another. Tomasi (1970) has tabulated some of these (Table 10-1) and has shown the wide variation in regional production thereby. In the mesenteric lymph of the dog Vaerman and Heremans (1970) have shown that 60–95% of the γA that is present is made by the plasma cells of the intestinal mucosa and that this pool contributes heavily to the γA in the total circulation. Using bovine serum albumin (BSA) as antigen in human studies Kriebel, Kraft, and Rothberg (1969) have found that anti-BSA antibodies in duodenal secretions are associated with γA, γM, and γD immunoglobulins whereas the γG that is present in 25/30 specimens is inactive with respect to BSA, thus indicating in yet another way the local selection and production of antibodies by one class or another.

γE-forming plasma cells are scarce in the more usual areas of γG production (the spleen and subcutaneous lymph nodes), but deposits of γE producers are contained in the respiratory and gastrointestinal mucosa, the regional lymph nodes, the tonsils, the adenoids, the broncheal passages, and the mesenteric lymph nodes (Tada and Ishizaka, 1970). The tonsils appear to contain the most

TABLE 10-1

Relative Regional Concentrations of Some Immunoglobulins in the Human

Region	Concentration per 100 ml*			Concentration Ratio	Cell Count Ratio
	γG	γA	γM	γG/γA	γG/γA
	mg	mg	mg		
Serum	1000	160	110	6	
Breast milk	30	600	0.50	0.05	
Parotid saliva	tr	10	tr	<0.1	
Nasal secretion	10	20	tr	0.5	1:6
Tears	tr	20	—	<0.1	
Bronchial					1:5
Gastric					1:16
Intestinal	140	150	—	0.9	1:22
Colon					1:23
Rectum					1:16
Appendix					1:1
Gallbladder bile	143	160	—	0.9	—

* tr = trace.
(From Tomasi, 1970.)

abundant number of γE-forming cells (Ishizaka and Ishizaka, 1970b) although in monkeys infested with parasitic mites the lungs and regional nodes are particularly prominent (Ishizaka, Ishizaka, and Tada, 1969). The significant role that γE plays in reaginic hypersensitivity (Ishizaka and Ishizaka, 1970) is a particularly fascinating and intriguing chapter in immunobiology, and one not completely confined to classical allergy (Heiner and Rose, 1970; Heiner, Goldstein, and Rose, 1970). The particularly insignificant role that γE plays in serum immunoblobulin dynamics (and vice versa) is emphasized by its mode of discovery (Ishizaka, Ishizaka, and Hornbrook, 1966) which occurred outside the realm of serology. In fact, when the atypical myeloma protein from patient N.D. (Johansson and Bennich, 1967) was found to have its counterpart as a very minor component, γND, in the normal serum of 62 blood donors (Johansson, Bennich, and Wide, 1968), a new class of immunoglobulin was thought to have been found until it was discovered that γND was none other than γE (Bennich, Ishizaka, Ishizaka, and Johansson, 1969).

In the proper and systematic study of the immune responses one would also need to include an extensive chapter on phylogenetic experimentation. One might begin with the hagfish, that most primitive of vertebrates, and explode the myth (Pollara, Swan, Finstad, and Good, 1968) concerning its lack of immunological vigor. As shown by Linthicum and Hildemann (1970), the Pacific hagfish "despite their 'most primitive vertebrate' status, are capable of vigorous production of antibodies to at least certain cellular and soluble antigens." These investigators were not even so sure that γM was the only antibody that might be obtained. They were reminded that it took Fidler, Clem, and Small (1969) 1 year to raise γG in nurse sharks to above detectable limits, only 30 days for γM, and that no one had as yet devised a way of keeping hagfish alive in captivity past 3 months even in constantly renewed ocean water. Exemplary studies that one would want to include in a phylogenetic chapter, in addition to those reviewed by Grey (1969) and similar works of more recent origin, would be the elegant immunodiffusion experiments of Coe (1970) on bullfrog antibody specificity and cross-reactivity for rabbit γG and egg albumin; the affinity and valence investigations of a teleost (grouper) antibody to dinitrophenyl bovine γ-immunoglobulin (DNP-BGG) (Clem and Small, 1970); the DNP-T4 neutralization kinetics exhibited by such primitive vertebrates as elasmobranchs (Leslie and Clem, 1969); the Sips and Scatchard plots of DNP binding data for nurse shark antibody (Voss, Russell, and Sigel, 1969) and for gray-snapper antibody (Russell, Voss, and Sigel, 1970); and the study of precipitins formed between leopard shark antibodies and hemocyanin antigens (Suran, Tarail, and Papermaster, 1967).

Another aspect of the immune responses to be explored is the molecular size of the immunizing antigen below which no measurable response can be expected. In spite of traditional thinking (and, unfortunately, teaching) to the contrary the lower limit appears to be not much larger than a single antigenic determinant. We have already discussed the fact that antibodies can be made against angiotensin, a peptide of 1031 molecular weight. Sela (1970) has assembled a table from the literature of some low molecular weight guinea pig immunogens that include not only angiotensin but also, among others, the synthetic α-DNP-hepta-L-lysine (mol. wt. 1080), Rp-hexa-L-tyrosine (mol. wt. 1200), and Rp-N-acetyl-L-tyrosine amide (mol. wt. 450). The fact that much higher molecular weights generally are required is probably more a profession of our ignorance of how to immunize with lesser sizes and how to recognize the immunization product once formed than it is of actual immunogenic requirements.

Molecular size is important to sequential determinants, but molecular shape is important to conformational ones. A discussion of the immune responses to conformational determinants, if adequately covered in immunobiology, must address itself to the paradox posed by traditional immunological thinking. If immunogens must be processed by degradative enzymatic processes in order to become recognizable as antigens in the selection process, how can the bulk of conformational determinants—which depend for their very existence upon preservation of molecular structures—become recognized? Sela, Schechter, Schechter, and Borek (1967) would rather reject traditions than to preserve paradoxes. "As the conformation of a protein determinant would be destroyed by proteolysis, it seems that the role of proteolysis is to destroy the antigen after the determinant has been 'recognized' at the site of biosynthesis." One of the most important conclusions to be drawn from the work of Sela and co-workers is that "antigenic determinants of proteins are controlled to a large extent by the secondary, tertiary, and quaternary structure of proteins." Any exposition of immunobiology and the immune responses that purports to have a contemporary flavor must take this very real conformational factor into serious account.

Probably of equal importance both to the practical conduct of immunological experimentation and to the comprehension of immunobiological theory is the schedule of immunization and bleeding— the art and science of raising antibodies. Dosage, route of administration, and physical state of the antigen; the timing between the initial administration, possible "boosters," and final bleeding; and age and species of the immunized recipient all enter into the final accounting. However, until the ideas of modern immunochemistry were applied by Eisen and Siskind (1964) to this area, there was, unfortunately, mostly opinionated art and very little objective science. Such art, combined with erroneous instructionist theories of antibody formation, more than any other factor, prevented the discipline of immunobiology from reaching the level of an acceptable theoretical science. After Eisen and Siskind (1964) described the variations in affinities of antibodies during the primary and secondary immune responses it was very apparent that an understanding of the science of raising antibodies could be reached through the avenue of immunochemistry. The work of Fujio and Karush (1966) that was described in Chapter 6 was a logical extension. The investigations by Paul, Siskind, Benacerraf, and Ovary (1967) were another. In the latter the secondary responses of rabbits to various DNP-protein conjugates after primary immunization with DNP-BGG were examined by carefully controlled studies in which the three variables—dosage, carrier type, and time of boosting—were recognized. The antibody concentrations in serum and the average intrinsic association constants of antibody were evaluated as parameters of the responses. Boosting with DNP upon homologous carrier increased the amount of antibody without affecting affinity to any great extent; boosting with DNP upon a carrier of limpet hemocyanin increased binding affinity by three orders of magnitude but had little effect upon increasing serum concentrations (i.e., titers). Many other excellent studies have been made, finally culminating in the theory of Siskind and Benacerraf (1969) concerning the mode of cell selection by antigen in the immune response—an essentially two-step process of antigen interaction with preexisting cell-associated antibody molecules followed by cell stimulation to proliferate and secrete or to become unresponsive (self-destruct?). Although not necessarily the last word in definitive theory the exposition is a model of what must be included in any modern theory—the nature of affinity, the effect of antigenic dosage upon the concentration and affinity of antibody, the mode of action of adjuvants and other immunogenic aids, the specificity of the cell proliferation process after stimulation, the feedback effect of humoral antibody upon response regulation, the real nature of cross-reacting antibodies, and the consequences of tolerance and unresponsiveness as the alternate outcome of any particular immune response. One might now add three additional features: the effect of monogamous bivalent binding in selection and feedback; the role of V_H gene products in selection vs. those under constant gene and subtype gene control; and the impact of the insertion-deletion hypothesis upon concepts of the nature and variety of clonal selection.

2. Affinity and clonal selection

The thesis advanced by Burnet (1967) and accepted here is that

" . . . no combining site is in any evolutionary sense adapted to a particular antigenic determinant. The pattern of the combining site is there and *if it happens to fit*, in the sense that the affinity of adsorption to a given antigenic determinant is above a certain value, immunologically significant reaction will be initiated."

Heterogeneity of the response results from the distribution pattern illustrated by Figure 10-1. Avidity (or affinity) which is measured by an affinity constant, K_a, must reach a certain value before an immunologically significant reaction will take place (involving either an immunocyte or an immunoglobulin). Beyond that point, for which there is no definite line of demarcation, specificity is obtained and a range of affinity constants is expressed.

Burnet advances his concept further with another type of diagram, the essence of which is contained in Figure 10-2. The relationship can

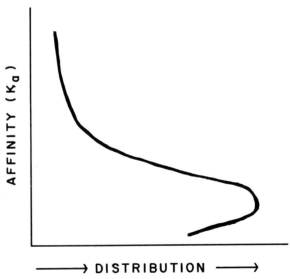

FIG. 10-1. Distribution of cells or molecules in a standard population of immunocytes or immunoglobulin molecules according to affinity for a given antigenic determinant as adapted from Burnet (1967). The convention of presenting the distribution parameter along the ordinate has been broken here in order to place affinity (avidity in Burnet's terms) in its more usual position.

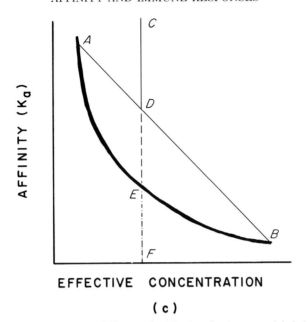

EFFECTIVE CONCENTRATION

(c)

FIG. 10-2. In the concept of Burnet (1967) the abscissa was labeled "effective concentration" and the ordinate was labeled "avidity (AD/CS)" where AD stood for antigenic determinant and CS for combining site. The avidity parameter obviously was not meant to represent the ratio of ligand to combining site, but rather to emphasize "the specific contact" of an antigenic determinant with its complementary binding site in an immunocyte, i.e., affinity. It is represented here by the association constant K_a. The concentration parameter, in order to be "effective", must represent the concentration of free ligand and is therefore represented here as c. According to Burnet the position of the diagonal (AB) is variable and represents the physiologic state of the immunocyte—to the far left, if thymus; to the middle, if progenitor. Above and to the right of the diagonal destruction of an immunocyte is likely to occur, e.g., CD. Below the curve (e.g., EF) no reaction takes place. Between the curve and the diagonal (e.g., ED) differentiation takes place in the case of thymus; commitment, in the case of progenitor immunocyte; and clonal cell proliferation and antibody production, in the case of the committed immunocyte.

be derived from the law of mass action. Starting with Equation 5.55b of Chapter 5 (which is also the Karush equation)

$$\alpha = (Kc)/(1 + Kc) \qquad (10.1)$$

one obtains by rearrangement

$$cK = \alpha/(1 - \alpha) \qquad (10.2)$$

where α is the extent of reaction, synonymous with the fraction b of bound antibody and $(1 - \alpha)$ is equal to the fraction a of unbound antibody. For a given fixed extent of reaction, an isoreaction line is obtained in the shape of a reciprocal curve when K and c are plotted against each other (Fig. 10-3). As the extent of reaction, α, becomes smaller, the family of isoreaction curves approaches the two axes (*curve AB*) and as α becomes very large the curves move away from both axes (*curve CD*). At half saturation of binding sites of antibody $cK = 1$ and a standard isoreaction curve is obtained. The lower limit of reaction according to the Burnet concept would be an isoreaction curve, such as *curve AB*. Below and to the left the immunocytes would remain physiologically unreactive. The upper limit of reaction would not be a diagonal but rather an isoreaction curve such as *curve CD*, above and to the right of which the extent of reaction would result in cell paralysis and/or destruction. Between AB and CD heter-

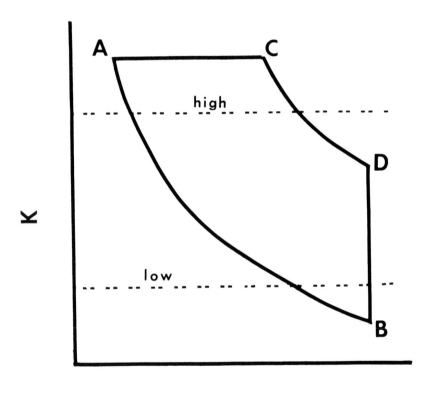

FIG. 10-3. Isoreaction *curves AB* and *CD* determine the lower and upper limits of an immunologic reaction. AC is the maximum affinity possible; BD, the maximum concentration of antigenic determinants. *Dashed lines* are examples of homogeneous binding.

ogeneous antibody formation and/or cell proliferation would take
place. Homogeneous binding at different energies would be a family
of lines parallel to the abscissa, and an upper limit of possible homogeneous binding, e.g., $K_a = 10^{12}$ M^{-1}, would set the upper ordinate
limit of the family of the isoreaction curves (*line AC*). An upper limit
of determinant concentration, essentially set by steric factors, would
set the upper abscissa limit of the family of isoreaction curves (*line
BD*). Within area *ABCD* immunological reactivity would be expected
to occur.

There is another aspect of cell reaction dynamics that derives from
the Karush equation which expresses the extent of reaction in two
ways, either (a) determinant concentration and degree of antibody
binding or (b) antibody binding site concentration and degree of
determinant coverage. Karush used the same symbols to designate
either state, but Equations 5.55b and 5.55a were used in this text
(Chapter 5) to distinguish one from the other. Thus,

$$\beta = Kd/(1 + Kd) \tag{10.3}$$

and

$$dK = \beta/(1 - \beta) \tag{10.4}$$

where β is the extent of reaction, synonymous with the fraction q of
bound antigen and $(1 - \beta)$ is equal to the fraction p of unbound antigenic determinants. For a given fixed extent of reaction, an isoreaction line is obtained in the shape of a reciprocal curve when K and d
are plotted against each other (Fig. 10-4). *Curves EF* and *GH* define
the lower and upper isoreaction limits of immunological reactivity,
line EG sets the upper limit of homogeneous binding (expressive
here of the highest degree of specificity attainable), and *line FH*
sets the upper limit of antibody or immunocyte binding site concentration. Within the area *EFGH* immunological reactivity would
be expected to occur.

Conceptually, then, the logical extension of Burnet's ideas through
the use of the two Karush equations is a three-dimensional picture
with K_a, c, and d as axes and with any particular extent of reaction
actually not within either the K-c or the K-d plane but somewhere
midway between them (Fig. 10-5). An isoreaction surface would be
formed by using K as the axis of revolution. One would have to know
the interrelationship between c and d and between α and β in order
to construct a meaningful surface, but somewhere in between the
two planes would be an isoreaction curve expressive of equivalence.
In the early development of an immune response the isoreactions
would be on the antigen excess side of equivalence and with continued

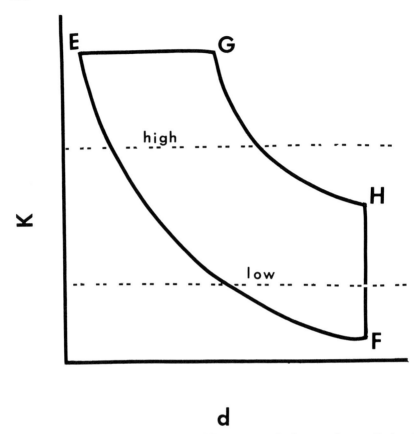

FIG. 10-4. Isoreaction *curves EF* and *GH* determine the lower and upper limits of an immunologic reaction. *EG* is the maximum affinity possible; *FH*, the maximum concentration of antibody binding sites. *Dashed lines* are examples of homogeneous binding.

development would sweep to the antibody excess side. Any particular homogeneous immune response that develops into a homogeneous clone with a given fixed association constant for a particular homogeneous antigen would trace two limiting curves in a plane parallel to the c-d plane and at a given fixed K_a level. Between the two curves a homogeneous positive immune response would occur; inside the inner limit, no response; outside the outer limit, paralysis and/or self-destruction.

The whole potential of a positive fully heterogeneous immune response would lie within a volume bounded by two physiological isoreaction surfaces (an inner hyporesponse limit and an outer hyperresponse limit) and two homogeneous immunochemical reaction

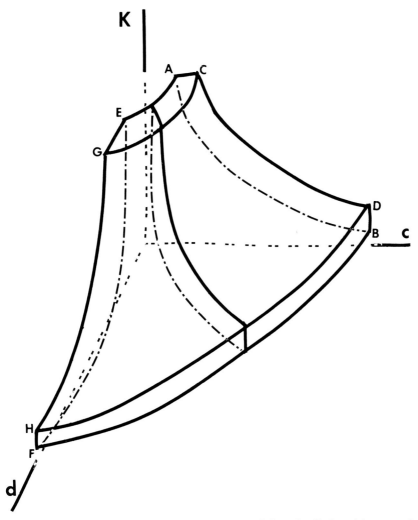

FIG. 10-5. Inner and outer isoreaction surfaces define the limits of hypo- and hyperreactivity between which immunologic responses result in clonal proliferation and antibody production.

planes (an upper plane of highest affinity and a lower ground level plane of lowest affinity). The density of the volume would resemble an atmosphere, according to Burnet's distribution curve (Fig. 10-1), which would be rarefied at highest affinity and denser at ground level, and which would vary from high to low pressure even at ground level depending upon the particular stage of the immune responses.

To the extent that the law of mass action and the concepts of affinity and concentration apply to immunological problems the relationships set forth here must be considered valid. It is now up to the immunobiologist to determine whether the physiological limits of immunocyte responses, as conceived by Burnet, are indeed governed by the law. Obviously, to obtain his answer the immunobiologist must know and test the law, not ignore it.

REFERENCES

Bennich, H., Ishizaka, K., Ishizaka, T., and Johansson, S. G. (1969). A comparative antigenic study of γE-globulin and myeloma-IgND. J. Immunol. *102:* 826–831.

Burnet, F. M. (1967). The impact on ideas of immunology. Symp. Quant. Biol. *32:* 1–8.

Cate, T. R., Rossen, R. D., Douglas, R. G., Jr., Butler, W. T., and Couch, R. B. (1967). The role of nasal secretion and serum antibody in the rhinovirus common cold. Am. J. Epidemiol. *84:* 352–363.

Clem, L. W., and Small, P. A., Jr. (1970). Phylogeny of immunoglobulin structure and function. V. Valence and association constants of teleost antibodies to a haptenic determinant. J. Exp. Med. *132:* 385–400.

Coe, J. E. (1970). Specificity of antibody produced in the bullfrog (*Rana catesbiana*). J. Immunol. *104:* 1166–1174.

Eisen, H. M., and Siskind, G. W. (1964). Variations in affinities of antibodies during the immune response. Biochemistry *3:* 996–1008.

Fidler, J. E., Clem, L. W., and Small, P. A., Jr. (1969). Immunoglobulin synthesis in neonatal nurse sharks (*Ginglymostoma cirratum*). Comp. Biochem. Physiol. *31:* 365–371.

Fujio, H., and Karush, F. (1966). Antibody affinity. II. Effect of immunization interval on antihapten antibody in the rabbit. Biochemistry *5:* 1856–1863.

Grey, H. M. (1969). Phylogeny of immunoglobulins. Adv. Immunol. *10:* 51–104.

Heiner, D. C., Goldstein, G. B., and Rose, B. (1970). Immunochemical studies of selected subjects with wheat intolerance. J. Allergy *45:* 333–346.

Heiner, D. C., and Rose, B. (1970). Elevated levels of γE (IgE) in conditions other than classical allergy. J. Allergy *45:* 30–42.

Ishizaka, K., and Ishizaka, T. (1970a). Significance of immunoglobulin E in reaginic hypersensitivity. Ann. Allergy *28:* 189–202.

Ishizaka, K., and Ishizaka, T. (1970b). Biological function of γE antibodies and mechanisms of reaginic hypersensitivity. Clin. Exp. Immunol. *6:* 25–42.

Ishizaka, K., Ishizaka, T., and Hornbrook, M. (1966). Physico-chemical properties of human reaginic antibody. IV. Presence of a unique immunoglobulin as a carrier of reaginic activity. J. Immunol. *97:* 75–85.

Ishizaka, K., Ishizaka, T., and Tada, T. (1969). Immunoglobulin E in the monkey. J. Immunol. *103:* 445–453.

Johansson, S. G. O., and Bennich, H. (1967). Immunological studies of an atypical (myeloma) immunoglobulin. Immunology *13:* 381–394.

Johansson, S. G. O., Bennich, H., and Wide, L. (1968). A new class of immunoglobulin in human serum. Immunology *14:* 265–272.

Kalff, M. W. (1970). A population study on serum immunoglobulin levels. Clin. Chim. Acta *28:* 277–289.

Kawakami, K., Tatsumi, H., Tatsumi, M., and Kono, R. (1966). Studies on poliovirus coproantibody. I. Neutralizing antibodies in feces of children following Sabin oral poliovirus vaccination. Am. J. Epidemiol. *83:* 1–23.

Keller, R., and Dwyer, J. E. (1968). Neutralization of polio-virus by IgA coproanti-bodies. J. Immunol. *101:* 192–202.

Kriebel, G. W., Jr., Kraft, S. C., and Rothberg, R. M. (1969). Locally produced anti-body in human gastrointestinal secretions. J. Immunol. *103:* 1268–1275.

Leslie, G. A., and Clem, L. W. (1969). Production of anti-hapten antibodies by several classes of lower vertebrates. J. Immunol. *103:* 613–617.

Linthicum, D. S., and Hildemann, W. H. (1970). Immunologic responses of Pacific hagfish. III. Serum antibodies to cellular antigens. J. Immunol. *105:* 912–918.

Lipton, M. M., and Steigman, A. J. (1963). Human coproantibody against polioviruses. J. Infect. Dis. *112:* 57–66.

Paul, W. E., Siskind, G. W., Benacerraf, B., and Ovary, Y. (1967). Secondary antibody responses in haptenic systems: cell population selection by antigen. J. Immunol. *99:* 760–770.

Pollara, B., Suran, A., Finstad, J., and Good, R. A. (1968). N-terminal amino acid sequences of immunoglobulin chains in *Polyodon spathula.* Proc. Natl. Acad. Sci. *59:* 1307–1312.

Russell, W. J., Voss, E. W., Jr., and Sigel, M. M. (1970). Some characteristics of anti-dinitrophenyl antibody of the gray snapper. J. Immunol. *105:* 262–264.

Sela, M. (1970). Structure and specificity of synthetic polypeptide antigens. Ann. N.Y. Acad. Sci. *169:* 23–35.

Sela, M., Schechter, B., Schechter, I., and Borek, F. (1967). Antibodies to sequential and conformational determinants. Symp. Quant. Biol. *32:* 537–545.

Siskind, G. W., and Benacerraf, B. (1969). Cell selection by antigen in the immune re-sponse. Adv. Immunol. *10:* 1–50.

Steigman, A. J., and Lipton, M. M. (1959). Polio-virus-neutralizing antibody in feces of poliomyelitic children. Lancet *2:* 272–273.

Suran, A. A., Tarail, M. H., and Papermaster, B. W. (1967). Immunoglobulins of the leopard shark. I. Isolation and characterization of 17S and 7S immunoglobulins with precipitating activity. J. Immunol. *99:* 679–686.

Tada, T., and Ishizaka, K. (1970). Distribution of γE-forming cells in lymphoid tissues of the human and monkey. J. Immunol. *104:* 377–387.

Tomasi, T. B., Jr. (1970). Structure and function of mucosal antibodies. Annu. Rev. Med. *21:* 281–298.

Vaerman, J.-P., and Heremans, J. F. (1970). Origin and molecular size of immuno-globulin-A in the mesenteric lymph of the dog. Immunology *18:* 27–38.

Voss, E. W., Jr., Russell, W. J., and Sigel, M. M. (1969). Purification and binding properties of nurse shark antibody. Biochemistry *8:* 4866–4872.

AUTHOR INDEX

Dorrington, K. J., 89, 95, 115, 116
Doty, P., 198, 261
Douglas, R. G., Jr., 389, 400
Dourmashkin, R. R., 99, 120
Dray, S., 21–23, 39, 40, 43, 56, 67, 68, 70, 159, 172, 175
Dreyer, W. J., 9, 11, 12, 21, 22, 26, 33, 35, 39, 40, 41, 46, 66
Dubiska, A., 21, 39
Dubiski, S., 21, 23, 38, 39, 58, 66
Dudley, M. A., 298, 308
Dudziak, Z., 21, 39
Dulbecco, R., 295, 308
Dwyer, J. E., 389, 401

Easley, C. W., 5, 7, 42, 43, 75, 120
Edelhoch, H., 111, 118
Edelman, G. M., 6–10, 12, 25, 30, 36, 39, 40, 42–49, 54, 62, 66, 67, 70–72, 75, 88, 109, 111–113, 116, 120, 123, 130, 171, 176, 233, 260
Edman, P., 25, 42, 64, 66, 232, 261
Edmundson, A. B., 105, 110, 116, 370, 371, 385
Edwards, M., 323, 352
Eichmann, K., 251, 260, 262
Eigen, M., 139, 171, 216, 261
Ein, D., 20, 38, 40, 85, 116
Eisen, H. N., 123, 135, 171, 173, 199, 200, 207–211, 213–215, 225, 229, 238, 239, 261–263, 265, 348, 350, 351, 356, 393, 400
Ely, K. R., 105, 110, 116
Englberger, F., 123, 157, 160, 172, 337, 341, 342, 355
Epperson, M. S., 375, 384
Epstein, S. I., 198, 261
Erlanger, B., 224, 266, 376, 385
Erspamer, V., 61, 65

Fahey, J. L., 20, 40, 53, 81, 116
Farr, R. S., 327, 347, 348, 353, 355, 356
Fasman, G. D., 149, 175
Fazekas de St. Groth, S., 274–294, 304, 308
Feigen, G. A., 344, 352
Feinstein, A., 21, 40, 56, 57, 66, 99, 100, 104, 105, 114, 116, 141, 171
Feizi, T., 253, 261
Fellows, R. E., Jr., 45–48, 50, 68
Fenton, J. W., II, 113, 117, 131, 171, 175
Fernandez-Moran, H., 379, 385
Fidler, J. E., 391, 400
Filitti-Wurmser, S., 95, 99, 100, 116
Finegold, I., 81, 116
Finstad, J., 63, 64, 69, 391, 401
Fisher, C. E., 67

Fitch, W. M., 17, 38, 40, 43, 63, 70
Fleischman, J. B., 7, 8, 10, 40, 75, 76, 80, 116, 130, 171, 251, 261
Fleming, J., 323, 356, 365, 387
Forssman, O., 86, 116
Fraenkel-Conrat, H., 267, 268, 308
Francis, T., 274, 275, 308, 309
Franek, F., 72, 83, 116, 171
Frangione, B., 10, 22, 28, 40, 42, 54, 55, 64, 65, 67, 69, 76, 83, 101, 116, 119, 120
Franklin, E. C., 8, 19, 40, 53–56, 66, 67, 80, 83, 101, 115, 116, 120, 122
Franklin, R. E., 268, 309
Fraser, K. J., 232, 261
Frauenberger, G., 213, 263, 321, 355
Freedman, M. H., 123, 124, 127, 158, 171, 378, 385
Freidin, R., 135, 173, 207, 263
Freychet, P., 348, 353
Fritz, R. B., 281, 284, 287, 289, 309, 334–341, 346, 348, 350, 353
Froese, A., 139, 171, 216–224, 261
Fruchter, R. G., 46–48, 58, 67
Fruton, J. S., 61, 66
Fuchs, S., 377, 385
Fudenberg, H. H., 19, 40, 50, 53–56, 60, 62, 63, 67, 70, 71, 90, 116
Fujio, H., 214, 215, 261, 393, 400
Fujita, N. J., 158, 159, 172, 230, 231, 263

Gaddone, S. M., 337, 341, 342, 355
Gall, W. E., 36, 39, 45, 48, 49, 66, 67, 105, 109, 111–113, 116, 120
Gallagher, J. S., 96, 116
Gally, J. A., 6, 25, 36, 39, 40
Gaspari, E. L., 323, 356
Gaudy, E., 324, 353
Gell, P. G. H., 21, 40
Gelzer, J., 154, 171
Genco, R. J., 377, 385
Gentou, C., 100, 116
Gerald, L., 21, 39
Gergely, J., 90, 116, 117
Gerwing, J., 369, 385
Geshickter, C. F., 4, 5, 39–42
Gill, T. J., III, 141, 142, 174
Gilman, A. M., 21, 40, 56, 67
Gilman-Sachs, A., 23, 40, 58, 68
Gindler, E. M., 140, 176
Ginsberg, B., 81, 121
Gitlin, D., 230, 261
Giustino, V., 101, 115
Givas, Sr. J., 372, 373, 385
Givol, D., 125, 168, 172, 175
Gleich, G. J., 101, 115
Godt, S. M., 208, 211, 212, 264

SUBJECT INDEX

MARSTON 8